UROLOGIC CLINICS
OF NORTH AMERICA

Erectile Dysfunction

GUEST EDITOR
Culley C. Carson, MD

CONSULTING EDITOR
Martin I. Resnick, MD

November 2005 • Volume 32 • Number 4

SAUNDERS

An Imprint of Elsevier, Inc.
PHILADELPHIA   LONDON   TORONTO   MONTREAL   SYDNEY   TOKYO

W.B. SAUNDERS COMPANY
A Division of Elsevier Inc.

1600 John F. Kennedy Boulevard • Suite 1800 • Philadelphia, Pennsylvania 19103-2899

http://www.theclinics.com

THE UROLOGIC CLINICS OF NORTH AMERICA   Volume 32, Number 4
November 2005   ISSN 0094-0143
Editor: Catherine Bewick   ISBN 1-4160-2803-X

The Urologic Clinics of North America (ISSN 0094-0143) is published quarterly by W.B. Saunders Company. Corporate and editorial offices: Elsevier, Inc., 1600 John F. Kennedy Blvd., Suite 1800, Phila-delphia, PA 19103-2899. Accounting and circulation offices: 6277 Sea Harbor Drive, Orlando, FL 32887-4800. Periodicals postage paid at Orlando, FL 32862, and additional mailing offices. Subscription prices are $210.00 per year (US individuals), $325.00 per year (US institutions), $240.00 per year (Canadian in-dividuals), $390.00 per year (Canadian institutions), $280.00 per year (foreign individuals), and $390.00 per year (foreign institutions). Foreign air speed delivery is included in all *Clinics* subscription prices. All prices are subject to change without notice. POSTMASTER: Send address changes to *The Urologic Clinics of North America*, W.B. Saunders Company, Periodicals Fulfillment, Orlando, FL 32887-4800. **Customer Service: 1-800-654-2452 (US). From outside the US, call 1-407-345-4000.**

The Urologic Clinics of North America is covered in *Index Medicus, Excerpta Medica, Current Contents/ Clinical Medicine, Science Citation Index,* and *ISI/BIOMED.*

Printed in the United States of America.

CONSULTING EDITOR

MARTIN I. RESNICK, MD, Lester Persky Professor and Chairman, Department of Urology,
   Case Western Reserve University, School of Medicine/University Hospitals, Cleveland, Ohio

GUEST EDITOR

CULLEY C. CARSON, MD, Rhodes Distinguished Professor and Chief, Division of Urology, Department
   of Surgery, University of North Carolina—Chapel Hill, Chapel Hill, North Carolina

CONTRIBUTORS

MELISSA BROWN, MPH, Clinical Coordinator, Department of Urology, College of Physicians and Surgeons,
   Columbia University, New York, New York,

CULLEY C. CARSON, MD, Rhodes Distinguished Professor and Chief, Division of Urology, Department
   of Surgery, University of North Carolina—Chapel Hill, Chapel Hill, North Carolina

JACKIE D. CORBIN, PhD, Professor of Molecular Physiology and Biophysics, Vanderbilt University School
   of Medicine, Nashville, Tennessee

ROBERT C. DEAN, MD, Clinical Fellow, Department of Urology, University of California—San Francisco,
   San Francisco Medical Center, San Francisco, California

SHARRON H. FRANCIS, PhD, Research Professor of Molecular Physiology and Biophysics, Vanderbilt University
   School of Medicine, Nashville, Tennessee

NOEL GENDRANO III, MPH, Department of Psychiatry, Robert Wood Johnson Medical School, Piscataway,
   New Jersey

JOHN L. GORE, MD, Resident, Department of Urology, David Geffen School of Medicine, University
   of California—Los Angeles, Los Angeles, California

JASON M. GREENFIELD, MD, Resident, Rush University Medical Center, Chicago, Illinois

WAYNE J.G. HELLSTROM, MD, FACS, Professor, Department of Urology, Chief, Section of Andrology, Tulane
   University Health Sciences Center, New Orleans, Louisiana

MUAMMER KENDIRCI, MD, Department of Urology, Tulane University Health Sciences Center, New Orleans,
   Louisiana

ROBERT A. KLONER, MD, PhD, Director of Research, Heart Institute, Good Samaritan Hospital; and Professor,
   Division of Cardiovascular Medicine, Keck School of Medicine, University of Southern California, Los Angeles,
   California

SARAH M. LAMBERT, MD, Postdoctoral Residency Fellow, Department of Urology, College of Physicians
   and Surgeons, Columbia University, New York, New York

LAURENCE A. LEVINE, MD, Professor of Urology, Rush University Medical Center, Chicago, Illinois

JOHN R. LOBO, MD, Department of Urology, Mayo Clinic, Rochester, Minnesota

TOM F. LUE, MD, Professor and Vice Chair, Emil Tanagho Endowed Chair, Department of Urology, University of California–San Francisco, San Francisco Medical Center, San Francisco, California

PUNEET MASSON, MD, Department of Urology, College of Physicians and Surgeons. Columbia University, New York, New York

AJAY NEHRA, MD, Professor of Urology, Mayo Clinic College of Medicine, Department of Urology, Mayo Clinic, Rochester, Minnesota

MICHAEL A. PERELMAN, PhD, Co-Director, Human Sexuality Program and Clinical Associate Professor of Psychiatry, Reproductive Medicine and Urology, The New York Presbyterian Hospital, Weill Medical College of Cornell University, New York, New York

JACOB RAJFER, MD, Professor, Department of Urology, David Geffen School of Medicine, University of California–Los Angeles, Los Angeles, California

RAYMOND C. ROSEN, PhD, Professor, Department of Psychiatry, Robert Wood Johnson Medical School, Piscataway, New Jersey

STEPHEN SCHNEIDER, MD, Professor, Department of Medicine, Robert Wood Johnson Medical School, New Brunswick, New Jersey

RIDWAN SHABSIGH, MD, Department of Urology, College of Physicians and Surgeons, Columbia University, New York, New York,

RONALD S. SWERDLOFF, MD, Professor, Division of Endocrinology, Department of Medicine, Harbor-UCLA Medical Center and Los Angeles Biomedical Research Institute, David Geffen School of Medicine, University of California-Los Angeles, Los Angeles, California

CHRIS TORNEHL, MD, Division of Urology, University of North Carolina–Chapel Hill, Chapel Hill, North Carolina

MELISSA M. WALLS, MD, Department of Urology, Tulane University Health Sciences Center, New Orleans, Louisiana

RENA WING, PhD, Professor, Department of Psychiatry & Human Behavior, Brown University School of Medicine, Providence, Rhode Island

CONTENTS

Foreword   xi
Martin I. Resnick

Preface   xiii
Culley C. Carson

Physiology of Penile Erection and Pathophysiology of Erectile Dysfunction   379
Robert C. Dean and Tom F. Lue

This article reviews the physiology of penile erection, the components of erectile function, and the pathophysiology of erectile dysfunction. The molecular and clinical understanding of erectile function continues to gain ground at a particularly fast rate. Advances in gene discovery have aided greatly in working knowledge of smooth muscle relaxation/contraction pathways. The understanding of the nitric oxide pathway has aided not only in the molecular understanding of the tumescence but also greatly in the therapy of erectile dysfunction.

Erectile Dysfunction and Cardiovascular Risk Factors   397
Robert A. Kloner

There are numerous causes of erectile dysfunction (ED), including psychogenic, organic, and mixed psychogenic/organic. Among the organic causes the most common include vascular, neurogenic, endocrine, structural, drug-induced, and others. Some have estimated that nearly one half of all causes of ED in men over 50 years of age are vascular in nature. This article reviews cardiovascular risk factors of ED.

**Epidemiology of Erectile Dysfunction: the Role of Medical Comorbidities
and Lifestyle Factors**   403
Raymond C. Rosen, Rena Wing, Stephen Schneider, and Noel Gendrano III

Erectile dysfunction (ED) is a highly prevalent condition in aging men with significant interpersonal and psychosocial consequences. Large-scale epidemiologic studies have demonstrated a consistent age-related loss of erectile function in men from different geographic and ethnic backgrounds, with approximately half of men over 70 years of age reporting moderate to severe symptoms. ED is associated strongly with specific comorbidities, such as cardiovascular disease and hypertension, diabetes mellitus, lower urinary tract symptoms, prostate cancer, and depression. Lifestyle factors, including obesity and exercise frequency, also have been implicated in recent studies.

Phosphodiesterase-5 Inhibition: the Molecular Biology of Erectile Function and Dysfunction

Sharron H. Francis and Jackie D. Corbin

419

This article discusses the role of phosphodiesterase-5 (PDE-5) inhibition in the molecular biology of erectile function and dysfunction. Commercially marketed PDE-5 inhibitors are highly specific for PDE-5, and in the face of continuing cyclic GMP (cGMP) synthesis, elevate cellular cGMP. This elevation results from direct competitive inhibition of PDE-5 and from blocking the negative feedback regulation of the enzyme. Elevation of cGMP activates cGMP-dependent protein kinase, which mediates the effects of the cGMP-signaling pathway to decrease smooth muscle tone and dilate penile vascular smooth muscle. By exploiting features of PDE-5 regulatory mechanisms that modulate PDE-5 function, the inhibitors enhance their own potencies.

Psychosocial Evaluation and Combination Treatment of Men with Erectile Dysfunction

Michael A. Perelman

431

The Sexual Tipping Point™ forms the foundation of a biopsychosocial model to help conceptualize a combination treatment, where sex coaching and sexual pharmaceuticals are integrated into a clinical approach, which addresses organic, psychologic, and cultural issues for men with erectile dysfunction (ED). At any moment in the intervention process, the clinician determines the most elegant solution, which focuses the majority of effort on fixing the predominant factor while not ignoring the others. Clinicians using this model, can fully conceptualize ED by understanding the predisposing, precipitating, and maintaining psychosocial aspects of their patient's diagnosis and management, as well as organic causes and risk factors. The sex status or focused sex history, and continuous reassessment based on follow-up are the core elements of this method. Restoration of lasting and satisfying sexual function requires a multidimensional understanding of all of the forces that created the dysfunction, whether a solo clinician or multidisciplinary team approach is used. Each clinician needs to carefully evaluate their own competence and interests when considering the treatment of a man's ED, so that regardless of the modality used, the patient receives optimized care to restore sexual function and satisfaction.

Clinical Evaluation of Erectile Dysfunction in the Era of PDE-5 Inhibitors

John R. Lobo and Ajay Nehra

447

Erectile dysfunction (ED) is a common disorder that has gained attention since the introduction of relatively safe treatment with phosphodiesterase-5 inhibitors. ED is a multifactorial disorder and a common presentation for several systemic illnesses, particularly vascular occlusive diseases. The clinical evaluation of ED should be thorough and systematic, with attention to the appropriate use of sexual symptom questionnaires and symptom scales, detailed medical and sexual history, physical examination, and basic screening laboratory tests. Patients should be referred for specialized evaluations when appropriate. The clinician must be familiar with the pathophysiologic mechanisms of ED, its associations with other systemic diseases, the indications for specialist referrals, and the role of specialized testing to diagnose and treat this disorder effectively.

Androgen Deficiency in the Etiology and Treatment of Erectile Dysfunction

John L. Gore, Ronald S. Swerdloff, and Jacob Rajfer

457

The evaluation and management of erectile dysfunction (ED) has evolved dramatically following the introduction of oral phosphodiesterase-5 inhibitors. Despite the limited role of directed diagnostic testing in the evaluation of the impotent patient, routine determination of a serum testosterone likely is indicated based on evidence that testosterone modulates erectile function, that hypogonadism is prevalent among elderly men and men with ED, and that symptomatology alone rarely detects hypogonadism. Forms of testosterone commonly used include oral, parenteral, transdermal, and implantable preparations, each with significant advantages and disadvantages. The risks and benefits of testosterone supplementation have been characterized incompletely and will require further validation before widespread use of testosterone as hormone replacement therapy in aging men.

Peyronie's Disease: Etiology, Epidemiology and Medical Treatment   469
Jason M. Greenfield and Laurence A. Levine

The investigation of medical options for the treatment of Peyronie's disease is lacking controlled clinical trials with uniform standardized assessments and objective measures of deformity, including curvature and circumference. A key to defining the beneficial effects of various medical therapies lies in standardizing the evaluation of the Peyronie's patient across various studies so that the proposed benefits can be confirmed and applied to all populations. Furthermore, basic science research into the pathophysiology of this disorder is likely to yield new insights into potential treatment options and direct future therapies.

Surgical Treatment of Peyronie's Disease   479
Chris Tornehl and Culley C. Carson

Peyronie's Disease (PD) is a sexually debilitating disease resulting in significant psychologic stress for many men. Urologists have an opportunity to help men suffering from PD to improve their lives. Appropriate treatment should be individualized and tailored to the patient's expectations, disease history, physical examination findings, and erectile function. This review is intended to share the experiences of other urologists in the surgical approach to PD.

Central Nervous System Agents in the Treatment of Erectile Dysfunction   487
Muammer Kendirci, Melissa M. Walls, and Wayne J.G. Hellstrom

In the last two decades, a better understanding of the mechanisms governing erectile function and the pathophysiologies underlying erectile dysfunction (ED) have led researchers to investigate novel treatment concepts. Selective type-5 phosphodiesterase inhibitors are recommended as first-line therapy because of their high efficacy, but 30% to 40% of patients who have ED do not respond adequately to these agents and require alternative methods. The central nervous system plays a fundamental role in sexual behavior. Animal models have advanced our understanding of the neuroanatomic and neuropharmacologic basis of centrally induced penile erections. Clinical research with apomorphine has demonstrated efficacy in men who have a range of ED. Recent interest has focused on other centrally acting agents for ED treatment, including the melanocortin receptor agonists.

Penile Prosthesis Implantation: Surgical Implants in the Era of Oral Medication   503
Culley C. Carson

In patients who are not satisfied with the results of oral agents (phosphodiesterase-5 inhibitors) or in whom oral agents or other medical treatment fails to produce an adequate response, penile prosthesis implantation is an excellent treatment modality for restoring erectile function. Patient/partner acceptance, use, and satisfaction rates of penile prostheses are better than for many other alternatives including pharmacologic injections. Inflatable penile prostheses are most frequently used and have the highest satisfaction rates. Complications of these multipiece prostheses continue to decline, and patient satisfaction rates, tolerability, and longevity continue to increase.

PDE-5 Inhibitors: Current Status and Future Trends

PDE-5 Inhibitors: Current Status and Future Trends 511

Puneet Masson, Sarah M. Lambert, Melissa Brown, and Ridwan Shabsigh

Phosphodiesterase-5 (PDE-5) inhibitors are a well-established, first-line therapy for erectile dysfunction (ED). Extensive clinical trials and clinical experience established the highly significant efficacy and the safety of this class of drugs in the treatment of ED. Furthermore, the efficacy of PDE-5 inhibitors has been established in men with ED with a broad range of etiologies and comorbidities. The future of PDE-5 inhibitors includes the expansion of indications such as the treatment of pulmonary hypertension and the potential of treatment of symptomatic BPH.

Cumulative Index 2005 527

GOAL STATEMENT

The goal of *Urologic Clinics of North America* is to keep practicing urologists and urology residents up to date with current clinical practice in urology by providing timely articles reviewing the state of the art in patient care.

ACCREDITATION

The *Urologic Clinics of North America* is planned and implemented in accordance with the Essential Areas and Policies of the Accreditation Council for Continuing Medical Education (ACCME) through the joint sponsorship of the University of Virginia School of Medicine and Elsevier. The University of Virginia School of Medicine is accredited by the ACCME to provide continuing medical education for physicians.

The University of Virginia School of Medicine designates this educational activity for a maximum of 60 category 1 credits per year, 15 category 1 credits per issue, toward the AMA Physician's Recognition Award. Each physician should claim only those credits that he/she actually spent in the activity.

The American Medical Association has determined that physicians not licensed in the US who participate in this CME activity are eligible for AMA PRA category 1 credit.

Category 1 credit can be earned by reading the text material, taking the CME examination online at http://www.theclinics.com/home/cme, and completing the evaluation. After taking the test, you will be required to review any and all incorrect answers. Following completion of the test and evaluation, your credit will be awarded and you may print your certificate.

FACULTY DISCLOSURE/CONFLICT OF INTEREST

The University of Virginia School of Medicine, as an ACCME accredited provider, endorses and strives to comply with the Accreditation Council for Continuing Medical Education (ACCME) Standards of Commercial Support, Commonwealth of Virginia statutes, University of Virginia policies and procedures, and associated federal and private regulations and guidelines on the need for disclosure and monitoring of proprietary and financial interests that may affect the scientific integrity and balance of content delivered in continuing medical education activities under our auspices.

The University of Virginia School of Medicine requires that all CME activities accredited through this institution be developed independently and be scientifically rigorous, balanced and objective in the presentation/discussion of its content, theories and practices.

All authors/editors participating in an accredited CME activity are expected to disclose to the readers relevant financial relationships with commercial entities occurring within the past 12 months (such as grants or research support, employee, consultant, stock holder, member of speakers bureau, etc.). The University of Virginia School of Medicine will employ appropriate mechanisms to resolve potential conflicts of interest to maintain the standards of fair and balanced education to the reader. Questions about specific strategies can be directed to the Office of Continuing Medical Education, University of Virginia School of Medicine, Charlottesville, Virginia.

The authors/editors listed below have identified no professional or financial affiliations for themselves or their spouse/partner:

Catherine Bewick, Acquisitions Editor; Cully C. Carson, MD, FACS; Robert C. Dean, MD; Sharron H. Francis, PhD; John L. Gore, MD; Jason M. Greenfield, MD; Ajay Neha, MD; Martin I. Resnick, MD; Christopher Tornehl, MD; and Rena R. Wing, PhD.

The authors/editors listed below identified the following professional or financial affiliations for themselves or their spouse/partner:

Noel C. Gendrano, III, MPH is an employee for Merck & Co. Inc.

Robert A. Kloner, MD, PhD serves as consultant/advisory committee for Pfizer, Lilly Icos, GSK, Kin, Schering Plough; he is on the speakers' bureau for Pfizer, Lilly. In addition, he has a grant from Eli Lilly.

Laurence A. Levine, MD serves as independent contractor, consultant, advisory board member and serves on the speakers' bureau for Pfizer, Lilly/ICOS; serves as an independent contractor, consultant, on the speakers' bureau for Bayer, Glaxo-Smith Kline, and Schering Plough; serves as independent contractor, consultant, advisory board member for Auxillium; serves as independent contractor and consultant for American Medical Systems.

Thomas F. Lue, MD is a consultant and speaker for Pfizer, Bayer, GlaxoSmithKline, Kos, and Lilly; he is an investigator doing basic drug research for Astellas, Rinat, and Biopharm; and he is a board member for Genix.

Michael A. Perelman, PhD serves as a consultant, advisory board member and is on the speakers' bureau for Pfizer, Bayer, Lilly ICOS, Sanofi-Aventis, Johnson & Johnson, GlaxoSmithKline; serves as consultant and advisory board member for Proctor and Gamble, Palatin Technologies, Inc., and Ortho-McNeil Pharmaceuticals; serves as consultant and on the speakers' bureau for Schering-Plough; and, serves as consultant for Alza.

Jacob Rajfer, MD independent contractor for Pfizer.

The authors listed below have not provided disclosure for themselves or their spouse/partner:

Melissa Brown, MPH; Jackie D. Corbin, PhD; Wayne J.G. Hellstrom, MD; Muhammer Kendirci, MD; Sarah M. Lambert, MD; John R. Lobo, MD; Puneet Masson, MD; Raymond C. Rosen, PhD; Stephen Schneider, MD; Ridwan Shabsigh, MD; Ronald S. Swerdloff, MD; and Melissa M. Walls, MD.

Disclosure of Discussion of non-FDA approved uses for pharmaceutical products and/or medical devices:

The University of Virginia School of Medicine, as an ACCME provider, requires that all faculty presenters identify and disclose any "off label" uses for pharmaceutical and medical device products. The University of Virginia School of Medicine recommends that each physician fully review all the available data on new products or procedures prior to instituting them with patients.

TO ENROLL

To enroll in the Urologic Clinics of North America Continuing Medical Education program, call customer service at 1-800-654-2452 or visit us online at www.theclinics.com/home/cme. The CME program is available to subscribers for an additional fee of $195.00

FORTHCOMING ISSUES

February 2006
> **Genitorurinary Trauma**
> Jack W. McAninch, MD, *Guest Editor*

May 2006
> **Urologic Imaging**
> Pat Fulgham, MD, *Guest Editor*

August 2006
> **Advanced Prostate Cancer**
> Joseph Smith Jr., MD, *Guest Editor*

RECENT ISSUES

August 2005
> **Office Management and Procedures**
> William F. Gee, MD, *Guest Editor*

May 2005
> **Contemporary Issues and
> Management of Bladder Cancer**
> John P. Stein, MD, FACS, *Guest Editor*

February 2005
> **Pelvic Neuromodulation**
> Firouz Daneshgari, MD, *Guest Editor*

THE CLINICS ARE NOW AVAILABLE ONLINE!

Access your subscription at:
http://www.theclinics.com

Urol Clin N Am 32 (2005) xi

UROLOGIC CLINICS of North America

Foreword

Erectile Dysfunction

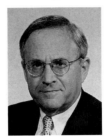

Martin I. Resnick, MD
Consulting Editor

In the not too distant past, erectile dysfunction was considered a consequence of aging and, although of great concern to the affected patient, little was available to evaluate or treat the problem. Over the ensuing years, much has been learned related to the various causes of erectile function and significant developments have occurred in patient evaluation and treatment. Cardiovascular disease, neurologic disorders, and the development of benign prostatic hyperplasia (with its associated urinary symptoms) have been associated with erectile problems. In addition, as noted in this issue of the *Urologic Clinics of North America*, increased recognition of the presence of Peyronie's disease and its impact on erectile function has been appreciated. The understanding of the physiology associated with penile tumescence and detumescence has allowed for better assessment of the disease so that appropriate treatment modalities can be specifically applied to a particular patient. Lastly, the development of phosphodiesterase-5 inhibitors in association with new prostheses and surgical procedures has been of great value to many.

Dr. Carson and associates are to be congratulated for developing an issue of the *Urologic Clinics of North America* that broadly and specifically addresses many of these issues. Erectile dysfunction is a common problem that is seen by urologists on a daily basis, and this issue should be of value in providing the most up-to-date information on patient evaluation and treatment.

Martin I. Resnick, MD
Lester Persky Professor and Chairman
Department of Urology
Case Western Reserve University
School of Medicine/University Hospitals
11100 Euclid Avenue
Cleveland, OH 44106-5046, USA

E-mail address: mir@po.cwru.edu

ELSEVIER
SAUNDERS

Urol Clin N Am 32 (2005) xiii

UROLOGIC
CLINICS
of North America

Preface

Erectile Dysfunction

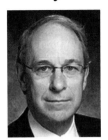

Culley C. Carson, MD
Guest Editor

It has been several years since *Urologic Clinics of North America* has discussed the topics associated with male sexual health. In the intervening years, there has been a revolution in the understanding of the basic and clinical sciences associated with erectile dysfunction (ED) and its treatment. At the same time, epidemiologic studies from throughout the world have confirmed the prevalence of ED and risk factors associated with this condition. Today, the physician and scientist understand that vascular disease and associated risk factors are the leading patient conditions associated with loss of erections. Newer risks including benign prostatic hyperplasia (BPH) associated with lower urinary tract symptoms (LUTS), depression, and hypogonadism can be single or additive risk factors for the development of ED. As more patients are treated for ED and men previously poorly functional become sexually active, more men are complaining of penile curvature associated with Peyronie's disease. The treatment of this incurable and difficult to treat condition continues to be controversial. Medical alternatives are few and only marginally effective while surgery is appropriate in only a limited number of men. Surgical treatment of Peyronie's disease is becoming more common and as the numbers increase, the success rates likewise improve.

In men in whom all conservative medical treatment fails, surgical implantation of penile prostheses continues to be a safe and effective strategy with excellent patient and partner acceptance and satisfaction. Newer implants with antibiotic coatings have significantly reduced morbidity and device failure.

In this issue of *Urologic Clinics of North America*, the contributors have endeavored to elucidate the latest data and clinical practice in the diagnosis of men with ED, review the risk factors and men who are at risk for ED. Finally, discussion of treatment of ED with PDE-5 inhibitors, newer central nervous system acting agents and surgery will give the reader a complete overview of the evaluation, diagnosis, and varied treatments available for men with sexual and erectile dysfunction.

It has been a great pleasure to edit this issue and work with so many outstanding authors. The efforts of the authors are evident throughout this issue with their lucid and complete discussions. I am indebted to the editorial staff of *Urologic Clinics* for their assistance, expertise and efficiency in publishing and outstanding issue.

Culley C. Carson, MD
Rhodes Distinguished Professor
Chief, Division of Urology
University of North Carolina at Chapel Hill
Chapel Hill, NC 27599-7235

doi:10.1016/j.ucl.2005.08.008

ELSEVIER
SAUNDERS

Urol Clin N Am 32 (2005) 379–395

UROLOGIC
CLINICS
of North America

Physiology of Penile Erection and Pathophysiology of Erectile Dysfunction

Robert C. Dean, MD, Tom F. Lue, MD*

Department of Urology, University of California–San Francisco, San Francisco Medical Center, 400 Parnassus Avenue, San Francisco, CA 94143-0738, USA

The molecular and clinical understanding of erectile function continues to gain ground at a particularly fast rate. Advances in gene discovery have aided greatly in working knowledge of smooth muscle relaxation/contraction pathways. Intensive research has yielded many advances. The understanding of the nitric oxide (NO) pathway has aided not only in the molecular understanding of the tumescence but also greatly in the therapy of erectile dysfunction (ED). As a man ages or undergoes surgery, preventative therapies to preserve erectile function have begun. All clinical interventions have derived from a full anatomic, molecular, and dynamic knowledge base of erectile function and dysfunction. In this article, the components of erectile function are explained.

Hemodynamics and mechanism of erection and detumescence

Corpora cavernosa

The penile erectile tissue (specifically, the cavernous smooth musculature and the smooth muscles of the arteriolar and arterial walls) plays a key role in the erectile process. In the flaccid state, these smooth muscles are tonically contracted, allowing only a small amount of arterial flow for nutritional purposes. The blood Po_2 is about 35 mmHg [1]. The flaccid penis is in a moderate state of contraction, as evidenced by further shrinkage in cold weather and after phenylephrine injection.

Sexual stimulation triggers the release of neurotransmitters from the cavernous nerve terminals, which results in relaxation of these smooth muscles and the following events:

1. Dilatation of the arterioles and arteries by increased blood flow in the diastolic and the systolic phases
2. Trapping of the incoming blood by the expanding sinusoids
3. Compression of the subtunical venular plexuses between the tunica albuginea and the peripheral sinusoids, reducing the venous outflow
4. Stretching of the tunica to its capacity, which occludes the emissary veins between the inner circular and the outer longitudinal layers and further decreases the venous outflow to a minimum
5. An increase in Po_2 (to about 90 mm Hg) and intracavernous pressure (around 100 mm Hg), which raises the penis from the dependent position to the erect state (the full-erection phase)
6. A further pressure increase (to several hundred millimeters of mercury) with contraction of the ischiocavernosus muscles (rigid-erection phase)

The angle of the erect penis is determined by its size and its attachment to the puboischial rami (the crura) and the anterior surface of the pubic bone (the suspensory and funiform ligaments). In men who have a long, heavy penis or a loose suspensory ligament, the angle is usually not greater than 90°, even with full rigidity.

Three phases of detumescence have been reported in an animal study [2]. The first entails a transient intracorporeal pressure increase, indicating the beginning of smooth muscle contraction

---

* Corresponding author.
E-mail address: tlue@urol.ucsf.edu (T.F. Lue).

doi:10.1016/j.ucl.2005.08.007

against a closed venous system. The second phase shows a slow pressure decrease, suggesting a slow reopening of the venous channels with resumption of the basal level of arterial flow. The third phase shows a fast pressure decrease with fully restored venous outflow capacity.

Erection thus involves sinusoidal relaxation, arterial dilatation, and venous compression [3]. The importance of smooth muscle relaxation has been demonstrated in animal and human studies [4,5].

Corpus spongiosum and glans penis

The hemodynamics of the corpus spongiosum and glans penis are somewhat different from those of the corpora cavernosa. During erection, the arterial flow increases in a similar manner; however, the pressure in the corpus spongiosum and glans is only one third to one half of the pressure in the corpora cavernosa because the tunical covering (thin over the corpus spongiosum and virtually absent over the glans) ensures minimal venous occlusion. During the full-erection phase, partial compression of the deep dorsal and circumflex veins between Buck's fascia and the engorged corpora cavernosa contribute to glanular tumescence, although the spongiosum and glans essentially function as a large arteriovenous shunt during this phase. In the rigid-erection phase, the ischiocavernosus and bulbocavernosus muscles forcefully compress the spongiosum and penile veins, which results in further engorgement and increased pressure in the glans and spongiosum.

Neuroanatomy and neurophysiology of penile erection

Peripheral pathways

The innervation of the penis is autonomic (sympathetic and parasympathetic) and somatic (sensory and motor). From the neurons in the spinal cord and peripheral ganglia, the sympathetic and parasympathetic nerves merge to form the cavernous nerves, which enter the corpora cavernosa and corpus spongiosum to affect the neurovascular events during erection and detumescence. The somatic nerves are primarily responsible for sensation and the contraction of the bulbocavernosus and ischiocavernosus muscles.

Autonomic pathways

The sympathetic pathway originates from the 11th thoracic to the second lumbar spinal segments and passes through the white rami to the sympathetic chain ganglia. Some fibers then travel through the lumbar splanchnic nerves to the inferior mesenteric and superior hypogastric plexuses, from which fibers travel in the hypogastric nerves to the pelvic plexus. In humans, the T10 through T12 segments are most often the origin of the sympathetic fibers, and the chain ganglia cells projecting to the penis are located in the sacral and caudal ganglia [6].

The parasympathetic pathway arises from neurons in the intermediolateral cell columns of the second, third, and fourth sacral spinal cord segments. The preganglionic fibers pass in the pelvic nerves to the pelvic plexus, where they are joined by the sympathetic nerves from the superior hypogastric plexus. The cavernous nerves are branches of the pelvic plexus that innervate the penis. Other branches of the pelvic plexus innervate the rectum, bladder, prostate, and sphincters. The cavernous nerves are easily damaged during radical excision of the rectum, bladder, and prostate. A clear understanding of the course of these nerves is essential to the prevention of iatrogenic ED [7]. Human cadaveric dissection has revealed medial and lateral branches of the cavernous nerves (the former accompany the urethra and the latter pierce the urogenital diaphragm 4 to 7 mm lateral to the sphincter) and multiple communications between the cavernous and the dorsal nerves [8].

Stimulation of the pelvic plexus and the cavernous nerves induces erection, whereas stimulation of the sympathetic trunk causes detumescence, clearly implying that the sacral parasympathetic input is responsible for tumescence and the thoracolumbar sympathetic pathway is responsible for detumescence. In experiments with cats and rats, removal of the spinal cord below the L4 or L5 level reportedly eliminated the reflex erectile response, but placement with a female in heat or electrical stimulation of the medial preoptic area produced marked erection [9,10]. Paick and Lee [11] also reported that apomorphine-induced erection is similar to psychogenic erection in the rat and can be induced by means of the thoracolumbar sympathetic pathway in case of injury to the sacral parasympathetic centers. In humans, many male patients who have sacral spinal cord injury retain psychogenic erectile ability even though reflexogenic erection is abolished. These cerebrally elicited erections are found more frequently in patients who have lower motoneuron lesions below the T12 level [12]. No psychogenic erection occurs in patients who have lesions above the T9 level;

the efferent sympathetic outflow is thus suggested to be at the levels T11 and T12 [13]. In patients who have psychogenic erections, lengthening and swelling of the penis are observed but rigidity is insufficient.

It is possible, therefore, that cerebral impulses normally travel through sympathetic (inhibiting norepinephrine release), parasympathetic (releasing NO and acetylcholine), and somatic (releasing acetylcholine) pathways to produce a normal rigid erection. In patients who have a sacral cord lesion, the cerebral impulses can still travel by means of the sympathetic pathway to inhibit norepinephrine release, and NO and acetylcholine can still be released through synapse with postganglionic parasympathetic and somatic neurons. Because the number of synapses between the thoracolumbar outflow and the postganglionic parasympathetic and somatic neurons is less than the sacral outflow, the resulting erection is not as strong.

Somatic pathways

The somatosensory pathway originates at the sensory receptors in the penile skin, glans, and urethra and within the corpus cavernosum. In the human glans penis are numerous afferent terminations: free nerve endings and corpuscular receptors, with a ratio of 10:1. The free nerve endings are derived from thin myelinated A_δ and unmyelinated C fibers and are unlike any other cutaneous area in the body [14]. The nerve fibers from the receptors converge to form bundles of the dorsal nerve of the penis, which joins other nerves to become the pudendal nerve. The latter enters the spinal cord by way of the S2 through S4 roots to terminate on spinal neurons and interneurons in the central, gray region of the lumbosacral segment [15]. Activation of these sensory neurons sends messages of pain, temperature, and touch by means of spinothalamic and spinoreticular pathways to the thalamus and sensory cortex for sensory perception. The dorsal nerve of the penis used to be regarded as a purely somatic nerve; however, nerve bundles testing positive for NO synthase, which is autonomic in origin, have been demonstrated in humans by Burnett and colleagues [16] and in the rat by Carrier and coworkers [17]. Giuliano and associates [18] also showed that stimulation of the sympathetic chain at the L4 to L5 level elicits an evoked discharge on the dorsal nerve of the penis and that stimulation of the dorsal nerve evokes a reflex discharge in the lumbosacral sympathetic chain of rats. These findings clearly demonstrate that the dorsal nerve is a mixed nerve, having somatic and autonomic components that enable it to regulate erectile and ejaculatory function.

Onuf's nucleus in the second to fourth sacral spinal segments is the center of somatomotor penile innervation. These nerves travel in the sacral nerves to the pudendal nerve to innervate the ischiocavernosus and bulbocavernosus muscles. Contraction of the ischiocavernosus muscles produces the rigid-erection phase. Rhythmic contraction of the bulbocavernosus muscle is necessary for ejaculation. In animal studies, direct innervation of the sacral spinal motoneurons by brain stem sympathetic centers (A5 catecholaminergic cell group and locus coeruleus) has been identified [19]. This adrenergic innervation of pudendal motoneurons may be involved in rhythmic contractions of perineal muscles during ejaculation. In addition, oxytocinergic and serotonergic innervation of lumbosacral nuclei, controlling penile erection and perineal muscles in the male rat, has also been demonstrated [20].

Depending on the intensity and nature of genital stimulation, several spinal reflexes can be elicited by stimulation of the genitalia. The best known is the bulbocavernosus reflex, which is the basis of genital neurologic examination and electrophysiologic latency testing. Although impairment of bulbocavernosus and ischiocavernosus muscles may impair penile erection, the significance of obtaining a bulbocavernosus reflex in overall sexual dysfunction assessment is controversial.

Supraspinal pathways and centers

Studies in animals have identified the medial preoptic area and the paraventricular nucleus of the hypothalamus and hippocampus as important integration centers for sexual function and penile erection: electrostimulation of this area induces erection, and lesions at this site limit copulation [21,22]. Marson and colleagues [22] injected pseudorabies virus into rat corpus cavernosum and traced labeled neurons from major pelvic ganglia to neurons in the spinal cord, brain stem, and hypothalamus. Mallick and coworkers also showed that stimulation of the dorsal nerve of the penis in the rat influenced the firing rate of about 80% of the neurons in the medial preoptic area but not in other areas of the hypothalamus [23]. Efferent pathways from the medial preoptic area enter the medial forebrain bundle and the midbrain tegmental region (near the substantia nigra).

Pathologic processes in these regions, such as Parkinson's disease or cerebrovascular accidents, are often associated with ED. Axonal tracing in monkeys, cats, and rats has shown direct projection from hypothalamic nuclei to the lumbosacral autonomic erection centers. The neurons in these hypothalamic nuclei contain peptidergic neurotransmitters including oxytocin and vasopressin, which may be involved in penile erection [21]. Several brain stem and medullary centers are also involved in sexual function. The A5 catecholamine cell group and locus ceruleus have been shown to provide adrenergic innervation to the hypothalamus, thalamus, neocortex, and spinal cord. Projections from the nucleus paragigantocellularis, which provides inhibitory serotonergic innervation, have also been demonstrated in the hypothalamus, limbic system, neocortex, and spinal cord.

Central neural activation during sexual arousal

Positron emission tomography (PET) and functional MRI (fMRI) have allowed a greater understanding of brain activation during human sexual arousal. PET and fMRI measure increases in regional cerebral blood flow or changes in regional cerebral activity during a particular moment in time. Using this technology, scanned brain images of young heterosexual male subjects taken during sexual arousal (triggered by showing sexually explicit pictures or videos) are compared with images taken when the subjects are shown sexually neutral images (relaxation, documentary, or humorous video clips). Brain activation centers and deactivation regions can be demonstrated. Although the simplicity of these study designs is elegant, multiple factors are involved in sexual arousal, especially arousal triggered by visual clues. The authors of these studies have placed many necessary conditions in an attempt to standardize the methods and participants; however, the complexity of human emotion and sexual response is extremely difficult to regulate.

In 1999, Stoleru and colleagues [24] studied eight healthy, right-handed, heterosexual males using PET during visually evoked sexual arousal. Regions of brain activation were correlated with testosterone plasma levels and penile tumescence. Significant activation during visually evoked sexual arousal was seen in the bilateral inferior temporal cortex, right insula, right inferior frontal cortex, and left anterior cingulate cortex. From this landmark study, a tentative model for brain function during sexual arousal was introduced.

The model suggests that there are three components of visually evoked sexual arousal associated with their neuroanatomic regions: (1) a perceptual-cognitive component that assesses the visual stimuli as sexual, performed in the bilateral inferior temporal cortex; (2) an emotional/motivational component that processes sensory information, with motivational states performed in the right insula, right inferior frontal cortex, and left cingulate cortex (paralimbic areas); and (3) a physiologic component that coordinates the endocrine and autonomic functions in the left anterior cingulate cortex.

Further investigations were performed using visual sexual stimuli and PET scanning. Bocher and colleagues [25] demonstrated increased activation in the inferior lateral occipital cortex, bilateral posterior temporal cortices (right greater than left), right inferior lateral prefrontal cortex, left postcentral gyrus, bilateral inferior parietal lobules, left superior parietal lobules, frontal pole (Brodmann's area 10), left prefrontal cortex, and midbrain regions. These investigators also noted deactivation in the medial frontal and anterior cingulate, contrary to Stoleru and colleague's [24] report. Visual association centers were again noted to be activated; in particular, posterior temporal cortices and the postcentral gyrus. It is of interest that the midbrain activation seen in this study correlates to the location of the dopaminergic neurons. The activation of the midbrain region was not demonstrated in other studies. This activation may be associated with prolonged provocation. The visual sexual stimulus used in this study was a 30-minute continuous video clip, whereas other studies used brief visual sexual stimuli (2–10 minutes).

Park and colleagues [26] studied 12 healthy male participants using fMRI. Viewing erotic film clips was alternated with viewing nonerotic clips. Regional brain activation was generally seen in the inferior frontal lobe, cingulate gyrus, insular gyrus, corpus collosum, thalamus, caudate nucleus, globus pallidus, and inferior temporal lobes. Some activation regions were similar to those found in other studies; in particular, the inferior frontal lobes, inferior temporal lobes, and insular gyrus.

In a well-designed study using fMRI and visual sexual stimuli correlated with penile turgidity, Arnow and coworkers [27] demonstrated a significant region of activation in the right subinsular/insula region including the claustrum. Activation of this region was similarly seen in previous studies using PET [24,28]. This region has been associated with sensory processing. Activation of the insula in this study may represent somatosensory processing and recognition of erection. Other brain regions that were activated during visual sexual stimuli were the right middle gyrus, right temporal gyrus, left caudate and putamen, bilateral cingulate gyri, right sensimotor, and premotor regions. In addition, a smaller activation was seen in the right hypothalamus. Dopamine is projected to the hypothalamus, and the evidence that dopamine facilitates male sexual behavior is substantial. Again, the right middle temporal gyrus was seen to be activated, which is probably associated with visual processing.

In 2003, Mouras and colleagues [29] studied eight men using fMRI. Instead of viewing video clips, the participants were quickly shown still photographs (neutral and sexually arousing). By using shorter visual sexual stimuli, these investigators believed that early neural responses would be generated instead of neural responses to the perception of penile tumescence. Again, activation of the middle and inferior occipital gyri was demonstrated, most likely linked to the visual stimuli and not necessarily to the sexual component. In addition to multiple brain centers that showed activation with visual sexual stimuli (bilateral parietal lobules, left inferior parietal lobule, right postcentral gyrus, right parietoccipital sulcus, left superior occipital gyrus, and bilateral precentral gyrus), the cerebellum demonstrated activation in three subjects and deactivation in four subjects. Multiple other reports have demonstrated activation of the cerebellum in response to erotic films and viewing pictures of love partners. It appears, therefore, that visual sexual stimuli create activation in regions within the cerebellum.

With the advances in fMRI technology, detailed comparisons of brain activation in response to visual sexual stimuli have been performed on varied groups. Stoleru and colleagues [30] studied healthy male subjects compared with men who had hypoactive sexual desire disorder (HSDD). The left gyrus rectus, a portion of the medial orbitofrontal cortex, remained activated in men who had HSDD, which contrasts with its deactivation in healthy men in response to visual sexual stimuli. This region is believed to mediate inhibitory control of motivated behavior. Continued activation of this region may help explain the pathophysiology of HSDD. Montorsi and coworkers [31] compared men who had psychogenic ED with potent controls following the administration

of apomorphine. In men who had psychogenic ED, extended activation of the cingulated gyrus, frontal mesial, and frontal basal cortex was seen during visual sexual stimuli. This extended activation may suggest an underlying organic etiology for psychogenic ED. With the administration of apomorphine, the fMRI images of psychogenic ED patients were similar to those of the potent controls. Apomorphine caused additional activation of foci in the psychogenic ED patient (seen in the nucleus accumbens, hypothalamus, and mesencephalon). In addition, the right hemisphere was significantly more activated than the left following apomorphine administration. Greater hemisphere activation in the right hemishphere is a common finding in studies of sexually evoked brain activation.

Brain scanning using PET and fMRI has become a powerful tool in the study of central activation of sexual arousal. Many brain regions of activation have been demonstrated in these reports. Some common brain centers of activation can now be described through these reports (Table 1). Psychogenic ED, premature ejaculation, sexual deviations, and orgasmic dysfunction are just a few conditions that may have an alteration in higher brain function and can perhaps now be studied. As we begin to understand brain function within the normal sexual response and arousal, the cause of sexual dysfunction conditions may be elucidated.

The structures discussed earlier are responsible for the three types of erection: psychogenic, reflexogenic, and nocturnal. Psychogenic erection

Table 1
Brain activation centers and corresponding function

Brain activation regions	Functional association
Bilateral inferior temporal cortex (right > left)	Visual association area
Right insula	Processes somatosensory information with motivational states
Right inferior frontal cortex	Processes sensory information
Left anterior cingulate cortex	Controls autonomic and neuroendocrine function
Right occipital gyrus	Visual processing
Right hypothalamus	Male copulatory behavior
Left caudate (the striatum)	Attentional processing and guide responsiveness to new environmental stimuli

is a result of audiovisual stimuli or fantasy. Impulses from the brain modulate the spinal erection centers (T11 through L2 and S2 through S4) to activate the erectile process. Reflexogenic erection is produced by tactile stimuli to the genital organs. The impulses reach the spinal erection centers; some follow the ascending tract, resulting in sensory perception, whereas others activate the autonomic nuclei to send messages by way of the cavernous nerves to the penis to induce erection. This type of erection is preserved in patients who have upper spinal cord injury. Nocturnal erection occurs mostly during rapid eye movement (REM) sleep. PET scanning of humans in REM sleep show increased activity in the pontine area, the amygdalas, and the anterior cingulate gyrus but decreased activity in the prefrontal and parietal cortex. The mechanism that triggers REM sleep is located in the pontine reticular formation. During REM sleep, the cholinergic neurons in the lateral pontine tegmentum are activated, whereas the adrenergic neurons in the locus ceruleus and the serontonergic neurons in the midbrain raphe are silent. This differential activation may be responsible for nocturnal erections during REM sleep.

Molecular mechanism of smooth muscle contraction and relaxation

Smooth muscle contraction and relaxation is regulated by cytosolic (sarcoplasmic) free Ca^{2+}. Norepinephrine from nerve endings and endothelins and prostaglandin $F_{2\alpha}$ from endothelium activate receptors on smooth muscle cells to increase inositol triphosphate and diacylglycerol, resulting in the release of calcium from intracellular stores (such as sarcoplasmic reticulum) or the opening of calcium channels on the smooth muscle cell membrane leading to an influx of calcium from extracellular space. This influx of calcium triggers a transient increase in cytosolic free Ca^{2+} from a resting level of 120 to 270 nmol/L to 500 to 700 nmol/L [32]. At the elevated level, Ca^{2+} binds to calmodulin and changes the latter's conformation to expose sites of interaction with myosin light-chain kinase. The resultant activation catalyzes phosphorylation of myosin light chains and triggers the cycling of myosin crossbridges (heads) along actin filaments and the development of force. In addition, phosphorylation of the light chain also activates myosin ATPase, which hydrolyzes ATP to provide energy for muscle contraction (Fig. 1).

After the cytosolic Ca^{2+} returns the basal levels, the calcium-sensitizing pathways take over. One such mechanism is by way of activation of excitatory receptors coupled to G proteins that can also cause contraction by increasing calcium sensitivity without any change in cytosolic Ca^{2+}. This pathway involves RhoA, a small, monomeric G protein that activates Rho-kinase. Activated Rho-kinase phosphorylates and thereby inhibits the regulatory subunit of smooth muscle myosin phosphatase and prevents dephosphorylation of myofilaments, thus maintaining contractile tone (Fig. 2) [33].

RhoA and Rho-kinase have been shown to be expressed in penile smooth muscle [34,35]. It is interesting that the amount of RhoA expressed in cavernosal smooth muscle is 17-fold higher than in vascular smooth muscle [35]. A selective inhibitor of Rho-kinase has been shown to elicit relaxation of human corpus cavernosum in vitro and to induce penile erection in animal models [36]. Anesthetized rats transfected with dominant negative RhoA exhibited an elevated erectile function compared with control animals [37]. The emerging consensus is that the phasic contraction of penile smooth muscle is regulated by an increase in cytosolic Ca^{2+} and the tonic contraction is governed by the calcium-sensitizing pathways [38].

In addition to the central role of myosin phosphorylation in smooth muscle contraction, other mechanisms may modulate or fine-tune the contractile state. For example, caldesmon may be involved in the latch state in which the force of contraction is maintained at a low level of myosin phosphorylation and with a low-energy expenditure.

Relaxation of the muscle follows a decrease of free Ca^{2+} in the sarcoplasma. Calmodulin dissociates from myosin light-chain kinase and inactivates it. When myosin is dephosphorylated by myosin light-chain phosphatase and detaches from the actin filament, the muscle relaxes [32]. Others suggest that the NO–cyclic GMP (cGMP) inhibitory pathway in corpus cavernosum smooth muscle is not simply a reversal of excitatory signal transduction mechanisms but that an unidentified mechanism may contribute to relaxation by decreasing the rate of crossbridge recruitment through phosphorylation.

Cyclic AMP (cAMP) and cGMP are the second messengers involved in smooth muscle relaxation. They activate cAMP- and cGMP-dependent protein kinases, which in turn phosphorylate certain proteins and ion channels, resulting

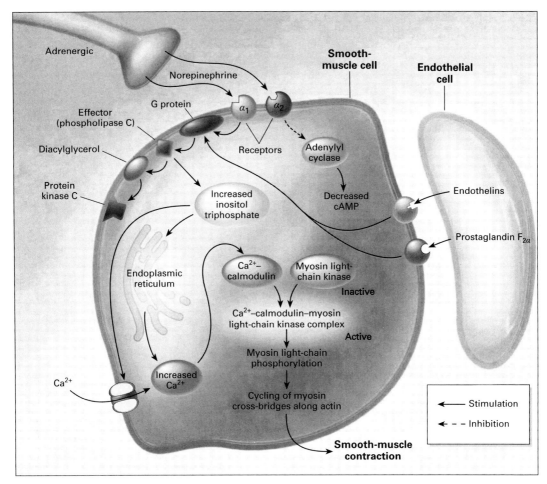

Fig. 1. Molecular mechanism of penile smooth muscle contraction. Norepinephrine from sympathetic nerve endings and endothelins and prostaglandin $F_{2\alpha}$ from the endothelium activate receptors on smooth muscle cells to initiate the cascade of reactions that eventually results in elevation of intracellular calcium concentrations and smooth muscle contraction. Protein kinase C is a regulatory component of the Ca^{2+}-independent, sustained phase of agonist-induced contractile responses. cAMP, cyclic AMP. (*From* Lue TF. Erectile dysfunction. N Engl J Med 2000;342:1804. Copyright © 2000 Massachusetts Medical Society. All rights reserved; with permission.)

in (1) opening of the potassium channels and hyperpolarization; (2) sequestration of intracellular calcium by the endoplasmic reticulum; and (3) inhibition of voltage-dependent calcium channels, blocking calcium influx. The consequence is a drop in cytosolic free Ca^{2+} and smooth muscle relaxation (Fig. 3).

Pathophysiology of erectile dysfunction

Classification

Many classifications have been proposed for ED. Some are based on the cause (diabetic,

iatrogenic, traumatic) and others on the neurovascular mechanism of the erectile process (failure to initiate [neurogenic], failure to fill [arterial], and failure to store [venous]). A classification recommended by the International Society of Impotence Research is shown in Box 1 [39].

Psychogenic

Previously, psychogenic impotence was believed to be the most common type, with 90% of impotent men thought to suffer from this condition [40]. This belief has given way to the realization that most men who have ED have

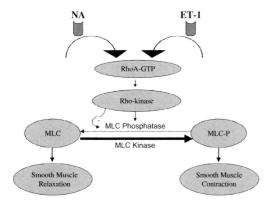

Fig. 2. RhoA/Rho-kinase pathway: the calcium sensitization pathway. ET-1, endothelin 1 receptor; GTP, guanosine triphosphate; MLC, myosin light chain; MLC-P, myosin light-chain phosphatase; NA, norepinephrine receptor.

a mixed condition that may be predominantly functional or predominantly physical.

Sexual behavior and penile erection are controlled by the hypothalamus, the limbic system, and the cerebral cortex. Therefore, stimulatory or inhibitory messages can be relayed to the spinal erection centers to facilitate or inhibit erection. Two possible mechanisms have been proposed to explain the inhibition of erection in psychogenic dysfunction: (1) direct inhibition of the spinal erection center by the brain as an exaggeration of the normal suprasacral inhibition and excessive sympathetic outflow or (2) elevated peripheral catecholamine levels, which may increase penile smooth muscle tone to prevent the relaxation necessary for erection [41]. Animal studies demonstrate that the stimulation of sympathetic nerves or systemic infusion of epinephrine causes detumescence of the erect penis [42,43]. Clinically, higher levels of serum norepinephrine have been reported in patients who have psychogenic ED compared with normal controls or patients who have vasculogenic ED [44].

Bancroft [45] theorized that male sexual response depends on the balance between excitatory and inhibitory impulses within the central nervous system. Investigation is underway that is testing sexual inhibitory and sexual excitatory questionnaires that may help identify whether a patient will have a more successful outcome with psychotherapy or pharmacologic treatment.

Neurogenic

It has been estimated that 10% to 19% of ED is of neurogenic origin [46,47]. If one includes

iatrogenic causes and mixed ED, then the prevalence of neurogenic ED is probably much higher. Although the presence of a neurologic disorder or neuropathy does not exclude other causes, confirming that ED is neurogenic in origin can be challenging. Because an erection is a neurovascular event, any disease or dysfunction affecting the brain, spinal cord, or cavernous and pudendal nerves can induce dysfunction.

The medial preoptic area, the paraventricular nucleus, and the hippocampus have been regarded as important integration centers for sexual drive and penile erection [21]. Pathologic processes in these regions, such as Parkinson's disease, stroke, encephalitis, or temporal lobe epilepsy, are often associated with ED. Parkinsonism's effect may be caused by the imbalance of the dopaminergic pathways [48]. Other lesions in the brain noted to be associated with ED are tumors, dementias, Alzheimer's disease, Shy-Drager syndrome, and trauma.

In men who have a spinal cord injury, their erectile function depends largely on the nature, location, and extent of the spinal lesion. In addition to ED, they may also have impaired ejaculation and orgasm. Reflexogenic erection is preserved in 95% of patients who have complete upper cord lesions, whereas only about 25% of those who have complete lower cord lesions can achieve an erection [49]. It appears that sacral parasympathetic neurons are important in the preservation of reflexogenic erection; however, the thoracolumbar pathway may compensate for loss of the sacral lesion through synaptic connections [10]. In these men, minimal tactile stimulation can trigger erection, albeit of short duration, requiring continuous stimulation to maintain erection. Other disorders at the spinal level (eg, spina bifida, disc herniation, syringomyelia, tumor, transverse myelitis, and multiple sclerosis) may affect the afferent or the efferent neural pathway in a similar manner.

Because of the close relationship between the cavernous nerves and the pelvic organs, surgery on these organs is a frequent cause of impotence. The incidence of iatrogenic impotence from various procedures has been reported as follows: radical prostatectomy, 43% to 100%; perineal prostatectomy for benign disease, 29%; abdominal perineal resection, 15% to 100%; and external sphincterotomy at the 3- and 9-o'clock positions, 2% to 49% [50–55].

An improved understanding of the neuroanatomy of the pelvic and cavernous nerves has resulted in modified surgery for cancer of the rectum,

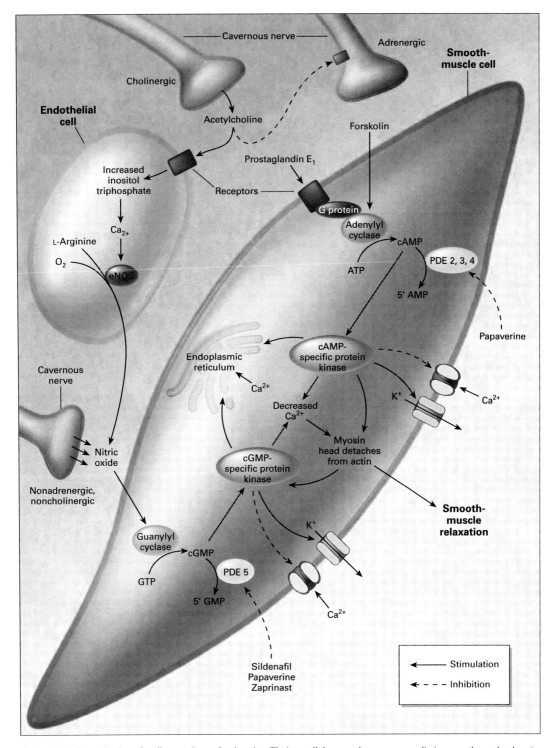

Fig. 3. Molecular mechanism of penile smooth muscle relaxation. The intracellular second messengers mediating smooth muscle relaxation (cAMP and cGMP) activate their specific protein kinases, which phosphorylate certain proteins to cause the opening of potassium channels, closing of calcium channels, and sequestration of intracellular calcium by the endoplasmic reticulum. The resultant fall in intracellular calcium leads to smooth muscle relaxation. Sildenafil inhibits the action of phosphodiesterase (PDE)-5 and thus increases the intracellular concentration of cGMP. Papaverine is a nonspecific phosphodiesterase inhibitor. eNOS, endothelial NO synthase. (*From* Lue TF. Erectile dysfunction. N Engl J Med 2000;342:1805. Copyright © 2000 Massachusetts Medical Society. All rights reserved; with permission.)

Box 1. Classification of male erectile dysfunction

Organic
Vasculogenic
    Arteriogenic
    Cavernosal
    Mixed
    Neurogenic
    Anatomic
    Endocrinologic

Psychogenic
Generalized
    Generalized unresponsiveness
    Primary lack of sexual arousability
    Aging-related decline in sexual
      arousability
    Generalized inhibition
    Chronic disorder of sexual intimacy
Situational
    Partner related
    Lack of arousability in specific
      relationship
    Lack of arousability owing to sexual
      object preference
    High central inhibition owing to
      partner conflict or threat
    Performance related
    Associated with other sexual
      dysfunction/s (eg, rapid ejaculation)
    Situational performance anxiety
      (eg, fear of failure)
    Psychologic distress related or
      adjustment related
    Associated with negative mood state
      (eg, depression) or major life stress
      (eg, death of partner)

---

bladder, and prostate, producing a lower incidence of iatrogenic impotence [52]. For example, the introduction of nerve-sparing radical prostatectomy has reduced the incidence of impotence from nearly 100% to between 30% and 50% [56,57]. Recovery of erectile function after radical pelvic surgery can take 6 to 24 months. Early treatment with intracavernous alprostadil or oral sildenafil has been shown to improve recovery of erectile function [58,59]. It is believed that the pharmacologically induced erections prevent the structural tissue changes associated with infrequent or no erections during the nerve recovery period.

In cases of pelvic fracture, ED can be a result of cavernous nerve injury, vascular insufficiency, or both. In an animal experiment in mature rats, alcoholism, vitamin deficiency, and diabetes may affect the cavernous nerve terminals and may result in deficiency of neurotransmitters. In diabetics, impairment of neurogenic and endothelium-dependent relaxation results in inadequate NO release [4]. Because there is no direct means to test the autonomic innervation of the penis, clinicians should be cautious in making the diagnosis of neurogenic ED. NADPH diaphorase staining of the nonadrenergic noncholinergic (NANC) nerve fibers in penile biopsy specimens has been proposed as an indicator of neurogenic status [60]. Stief and associates [61] also proposed single potential analysis of cavernous electrical activity for assessment of cavernous nerve function. Further studies are needed before these tests can routinely be used in clinical practice.

Bemelmans and colleagues [62] performed somatosensory-evoked potentials and sacral-reflex latencies on impotent patients who had no clinically overt neurologic disease and found that 47% had at least one abnormal neurophysiologic measurement and that an abnormality was found more often in older patients. A decrease in penile tactile sensitivity with increasing age was also reported by Rowland and coworkers [63]. Sensory input from the genitalia is essential in achieving and maintaining reflexogenic erection, and the input becomes even more important when older people gradually lose psychogenic erection. Therefore, sensory evaluation should be an integral part of the evaluation for ED in all patients who have or do not have an apparent neurologic disorder.

Endocrinologic

Hypogonadism is a frequent finding in the impotent population. Androgens influence the growth and development of the male reproductive tract and secondary sex characteristics; their effects on libido and sexual behavior are well established. In a review of published articles from 1975 to 1992, Mulligan and Schmitt [64] concluded that (1) testosterone enhances sexual interest, (2) testosterone increases the frequency of sexual acts, and (3) testosterone increases the frequency of nocturnal erections but has little or no effect on fantasy-induced or visually induced erections. A study correlating testosterone levels and nocturnal erections in men reported that the threshold testosterone level for normal nocturnal erections is about 200 ng/dL [65]. Men who have lower serum testosterone levels often have abnormal nocturnal erection parameters compared with men who have normal levels of testosterone. Exogenous testosterone therapy in impotent men who have borderline low testosterone levels, however, reportedly has little effect on potency [66].

Several investigators have examined the mechanism of androgen's effect. Beyer and Gonzales-Mariscal [67] reported that testosterone and dihydrotestosterone are responsible for male pelvic thrusting and estradiol or testosterone is responsible for female pelvic thrusting during copulation. In rats, castration has been reported to decrease arterial flow, induce venous leakage, and reduce about half of the erectile response to stimulation of the cavernous nerve [68,69]. Treatment with flutamide, estradiol, or a gonadotropin-releasing hormone antagonist, in addition to castration, further depresses the erectile response. Although penile NO synthase activity is reduced in these animals, the contents of neuronal NO synthase and endothelial NO synthase are not significantly reduced by the treatment. Castration also increases α-adrenergic responsiveness of penile smooth muscle, increases apoptosis in the corpus cavernosum in rats, and reduces trabecular smooth muscle content in rabbits [70–72]. Clinically, many men on long-term androgen ablation therapy for prostate cancer have reported poor libido and ED.

Any dysfunction of the hypothalamic-pituitary axis can result in hypogonadism. Hypogonadotropic hypogonadism can be congenital or caused by a tumor or injury; hypergonadotropic hypogonadism may result from a tumor, an injury, or surgery to the testis or from mumps orchitis.

Hyperprolactinemia, whether from a pituitary adenoma or drugs, results in reproductive and sexual dysfunction. Symptoms may include loss of libido, ED, galactorrhea, gynecomastia, and infertility. Hyperprolactinemia is associated with low circulating levels of testosterone, which appear to be secondary to inhibition of gonadotropin-releasing hormone secretion by the elevated prolactin levels [73].

ED also may be associated with the hyperthyroid and the hypothyroid state. Hyperthyroidism is commonly associated with diminished libido, which may be caused by the increased circulating estrogen levels, and less often with ED. In hypothyroidism, low testosterone secretion and elevated prolactin levels contribute to ED.

Arteriogenic

Atherosclerotic or traumatic arterial occlusive disease of the hypogastric-cavernous-helicine arterial tree can decrease the perfusion pressure and arterial flow to the sinusoidal spaces, thus increasing the time to maximal erection and decreasing the rigidity of the erect penis. In most patients who have arteriogenic ED, the impaired penile perfusion is a component of the generalized atherosclerotic process. Michal and Ruzbarsky [74] found that the incidence and age at onset of coronary disease and ED are parallel. Common risk factors associated with arterial insufficiency include hypertension, hyperlipidemia, cigarette smoking, diabetes mellitus, blunt perineal or pelvic trauma, and pelvic irradiation [75–77]. Shabsigh and associates [78] reported that abnormal penile vascular findings increase significantly as the number of risk factors for ED increase. On arteriography, bilateral diffuse disease of the internal pudendal, common penile, and cavernous arteries has been found in impotent patients who have atherosclerosis. Focal stenosis of the common penile or cavernous artery is most often seen in young patients who have sustained blunt pelvic or perineal trauma [76]. Long-distance cycling is also a risk factor for vasculogenic and neurogenic ED [79,80].

In one report, older men and men who had diabetes had a high incidence of fibrotic lesions of the cavernous artery, with intimal proliferation, calcification, and luminal stenosis [74]. Nicotine may adversely affect erectile function not only by decreasing arterial flow to the penis but also by blocking corporeal smooth muscle relaxation and thus preventing normal venous occlusion [81,82].

ED and cardiovascular disease share the same risk factors such as hypertension, diabetes mellitus, hypercholesterolemia, and smoking [83,84]. Lesions in the pudendal arteries are much more common in impotent men than in similarly aged men in the general population [85]. ED can therefore be a manifestation of generalized or focal arterial disease [86].

Structural changes

In ED, due to arterial insufficiency, there is a decrease in oxygen tension in corpus cavernosum blood compared with oxygen tension measured in patients who have psychogenic ED [87]. Because prostaglandin E_1 and prostaglandin E_2 formation is oxygen dependent, an increase in oxygen tension is associated with elevation of prostaglandin E_2 and suppression of transforming growth factor β1–induced collagen synthesis in rabbit and human corpus cavernosum [88,89]. Conversely, a decrease in oxygen tension may diminish cavernous trabecular smooth muscle content and lead to diffuse venous leakage [90,91].

A narrowed lumen or increased wall-to-lumen ratio in the arteries contributes to increased peripheral vascular resistance in hypertension [92]. An increased resistance was also found in the penile vasculature of spontaneously hypertensive rats (SHR), and these alterations were ascribed to structural changes of the arterial and erectile tissue [93–95]. The increase in extracellular matrix expansion affects the interstitium and neural structures of the penis.

Vasoconstriction

Enhanced basal and myogenic tone has been observed in arteries of hypertensive rats. Enhanced sympathetic nerve activity accompanying hypertension has also been reported in humans and hypertensive animals [96,97]. The enhanced vasoconstriction of the penile vasculature in SHR induced by infusion of phenylephrine was attributed to hypertrophy of the vascular wall but not to the alteration of sympathetic neurotransmitters [93].

Impaired endothelium-dependent vasodilatation

In patients who have essential hypertension, the endothelium-dependent vasodilatation elicited by the infusion of agonists (acetylcholine, bradykinin), or by vascular flow is diminished [98–100]. Recent evidence indicates that profound endothelial dysfunction in the coronary circulation can predict major coronary events [101,102].

Endothelial dysfunction, measured as blunted acetylcholine-induced vasorelaxation, is evident in small arteries from patients who have renovascular hypertension [103,104]; however, there is a lack of studies on penile endothelial function in hypertensive men.

In the SHR, the relaxing effect of acetylcholine is blunted in large and small arteries, and endothelial dysfunction appears to develop with the appearance of hypertension [105]. Endothelium-dependent relaxation evoked by acetylcholine is also impaired in corporal strips from SHR, and these relaxations are restored in the presence of indomethacin [106]. Impairment of endothelium-dependent relaxation could be ascribed to angiotensin II thromboxane and superoxide in arteries

from SHR or to high blood pressure per se [107–111].

Cavernosal (venogenic)

Failure of adequate venous occlusion has been proposed as one of the most common causes of vasculogenic impotence [112]. Veno-occlusive dysfunction may result from the following pathophysiologic processes:

1. The presence or development of large venous channels can drain the corpora cavernosa.
2. Degenerative changes (Peyronie's disease, old age, and diabetes) or traumatic injury to the tunica albuginea (penile fracture) can result in inadequate compression of the subtunical and emissary veins. In Peyronie's disease, the inelastic tunica albuginea may prevent the emissary veins from closing [113]. Iacono and coworkers [114,115] postulated that a decrease in elastic fibers in the tunica albuginea and an alteration of microarchitecture may contribute to impotence in some men. Changes in the subtunical areolar layer may impair the veno-occlusive mechanism, as is occasionally seen in patients after surgery for Peyronie's disease [116].
3. Structural alterations in the fibroelastic components of the trabeculae, cavernous smooth muscle, and endothelium may result in venous leak.
4. Insufficient trabecular smooth muscle relaxation, causing inadequate sinusoidal expansion and insufficient compression of the subtunical venules, may occur in an anxious individual who has excessive adrenergic tone or in a patient who has inadequate neurotransmitter release. It has been shown that alteration of an α-adrenoceptor or a decrease in NO release may heighten the smooth muscle tone and impair the relaxation in response to an endogenous muscle relaxant [117].
5. Acquired venous shunts—the result of operative correction of priapism—may cause persistent glans/cavernosum or cavernosum/spongiosum shunting.

Fibroelastic component

Loss of compliance of the penile sinusoids associated with increased deposition of collagen and decreased elastic fibers may be seen in diabetes, hypercholesterolemia, vascular disease, penile injury, or old age [118,119]. Sattar and colleagues [120] reported a significant difference in the mean percentage of elastic fibers in the penis: 9% in normal men, 5.1% in patients who had venous leakage, and 4.3% in patients who had arterial disease. In an animal model of vasculogenic ED, Nehra and associates [91] demonstrated that cavernosal expandability correlates with smooth muscle content and may be used to predict trabecular histology. Moreland and colleagues [88] showed that prostaglandin E_1 suppresses collagen synthesis by decreasing transforming growth factor $\beta 1$ in human cavernous smooth muscle, which implies that intracavernous injection of prostaglandin E_1 may be beneficial in preventing intracavernous fibrosis.

Smooth muscle

Because corporeal smooth muscle controls the vascular event leading to erection, change of smooth muscle content and ultrastructure can be expected to affect erectile response. In a study of human penile tissue, Sattar and associates [120] demonstrated a significant difference between the mean percentage of cavernous smooth muscle (stained with antidesmin [38.5%] or antiactin [45.2%]) in normal potent men and the venous group (antidesmin, 27.4%; antiactin, 34.2%) or arteriogenic group (antidesmin, 23.7%, antiactin, 28.9%). An in vitro biochemical study has shown impaired neurogenic and endothelium-related relaxation of penile smooth muscle in impotent men who had diabetes [4]. In vasculogenic and neurogenic ED, the damaged smooth muscle can be a key factor, aggravating the primary cause [121]. Pickard and coworkers [122] also showed impairment of nerve-evoked relaxation and α-adrenergic–stimulated contraction of cavernous muscle and reduced muscle content in men who had venous or mixed venous/arterial impotence.

Ion channels are intimately involved in the biochemical events of muscle function, and an alteration of ion channels may have a profound effect on muscle function. Fan and colleagues [123] reported an alteration of the maxi-K^+ channel in cells from impotent patients and suggested that impairment in the function or regulation of potassium channels might contribute to the decreased hyperpolarizing ability, altered calcium homeostasis, and impaired smooth muscle relaxation in impotent patients. In animal studies, Junemann and coworkers [81] showed significant smooth muscle degeneration with loss of cell-to-cell contact in rabbits fed a high-cholesterol diet

for 3 months. In a rabbit model of vasculogenic impotence, Azadzoi and associates [124] demonstrated that veno-occlusive dysfunction could be induced by cavernosal ischemia.

Gap junction

These intercellular communication channels are responsible for the synchronized and coordinated erectile response, although their pathophysiologic impact has yet to be clarified [125,126]. In severe arterial disease, a loss or reduction of membrane contact is seen because of the presence of collagen fibers between cellular membranes [127]. These findings imply that a malfunction or loss of gap junctions may alter the coordinated smooth muscle activity.

Endothelium

By release of vasoactive agents, the endothelium of the corpus cavernosum can modify the tone of adjacent smooth muscle and affect the development or inhibition of an erection. NO, prostaglandin, and the polypeptide endothelins have been identified in the endothelial cell [5,90]. Activation of cholinergic receptors on the endothelial cell by acetylcholine or stretching of the endothelial cells as a result of increased blood flow may elicit underlying smooth muscle relaxation through the release of NO. Diabetes and hypercholesterolemia have been shown to alter the function of endothelium-mediated relaxation of the cavernous muscle and to impair erection [128].

In summary, considerable events can cause ED. In addition, no one cause may be involved independently. A cascade of issues (including psychologic and organic) can lead the to the impotent state. A continued understanding of the organic causes of ED will allow the physician to discover therapies for correction and provide reassurance to the patient.

References

[1] Sattar AA, Salpigides G, Vanderhaeghen JJ, et al. Cavernous oxygen tension and smooth muscle fibers: relation and function. J Urol 1995;154:1736.

[2] Bosch RJ, Benard F, Aboseif SR, et al. Penile detumescence: characterization of three phases. J Urol 1991;146:867.

[3] Lue TF, Takamura T, Schmidt RA, et al. Hemodynamics of erection in the monkey. J Urol 1983;130:1237.

[4] Saenz de Tejada I, Goldstein I, Azadzoi K, et al. Impaired neurogenic and endothelium-mediated

relaxation of penile smooth muscle from diabetic men with impotence. N Engl J Med 1989;320:1025.

[5] Ignarro LJ, Bush PA, Buga GM, et al. Nitric oxide and cyclic GMP formation upon electrical field stimulation cause relaxation of corpus cavernosum smooth muscle. Biochem Biophys Res Commun 1990;170:843.

[6] De Groat W, Booth A. Neural control of penile erection. London: Harwood; 1993.

[7] Walsh PC, Brendler CB, Chang T, et al. Preservation of sexual function in men during radical pelvic surgery. MD Med J 1990;39:389.

[8] Paick JS, Donatucci CF, Lue TF. Anatomy of cavernous nerves distal to prostate: microdissection study in adult male cadavers. Urology 1993;42:145.

[9] Root W, Bard P. The mediation of feline erection through sympathetic pathways with some reference on sexual behavior after deafferentation of the gentalia. Am J Physiol 1947;151:80.

[10] Courtois FJ, Macdougall JC, Sachs BD. Erectile mechanism in paraplegia. Physiol Behav 1993;53: 721.

[11] Paick JS, Lee SW. The neural mechanism of apomorphine-induced erection: an experimental study by comparison with electrostimulation-induced erection in the rat model. J Urol 1994;152:2125.

[12] Bors E, Camarr A. Neurological distubances in sexual function with special reference to 529 patients with spinal cord injury. Urol Surv 1960; 10:191.

[13] Chapelle PA, Durand J, Lacert P. Penile erection following complete spinal cord injury in man. Br J Urol 1980;52:216.

[14] Halata Z, Munger BL. The neuroanatomical basis for the protopathic sensibility of the human glans penis. Brain Res 1986;371:205.

[15] McKenna KE. Central control of penile erection. Int J Impot Res 1998;10(Suppl 1):S25.

[16] Burnett AL, Tillman SL, Chang TS, et al. Immunohistochemical localization of nitric oxide synthase in the autonomic innervation of the human penis. J Urol 1993;150:73.

[17] Carrier S, Zvara P, Nunes L, et al. Regeneration of nitric oxide synthase-containing nerves after cavernous nerve neurotomy in the rat. J Urol 1995; 153:1722.

[18] Giuliano F, Rampin O, Jardin A, et al. Electrophysiological study of relations between the dorsal nerve of the penis and the lumbar sympathetic chain in the rat. J Urol 1993;150:1960.

[19] Marson L, McKenna KE. CNS cell groups involved in the control of the ischiocavernosus and bulbospongiosus muscles: a transneuronal tracing study using pseudorabies virus. J Comp Neurol 1996;374:161.

[20] Tang Y, Rampin O, Calas A, et al. Oxytocinergic and serotonergic innervation of identified lumbosacral nuclei controlling penile erection in the male rat. Neuroscience 1998;82:241.

[21] Sachs B, Meisel R. The physiology of male sexual behavior. In: Knobil E, Neill J, Ewing L, editors. The physiology of reproduction. New York: Raven Press; 1988. p. 1393–423.

[22] Marson L, Platt KB, McKenna KE. Central nervous system innervation of the penis as revealed by the transneuronal transport of pseudorabies virus. Neuroscience 1993;55:263.

[23] Mallick HN, Manchanda SK, Kumar VM. Sensory modulation of the medial preoptic area neuronal activity by dorsal penile nerve stimulation in rats. J Urol 1994;151:759.

[24] Stoleru S, Gregoire MC, Gerard D, et al. Neuroanatomical correlates of visually evoked sexual arousal in human males. Arch Sex Behav 1999;28:1.

[25] Bocher M, Chisin R, Parag Y, et al. Cerebral activation associated with sexual arousal in response to a pornographic clip: a 15O-H2O PET study in heterosexual men. Neuroimage 2001;14:105.

[26] Park K, Seo JJ, Kang HK, et al. A new potential of blood oxygenation level dependent (BOLD) functional MRI for evaluating cerebral centers of penile erection. Int J Impot Res 2001;13:73.

[27] Arnow BA, Desmond JE, Banner LL, et al. Brain activation and sexual arousal in healthy, heterosexual males. Brain 2002;125:1014.

[28] Redoute J, Stoleru S, Gregoire MC, et al. Brain processing of visual sexual stimuli in human males. Hum Brain Mapp 2000;11:162.

[29] Mouras H, Stoleru S, Bittoun J, et al. Brain processing of visual sexual stimuli in healthy men: a functional magnetic resonance imaging study. Neuroimage 2003;20:855.

[30] Stoleru S, Redoute J, Costes N, et al. Brain processing of visual sexual stimuli in men with hypoactive sexual desire disorder. Psychiatry Res 2003; 124:67.

[31] Montorsi F, Perani D, Anchisi D, et al. Brain activation patterns during video sexual stimulation following the administration of apomorphine: results of a placebo-controlled study. Eur Urol 2003;43: 405.

[32] Walsh MP. The Ayerst Award Lecture 1990. Calcium-dependent mechanisms of regulation of smooth muscle contraction. Biochem Cell Biol 1991;69:771.

[33] Somlyo AP, Somlyo AV. Signal transduction by G-proteins, rho-kinase and protein phosphatase to smooth muscle and non-muscle myosin II. J Physiol 2000;522(Pt 2):177.

[34] Rees RW, Ziessen T, Ralph DJ, et al. Human and rabbit cavernosal smooth muscle cells express Rho-kinase. Int J Impot Res 2002;14:1.

[35] Wang H, Eto M, Steers WD, et al. RhoA-mediated Ca2+ sensitization in erectile function. J Biol Chem 2002;277:30614.

[36] Rees RW, Ralph DJ, Royle M, et al. Y-27632, an inhibitor of Rho-kinase, antagonizes noradrenergic contractions in the rabbit and human penile corpus cavernosum. Br J Pharmacol 2001;133:455.

[37] Chitaley K, Bivalacqua TJ, Champion HC, et al. Adeno-associated viral gene transfer of dominant negative RhoA enhances erectile function in rats. Biochem Biophys Res Commun 2002;298:427.

[38] Cellek S, Rees RW, Kalsi J. A Rho-kinase inhibitor, soluble guanylate cyclase activator and nitric oxide-releasing PDE5 inhibitor: novel approaches to erectile dysfunction. Expert Opin Investig Drugs 2002;11:1563.

[39] Lizza EF, Rosen RC. Definition and classification of erectile dysfunction: report of the Nomenclature Committee of the International Society of Impotence Research. Int J Impot Res 1999;11:141.

[40] Masters W, Johnson V. Human sexual response. Boston: Little Brown; 1970.

[41] Steers WD. Neural control of penile erection. Semin Urol 1990;8:66.

[42] Diederichs W, Stief CG, Benard F, et al. The sympathetic role as an antagonist of erection. Urol Res 1991;19:123.

[43] Diederichs W, Stief CG, Lue TF, et al. Sympathetic inhibition of papaverine induced erection. J Urol 1991;146:195.

[44] Kim SC, Oh MM. Norepinephrine involvement in response to intracorporeal injection of papaverine in psychogenic impotence. J Urol 1992;147:1530.

[45] Bancroft J. Lecture 4: psychogenic erectile dysfunction-a theoretical approach. Int J Impot Res 2000; 12(Suppl 3):S46.

[46] Abicht J. Testing the autonomic system. In: Jonas U, Thoh W, Steif C, editors. Erectile dysfunction. Berlin: SpringerVerlag; 1991. p. 187–94.

[47] Aboseif S, Shinohara K, Borirakchanyavat S, et al. The effect of cryosurgical ablation of the prostate on erectile function. Br J Urol 1997;80:918.

[48] Wermuth L, Stenager E. Sexual aspects of Parkinson's disease. Semin Neurol 1992;12:125.

[49] Eardley I, Kirby R. Neurogenic impotence. In: Kirby R, Carson C, Webster G, editors. Impotence: diagnosis and management of male erectile dysfunction. Oxford, England: Butterworth-Heinemann; 1991. p. 227–31.

[50] Veenema RJ, Gursel EO, Lattimer JK. Radical retropubic prostatectomy for cancer: a 20-year experience. J Urol 1977;117:330.

[51] Finkle AL, Taylor SP. Sexual potency after radical prostatectomy. J Urol 1981;125:350.

[52] Walsh PC, Donker PJ. Impotence following radical prostatectomy: insight into etiology and prevention. J Urol 1982;128:492.

[53] Weinstein M, Roberts M. Sexual potency following surgery for rectal carcinoma. A followup of 44 patients. Ann Surg 1977;185:295.

[54] Yeager ES, Van Heerden JA. Sexual dysfunction following proctocolectomy and abdominoperineal resection. Ann Surg 1980;191:169.

[55] McDermott DW, Bates RJ, Heney NM, et al. Erectile impotence as complication of direct vision cold knife urethrotomy. Urology 1981;18:467.

[56] Catalona WJ, Bigg SW. Nerve-sparing radical prostatectomy: evaluation of results after 250 patients. J Urol 1990;143:538.

[57] Quinlan DM, Epstein JI, Carter BS, et al. Sexual function following radical prostatectomy: influence of preservation of neurovascular bundles. J Urol 1991;145:998.

[58] Montorsi F, Guazzoni G, Strambi LF, et al. Recovery of spontaneous erectile function after nerve-sparing radical retropubic prostatectomy with and without early intracavernous injections of alprostadil: results of a prospective, randomized trial. J Urol 1997;158:1408.

[59] Padma-Nathan H, McCullough A, Forest C. Erectile dysfunction secondary to nerve-sparing radical retropubic prostatectomy: comparative phosphodiesterase-5 inhibitor efficacy for therapy and novel prevention strategies. Curr Urol Rep 2004;5:467.

[60] Brock G, Nunes L, Padma-Nathan H, et al. Nitric oxide synthase: a new diagnostic tool for neurogenic impotence. Urology 1993;42:412.

[61] Stief CG, Djamilian M, Anton P, et al. Single potential analysis of cavernous electrical activity in impotent patients: a possible diagnostic method for autonomic cavernous dysfunction and cavernous smooth muscle degeneration. J Urol 1991;146:771.

[62] Bemelmans BL, Meuleman EJ, Anten BW, et al. Penile sensory disorders in erectile dysfunction: results of a comprehensive neuro-urophysiological diagnostic evaluation in 123 patients. J Urol 1991; 146:777.

[63] Rowland DL, Greenleaf WJ, Dorfman LJ, et al. Aging and sexual function in men. Arch Sex Behav 1993;22:545.

[64] Mulligan T, Schmitt B. Testosterone for erectile failure. J Gen Intern Med 1993;8:517.

[65] Granata AR, Rochira V, Lerchl A, et al. Relationship between sleep-related erections and testosterone levels in men. J Androl 1997; 18:522.

[66] Graham C, Regan J. Blinded clinical trial of testosterone enanthate in impotent men with low or low-normal serum testosterone levels. Int J Impot Res 1992;4:144.

[67] Beyer C, Gonzalez-Mariscal G. Effects of sex steroids on sensory and motor spinal mechanisms. Psychoneuroendocrinology 1994;19:517.

[68] Mills TM, Stopper VS, Wiedmeier VT. Effects of castration and androgen replacement on the hemodynamics of penile erection in the rat. Biol Reprod 1994;51:234.

[69] Penson DF, Ng C, Cai L, et al. Androgen and pituitary control of penile nitric oxide synthase and erectile function in the rat. Biol Reprod 1996;55: 567.

[70] Reilly CM, Lewis RW, Stopper VS, et al. Androgenic maintenance of the rat erectile response via a non-nitric-oxide-dependent pathway. J Androl 1997;18:588.

[71] Shabsigh R. The effects of testosterone on the cavernous tissue and erectile function. World J Urol 1997;15:21.

[72] Traish AM, Park K, Dhir V, et al. Effects of castration and androgen replacement on erectile function in a rabbit model. Endocrinology 1999; 140:1861.

[73] Leonard MP, Nickel CJ, Morales A. Hyperprolactinemia and impotence: why, when and how to investigate. J Urol 1989;142:992.

[74] Michal V, Ruzbarsky V. Histological changes in the penile artial bed with aging and diabetes. In: Zorgniotti A, Rossi G, editors. Vasculogenic impotence. Proceedings of the First International Conference on Corpus Cavernosum Revascularization. Springfield (IL): Charles C. Thomas; 1980. p. 113–9.

[75] Goldstein I, Feldman MI, Deckers PJ, et al. Radiation-associated impotence. A clinical study of its mechanism. JAMA 1984;251:903.

[76] Levine FJ, Greenfield AJ, Goldstein I. Arteriographically determined occlusive disease within the hypogastric-cavernous bed in impotent patients following blunt perineal and pelvic trauma. J Urol 1990;144:1147.

[77] Rosen MP, Greenfield AJ, Walker TG, et al. Arteriogenic impotence: findings in 195 impotent men examined with selective internal pudendal angiography. Young Investigator's Award. Radiology 1990;174:1043.

[78] Shabsigh R, Fishman IJ, Schum C, et al. Cigarette smoking and other vascular risk factors in vasculogenic impotence. Urology 1991;38:227.

[79] Andersen KV, Bovim G. Impotence and nerve entrapment in long distance amateur cyclists. Acta Neurol Scand 1997;95:233.

[80] Ricchiuti VS, Haas CA, Seftel AD, et al. Pudendal nerve injury associated with avid bicycling. J Urol 1999;162:2099.

[81] Junemann KP, Aufenanger J, Konrad T, et al. The effect of impaired lipid metabolism on the smooth muscle cells of rabbits. Urol Res 1991; 19:271.

[82] Rosen MP, Greenfield AJ, Walker TG, et al. Cigarette smoking: an independent risk factor for atherosclerosis in the hypogastric-cavernous arterial bed of men with arteriogenic impotence. J Urol 1991;145:759.

[83] Martin-Morales A, Sanchez-Cruz JJ, Saenz de Tejada I, et al. Prevalence and independent risk factors for erectile dysfunction in Spain: results of the Epidemiologia de la Disfuncion Erectil Masculina Study. J Urol 2001;166:569.

[84] Feldman HA, Goldstein I, Hatzichristou DG, et al. Impotence and its medical and psychosocial correlates: results of the Massachusetts Male Aging Study. J Urol 1994;151:54.

[85] Virag R, Bouilly P, Frydman D. Is impotence an arterial disorder? A study of arterial risk factors in 440 impotent men. Lancet 1985;1:181.

[86] Sullivan ME, Thompson CS, Dashwood MR, et al. Nitric oxide and penile erection: is erectile dysfunction another manifestation of vascular disease? Cardiovasc Res 1999;43:658.

[87] Tarhan F, Kuyumcuoglu U, Kolsuz A, et al. Cavernous oxygen tension in the patients with erectile dysfunction. Int J Impot Res 1997;9:149.

[88] Moreland RB, Traish A, McMillin MA, et al. PGE1 suppresses the induction of collagen synthesis by transforming growth factor-beta 1 in human corpus cavernosum smooth muscle. J Urol 1995; 153:826.

[89] Nehra A, Gettman MT, Nugent M, et al. Transforming growth factor-beta1 (TGF-beta1) is sufficient to induce fibrosis of rabbit corpus cavernosum in vivo. J Urol 1999;162:910.

[90] Saenz de Tejada I, Moroukian P, Tessier J, et al. Trabecular smooth muscle modulates the capacitor function of the penis. Studies on a rabbit model. Am J Physiol 1991;260:H1590.

[91] Nehra A, Azadzoi KM, Moreland RB, et al. Cavernosal expandability is an erectile tissue mechanical property which predicts trabecular histology in an animal model of vasculogenic erectile dysfunction. J Urol 1998;159:2229.

[92] Mulvany MJ. Small artery remodeling in hypertension. Curr Hypertens Rep 2002;4:49.

[93] Okabe H, Hale TM, Kumon H, et al. The penis is not protected—in hypertension there are vascular changes in the penis which are similar to those in other vascular beds. Int J Impot Res 1999;11:133.

[94] Toblli JE, Stella I, Inserra F, et al. Morphological changes in cavernous tissue in spontaneously hypertensive rats. Am J Hypertens 2000;13:686.

[95] Hale TM, Okabe H, Heaton JP, et al. Antihypertensive drugs induce structural remodeling of the penile vasculature. J Urol 2001;166:739.

[96] Norman RA Jr, Dzielak DJ. Immunological dysfunction and enhanced sympathetic activity contribute to the pathogenesis of spontaneous hypertension. J Hypertens Suppl 1986;4:S437.

[97] Mancia G, Grassi G, Giannattasio C, et al. Sympathetic activation in the pathogenesis of hypertension and progression of organ damage. Hypertension 1999;34:724.

[98] Panza JA, Quyyumi AA, Brush JE Jr, et al. Abnormal endothelium-dependent vascular relaxation in patients with essential hypertension. N Engl J Med 1990;323:22.

[99] Taddei S, Virdis A, Ghiadoni L, et al. Vitamin C improves endothelium-dependent vasodilation by restoring nitric oxide activity in essential hypertension. Circulation 1998;97:2222.

[100] Cai H, Harrison DG. Endothelial dysfunction in cardiovascular diseases: the role of oxidant stress. Circ Res 2000;87:840.

[101] Suwaidi JA, Hamasaki S, Higano ST, et al. Long-term follow-up of patients with mild coronary

artery disease and endothelial dysfunction. Circulation 2000;101:948.

[102] Schachinger V, Britten MB, Zeiher AM. Prognostic impact of coronary vasodilator dysfunction on adverse long-term outcome of coronary heart disease. Circulation 2000;101:1899.

[103] Rizzoni D, Porteri E, Castellano M, et al. Endothelial dysfunction in hypertension is independent from the etiology and from vascular structure. Hypertension 1998;31:335.

[104] Rizzoni D, Porteri E, Castellano M, et al. Vascular hypertrophy and remodeling in secondary hypertension. Hypertension 1996;28:785.

[105] Konishi M, Su C. Role of endothelium in dilator responses of spontaneously hypertensive rat arteries. Hypertension 1983;5:881.

[106] Behr-Roussel D, Chamiot-Clerc P, Bernabe J, et al. Erectile dysfunction in spontaneously hypertensive rats: pathophysiological mechanisms. Am J Physiol Regul Integr Comp Physiol 2003;284:R682.

[107] Rajagopalan S, Kurz S, Munzel T, et al. Angiotensin II-mediated hypertension in the rat increases vascular superoxide production via membrane NADH/NADPH oxidase activation. Contribution to alterations of vasomotor tone. J Clin Invest 1996; 97:1916.

[108] Heitzer T, Wenzel U, Hink U, et al. Increased NAD(P)H oxidase-mediated superoxide production in renovascular hypertension: evidence for an involvement of protein kinase C. Kidney Int 1999;55:252.

[109] Cosentino F, Patton S, d'Uscio LV, et al. Tetrahydrobiopterin alters superoxide and nitric oxide release in prehypertensive rats. J Clin Invest 1998;101:1530.

[110] Yang D, Feletou M, Boulanger CM, et al. Oxygen-derived free radicals mediate endothelium-dependent contractions to acetylcholine in aortas from spontaneously hypertensive rats. Br J Pharmacol 2002;136:104.

[111] Paniagua OA, Bryant MB, Panza JA. Transient hypertension directly impairs endothelium-dependent vasodilation of the human microvasculature. Hypertension 2000;36:941.

[112] Rajfer J, Rosciszewski A, Mehringer M. Prevalence of corporeal venous leakage in impotent men. J Urol 1988;140:69.

[113] Metz P, Ebbehoj J, Uhrenholdt A, et al. Peyronie's disease and erectile failure. J Urol 1983;130:1103.

[114] Iacono F, Barra S, de Rosa G, et al. Microstructural disorders of tunica albuginea in patients affected by impotence. Eur Urol 1994;26:233.

[115] Iacono F, Barra S, De Rosa G, et al. Microstructural disorders of tunica albuginea in patients affected by Peyronie's disease with or without erection dysfunction. J Urol 1993;150:1806.

[116] Dalkin BL, Carter MF. Venogenic impotence following dermal graft repair for Peyronie's disease. J Urol 1991;146:849.

[117] Christ GJ, Maayani S, Valcic M, et al. Pharmacological studies of human erectile tissue: characteristics of spontaneous contractions and alterations in alpha-adrenoceptor responsiveness with age and disease in isolated tissues. Br J Pharmacol 1990;101:375.

[118] Cerami A, Vlassara H, Brownlee M. Glucose and aging. Sci Am 1987;256:90.

[119] Hayashi K, Takamizawa K, Nakamura T, et al. Effects of elastase on the stiffness and elastic properties of arterial walls in cholesterol-fed rabbits. Atherosclerosis 1987;66:259.

[120] Sattar AA, Haot J, Schulman CC, et al. Comparison of anti-desmin and anti-actin staining for the computerized analysis of cavernous smooth muscle density. Br J Urol 1996;77:266.

[121] Mersdorf A, Goldsmith PC, Diederichs W, et al. Ultrastructural changes in impotent penile tissue: a comparison of 65 patients. J Urol 1991;145:749.

[122] Pickard RS, King P, Zar MA, et al. Corpus cavernosal relaxation in impotent men. Br J Urol 1994; 74:485.

[123] Fan SF, Brink PR, Melman A, et al. An analysis of the Maxi-K+ (KCa) channel in cultured human corporal smooth muscle cells. J Urol 1995;153:818.

[124] Azadzoi KM, Park K, Andry C, et al. Relationship between cavernosal ischemia and corporal veno-occlusive dysfunction in an animal model. J Urol 1997;157:1011.

[125] Christ GJ, Moreno AP, Parker ME, et al. Intercellular communication through gap junctions: a potential role in pharmacomechanical coupling and syncytial tissue contraction in vascular smooth muscle isolated from the human corpus cavernosum. Life Sci 1991;49:PL195.

[126] Lerner SE, Melman A, Christ GJ. A review of erectile dysfunction: new insights and more questions. J Urol 1993;149:1246.

[127] Persson C, Diederichs W, Lue TF, et al. Correlation of altered penile ultrastructure with clinical arterial evaluation. J Urol 1989;142:1462.

[128] Azadzoi KM, Saenz de Tejada I. Hypercholesterolemia impairs endothelium-dependent relaxation of rabbit corpus cavernosum smooth muscle. J Urol 1991;146:238.

ELSEVIER
SAUNDERS

Urol Clin N Am 32 (2005) 397–402

UROLOGIC
CLINICS
of North America

Erectile Dysfunction and Cardiovascular Risk Factors

Robert A. Kloner, MD, PhD[a,b,*]

aHeart Institute, Good Samaritan Hospital, 1225 Wilshire Boulevard, Los Angeles, CA 90017, USA
bDivision of Cardiovascular Medicine, Keck School of Medicine,
University of Southern California, Ambulatory Health Center, 1355 San Pablo Street,
AHC 117, Los Angeles, CA 90089, USA

There are numerous causes of erectile dysfunction (ED), including psychogenic, organic, and mixed psychogenic/organic. Among the organic causes the most common include vascular (including endothelial dysfunction and frank obstructive atherosclerosis), neurogenic (such as stroke, multiple sclerosis, spinal cord injury), endocrine (diabetes mellitus, hypothyroidism, hyperthyroidism, hyperprolactinemia), structural (trauma, Peyronie's disease), drug-induced, and others [1]. Some have estimated that nearly one half of all causes of ED in men over 50 years of age are vascular in nature [2,3].

Endothelial dysfunction and erectile dysfunction

For an erection to occur there must be adequate dilatation of the arteries and arterioles that bring blood into the corpus cavernosum of the penis and adequate dilatation of the sinusoids that are present in this structure [1]. Blood flow can be impeded by failure of nonobstructed blood vessels to dilate normally, and by mechanical obstruction caused by atherosclerotic plaques.

Endothelial dysfunction is one of the earliest manifestations of atherosclerotic vascular disease and can be detected in damaged blood vessels at a much earlier stage than the physical blockage of blood flow by atherosclerotic plaques. Endothelial dysfunction refers to physiological dysfunction of the normal biochemical processes of the cells that line the inner surface of blood vessels. Normally, blood vessels dilate in response to endothelial-dependent stimulation in which the endothelium releases substances (nitric oxide [NO]) that cause the surrounding smooth muscle to relax [4]. An example of a stimulus that causes NO release from the endothelium is changes in shear stress related to induction of reactive hyperemia by occluding and then reperfusing a blood vessel.

The flow-mediated vasodilatation that occurs upon release of an occluded vessel can be measured with high-resolution ultrasound and is used as a test of endothelial function. Typically, endothelial dysfunction is tested in the brachial arteries by inflating a blood pressure cuff to stop flow for several minutes and then releasing the cuff. The normal postischemic response is dilatation of the brachial artery (reactive hyperemia) for several minutes while the oxygen debt is paid back. In patients with endothelial dysfunction the vasodilator response is blunted.

Endothelial dysfunction also can be tested by infusing a blood vessel with acetylcholine. In normal vessels, acetylcholine causes the vessel to dilate. In vessels with endothelial dysfunction, there is a lack of dilatation or even vasoconstriction. Although the term *endothelial dysfunction* is used to describe this phenomenon, presumably related to hindered production or release of NO (endothelial-derived relaxing substance), it is also possible that blunted vasodilation can be related to an abnormality of the smooth muscle cells in

* Heart Institute, Good Samaritan Hospital, 1225 Wilshire Boulevard, Los Angeles, CA 90017, USA.
E-mail address: rkloner@goodsam.org

the wall of the blood vessels. Use of nonendothelial-dependent substances that dilate the arteries through a more direct effect on the smooth muscles (nitrates) can be considered to test for this concept.

Early experimental studies showed that rabbits fed an atherosclerotic diet failed to achieve normal erections following intracavernous injections of vasodilators, even before the development of obstructive atherosclerotic lesions in the blood vessels supplying the penis [5]. This observation suggests that a high-cholesterol diet, known to induce endothelial dysfunction, caused enough early functional damage to the blood vessels to hinder the vasodilatory response needed for erection.

Evidence that erectile dysfunction is an early marker of vascular disease

Kaiser and colleagues [6] recently reported that men who had ED and no other clinical cardiovascular disease demonstrated reduced brachial artery endothelium-dependent and -independent vasodilation. They studied 30 patients who had ED and 27 age-matched, normal control subjects. None of these patients had histories or physical findings of cardiovascular disease. The men who had ED had objective evidence of penile vascular disease. Mean peak systolic velocity of penile blood flow assessed by Doppler was 28 m/sec, whereas normal is greater than 35 m/sec. Brachial artery flow-mediated vasodilatation was reduced in ED patients (1.3%) compared with controls (2.4% at 90 seconds after cuff relief; $P = .014$). In addition to reduced flow-mediated vasodilatation of the brachial arteries, suggesting endothelial dysfunction, in the ED patients there was also a decrease in vasodilator response to sublingual nitroglycerin (13% in ED patients versus 18% in normal subjects, $P = .02$).

The latter finding suggests that endothelial-independent vasodilatation also was impaired in ED patients, suggesting that there is a possible problem with the smooth muscle cells of these patients involving the NO–cyclic GMP pathways. Of importance, the patients in this study had coronary calcium scores (rapid CT scanning) similar to the normal subjects. An accompanying editorial stated that ED should alert the physician to the presence or future presence of vascular problems elsewhere [7].

Other studies have suggested that the presence of ED may be an early marker for vascular disease [8–10]. Prior ED was present in 64% of patients who presented with myocardial infarction (MI). The ED occurred before the patient had known cardiovascular disease. Prior ED was present in 57% of men who required coronary artery bypass surgery [11]. ED may present before manifestations of coronary artery disease in some patients because the arteries supplying the penis are smaller than the coronary arteries. The penile arteries are typically 1 to 2 mm in diameter compared with the proximal left anterior descending coronary artery, which is 3 to 4 mm in diameter. Thus, the same plaque burden might limit flow in the penile artery, but not in a larger artery [8]. In addition, certain biochemical markers of endothelial cell activation were higher in men who had ED and no overt cardiovascular disease compared with healthy subjects, including soluble P-selectin, intercellular adhesion molecule–1, vascular cell adhesion molecule–1, and endothelin levels [12].

In a preliminary study, Pritzker and colleagues [13] described the results of stress testing, risk profile analysis, and, where available, angiography in 50 asymptomatic (cardiac) men 40 to 60 years of age who had ED. Eighty percent of the men had multiple cardiovascular risk factors, including smoking, high cholesterol levels, hypertension, diabetes mellitus, positive family history, and sedentary lifestyle. Exercise stress testing was positive for ECG evidence of ischemia in 28 of 50 patients. Twenty patients underwent coronary angiography. Six patients had left main coronary artery disease or severe three-vessel disease, seven patients had two-vessel disease, and seven patients had single-vessel disease. The investigators concluded that there was a high prevalence of risk factors and coronary artery disease in these cardiac asymptomatic men who had ED and coined the term *the Penile Stress Test* as a "Window to the Hearts of Man."

Gazzaruso and colleagues [14] studied the prevalence of ED in 133 diabetic men with angiographically documented silent coronary artery disease and 127 diabetic men without ischemia (documented by exercise ECG and echocardiographic stress testing as well as 48-hour ambulatory electrocardiographic monitoring). Patients were screened for ED by use of the validated International Index of Erectile Function questionnaire. ED was present in 33.8% of the male diabetic patients with angiographically detected silent coronary artery disease versus 4.7% of patients with no silent cardiac ischemia ($P = .0000$). Even when taking into account other known cardiovascular risk factors, ED was the best predictor of the presence of silent coronary artery disease. The investigators concluded that ED is associated strongly and independently with angiographically proven silent coronary artery disease in the type-2 diabetic men. ED prevalence was approximately eightfold higher in patients who had than who did not have silent coronary artery disease. Thus, ED should be considered a strong predictor of silent coronary artery disease in diabetic men.

Blumentals and colleagues [15] studied whether ED should be considered a marker for future acute MI. In a retrospective manner, they studied a database in which there were 12,825 patients who had ED and an equal number of men without ED. Each MI patient was followed from the first date of ED diagnosis until first diagnosis of acute MI. The average follow-up period was 1 year. The men who had ED had a twofold increase in the risk for MI after adjusting for confounding variables: age, smoking, obesity, and use of cardiovascular drugs. This increased risk became more prominent with age. The investigators concluded that cardiologists and internists should monitor ED patients who may not necessarily present with cardiovascular symptoms [15].

The Massachusetts Male Aging study [16] was one of the first studies to document the association between cardiovascular risk factors and ED. They observed that after adjustment for age, ED correlated with the presence of heart disease, hypertension, diabetes mellitus, smoking, and inversely with high-density lipoprotein (HDL) cholesterol. Virag and colleagues [17] showed that men who smoked, had lipid abnormalities, and diabetes mellitus were more likely to demonstrate ED than the general male population. Other studies have verified that many of the same risk factors that we associate with coronary artery disease are also risk factors for ED [18]. This makes sense because hypertension, diabetes mellitus, smoking, and cholesterol abnormalities can damage the endothelium, leading to endothelial dysfunction and acceleration of atherosclerosis. Atherosclerotic plaques extend beyond the intima and may involve the media as well as abnormalities in smooth muscle cells that may contribute to ED.

Initial workup for patient who has erectile dysfunction in relation to cardiac disease

The studies discussed suggest that ED may be an early warning sign for cardiovascular disease or that the patient has cardiovascular risk factors. When patients present to their health care provider with ED they should be questioned about their cardiovascular health. Do they have any cardiac symptoms: chest pain, dyspnea, orthopnea, fatigue, palpitations, syncope, and edema? Do they have modifiable cardiovascular risk factors: smoking, diabetes mellitus, hypertension, dyslipidemia (including elevated low-density lipoprotein [LDL] cholesterol and reduced levels of HDL cholesterol), physical inactivity, or obesity? Are they taking any cardiovascular medicines (eg, thiazide diuretics, beta-blockers, and other antihypertensives that may worsen erectile function)?

On physical examination, palpate the peripheral pulses and listen for carotid and abdominal bruits. Take an accurate blood pressure reading sitting and standing. Does the lung examination suggest chronic obstructive pulmonary disease and past smoking; are there rales, suggesting congestive heart failure? Are the nail beds stained yellow from heavy smoking? Is there clubbing? Check the jugular veins for evidence of distension (right-sided heart failure). A dyskinetic apex may reflect an MI. Are heart sounds normal? Pathologic fourth heart sounds are common in patients who have coronary heart disease or hypertension, whereas pathologic third heart sounds suggest volume overload or congestive heart failure. A mitral regurgitation murmur might reflect papillary muscle dysfunction caused by ischemic heart disease and scarring. Are there skin changes or ulcers on the extremities suggesting diabetes mellitus? Consider ordering a fasting blood sugar, hemoglobin A1C, lipid panel, and other laboratory tests to work up risk factors.

If cardiovascular risk factors are identified, they should be worked up and treated. In some cases, additional work-up may be indicated, such as a cardiac stress test, echocardiography, or coronary angiogram. There are excellent medicines that can control hypertension, lipid abnormalities, and diabetes mellitus and curb the use of cigarettes. Lifestyle modification always is indicated, and there is evidence that physical activity might improve ED. Although there is some controversy in the literature, treating risk factors may improve erectile function or may improve the responsiveness of men who have ED to therapies such as phosphodiesterase-5 inhibitors [10]. Furthermore, control of such risk factors as hypertension and hyperlipidemia reduce major cardiovascular and cerebrovascular events. Therefore, identifying and treating cardiovascular risk factors in the patient presenting with ED may not only improve the patient's ED, it may save the patient's life.

How common is erectile dysfunction in the patient with known coronary artery disease?

How common is ED in the patient who has documented coronary artery disease? According to a recent study from the author's research group, it is very common [19]. The author distributed the validated Sexual Health Inventory for men (SHIM), a five-item questionnaire derived from the International Index of Erectile Function questionnaire, which focuses on a man's ability to attain and then maintain an erection, to 76 men who had chronic stable coronary artery disease. These men were seeing their cardiologists for a routine outpatient visit. Most of these men had not discussed their sexual health with either their cardiologists or primary care providers. The mean age of the patients was 64 years with a range of 40 to 82 years. Twenty-four men had undergone coronary artery bypass surgery; 29 had undergone percutaneous transluminal coronary angioplasty with or without stenting. Hypertension was present in 17 patients and 11 had diabetes mellitus. Forty-seven percent of the men were taking beta-blockers, 92% were on statins, and 28% were on diuretics. Fifty-three of 76 (70%) men had a SHIM score of 21 or less, indicating a diagnosis of ED. Of those with a SHIM score of 21 or less, 25% had severe ED: a SHIM score of 7 or less. According to question 2 of the SHIM, 75% of the men had some difficulty achieving erections; according to question 3 of the SHIM, 67% had some difficulty maintaining an erection following penetration. Four men who were using sildenafil had SHIM scores of 23 to 25, reflecting successful therapy. Before their use of sildenafil they had histories of ED. When these four men are included in the category of having had ED, then 57 of 76 (75%) of the cohort had ED or a recent history of ED. Therefore, ED is common in men who have chronic stable coronary artery disease. Cardiologists and internists need to be aware of this connection and ask patients with coronary disease and risk factors for coronary artery disease about their sexual health.

Can phosphodiesterase-5 inhibitors improve vascular function?

The phosphodiesterase-5 inhibitors, including sildenafil, vardenafil, and tadalafil, are effective oral agents for the treatment of ED. How do they work? During sexual stimulation, there is release of NO from nerve cells and endothelial cells of the vasculature of the corpus cavernosum. Within the smooth muscle cell, NO stimulates the enzyme guanylate cyclase, which catalyzes the formation of cyclic GMP (cGMP), the substance that ultimately causes relaxation of the smooth muscle cells of the vasculature of the corpus cavernosum. The blood vessels and sinusoids of the corpus cavernosum dilate, resulting in a penile erection. In some men who have ED, cGMP levels are not adequate for normal erection. Phosphodiesterase-5 inhibitors prevent the breakdown of cGMP. cGMP then accumulates in the corpus cavernosum, resulting in improved dilatation of the vasculature and a better erection.

Because phosphodiesterase-5 is found not only in the vasculature of the genitals but also in systemic arteries and veins, there is a potential for phosphodiesterase-5 inhibitors to enhance vasodilatation in systemic vessels with functional or structural abnormalities. Katz and colleagues [20] studied the effect of sildenafil on flow-mediated vasodilation of the brachial artery in patients who had stable Class-II or -III heart failure. High-resolution two-dimensional ultrasound imaging was used to measure brachial artery diameter 60 to 75 seconds after release of a 1-, 3-, and 5-minute cuff occlusion of the artery. Patients received placebo or sildenafil 1 hour before the cuff inflation. There was a greater flow-mediated vasodilatation in patients receiving sildenafil than in the placebo group. Sildenafil was associated with a 3.3% to 4.1% increase in diameter versus a 0.2% to 0.7% increase in the placebo group. Therefore, sildenafil increased flow-mediated vasodilatation in patients who had stable heart failure.

Halcox and colleagues [21] studied the effects of sildenafil on epicardial coronary arteries. Sildenafil caused approximately 7% dilatation of these arteries in patients with and without coronary artery disease. Sildenafil enhanced coronary response to acetylcholine (endothelial-dependent) with greater enhancement in patients who had coronary artery disease. Sildenafil did not increase peak flow-mediated dilatation of the brachial artery, but did result in a longer duration of brachial artery vasodilatation. The investigators concluded that sildenafil not only dilates epicardial coronary arteries but also improves endothelial dysfunction.

Gori [22] presented recent studies that investigated whether sildenafil could prevent the impairment in endothelium-dependent vasodilatation that occurred following a 15-minute period of brachial artery ischemia. Gori showed that a 15-minute occlusion/reperfusion sequence of the brachial artery using a pneumatic cuff induced an abnormality in flow-mediated vasodilation of the radical artery. Radial artery diameter was assessed using B-mode ultrasound. A pneumatic cuff was placed at the wrist and inflated for 4.5 minutes and then deflated. The percent maximum increase in radial artery diameter was measured over 3.5 minutes. Before the 15-minute ischemia/reperfusion of the brachial artery, the degree of flow-mediated dilatation of the radial artery (percent increase in radial diameter during reactive hyperemia following a 4.5-minute inflation) was approximately 8%. After the 15-minute ischemia/reperfusion of the brachial artery, flow-mediated dilatation of the radial artery was approximately 1%. Sildenafil given 2 hours before brachial artery occlusion restored flow-mediated dilatation after brachial artery ischemia to 6.2%. The protective effect of sildenafil was prevented by prior administration of the K_{ATP} channel blocker, glibenclamide. The investigators concluded that sildenafil protected against ischemia/reperfusion-induced endothelial dysfunction by opening K_{ATP} channels. DeSouza and colleagues [23] showed that sildenafil had acute and chronic benefits on brachial artery flow-mediated vasodilation in type 2 diabetics.

A recent study suggested that the long-acting phosphodiesterase-5 inhibitor tadalafil also can improve endothelial function. Rosano and colleagues [24] randomized 32 patients with more than two cardiovascular risk factors to tadalafil, 20 mg, on alternate days or placebo for 4 weeks. Patients underwent assessment of endothelial function by assessing flow-mediated dilatation of the brachial artery with a 3-minute pneumatic tourniquet occlusion and measurements of brachial artery diameter at rest, during reactive hyperemia, and after 10 minutes of recovery. Assessment of endothelial function was performed at baseline, at the end of 4 weeks of treatment, and after 2 weeks of follow-up. Placebo had no effect on flow-mediated vasodilatation, whereas tadalafil increased it from 4.2% at baseline to 9.3% after 4 weeks of therapy ($P < .01$). Of interest, the benefit in flow-mediated vasodilatation was still present in tadalafil-treated patients 2 weeks after cessation of therapy. Thus the benefit of therapy was sustained and the investigators postulated that this effect might be related to an induction of NO production. Tadalafil therapy also was associated with an increase in nitrite/nitrate levels and a reduction in endothelin levels.

Although the phosphodiesterase-5 inhibitors initially were studied as possible cardiovascular drugs (specifically, sildenafil was studied for possible antianginal properties), they eventually were approved for therapy for ED. Now interest in these drugs as possible therapies for cardiovascular disease has come full circle as they are being explored for treating pulmonary hypertension, congestive heart failure, ischemic heart disease, and endothelial dysfunction [25].

Summary

ED is common in men who have chronic stable coronary artery disease. Cardiologists and internists need to be aware of this connection and ask patients with coronary disease and risk factors for coronary artery disease about their sexual health. Identifying and treating cardiovascular risk factors in the patient presenting with ED may not only improve the patient's ED, it may save the patient's life.

References

[1] Anastasiadis A, Droggin D, Burchardt M, et al. Physiology of erection and causes of erectile dysfunction in contemporary cardiology. In: Kloner RA, editor. Heart disease and erectile dysfunction. Totowa (NJ): Humana Press Inc.; 2004. p. 1–18.

[2] Benet AE, Melman A. The epidemiology of erectile dysfunction. Urol Clin North Am 1995;22:699–709.

[3] Sullivan ME, Keoghane SR, Miller MA. Vascular risk factors and erectile dysfunction. BJU Int 2001; 87:838–45.

[4] Weisberg PL, Rudd JHF. Atherosclerotic biology and epidemiology of disease. In: Topol EJ, editor. Textbook of cardiovascular medicine. 2nd edition. Philadelphia: Lippincott Williams and Wilkins; 2002. p. 3–14.

[5] Azadzoi KM, Siroky MB, Goldstein I. Study of etiologic relationship of arterial atherosclerosis to corporal veno-occlusive dysfunction in the rabbit J Urol 1996;155:1795–800.

[6] Kaiser DR, Billups K, Mason C, et al. Impaired brachial artery endothelium dependent and independent vasodilation in men with erectile dysfunction and no other clinical cardiovascular disease. J Am Coll Cardiol 2004;43:179–84.

[7] Cheitlin MD. Erectile dysfunction: the earliest sign of generalized vascular disease? J Am Coll Cardiol 2004;43:185–6.

[8] Montorsi P, Montorsi F, Schulman CC. Is erectile dysfunction the "tip of the iceberg" of a systemic vascular disorder? Eur Urol 2003;44:352–4.

[9] Bivalacqua TJ, Usta MF, Champion HC, et al. Endothelial dysfunction in erectile dysfunction. Role of the endothelium in erectile physiology and disease J Androl 2003;24(6 Suppl):S17–37.

[10] Billups KL. Endothelial dysfunction as a common link between erectile dysfunction and cardiovascular disease. Current Sexual Health Reports 2004;1: 137–41.

[11] Morley JE, Korenman SG, Kaiser FE, et al. Relationship of penile brachial pressure index to myocardial infarction and cerebrovascular accidents in older men. Am J Med 1988;84:445–58.

[12] Bocchio M, Desideri G, Scarpelli P, et al. Endothelial cell activation in men with erectile dysfunction without cardiovascular risk factors and overt vascular damage. J Urol 2004;171:1601–4.

[13] Pritzker MR. The penile stress test: a window to the hearts of man? Circulation 1999;100(Suppl I):I–711.

[14] Gazzaruso C, Giordanetti S, De Amici E, et al. Relationship between erectile dysfunction and silent myocardial ischemia in apparently uncomplicated Type 2 diabetic patients. Circulation 2004; 110:22–6.

[15] Blumentals WA, Gomez-Caminero A, Joo S, et al. Should erectile dysfunction be considered as a marker for acute myocardial infarction? Results from a retrospective cohort study. Int J Impot Res 2004;16:350–3.

[16] Feldman HA, Goldstein I, Hatzichristou DG, et al. Impotence and its medical psychosocial correlates: results of the Massachusetts Male Aging Study J Urol 1994;151:54–61.

[17] Virag R, Bouilly P, Frydman D. Is impotence an arterial disorder? A study of arterial risk factors in 440 impotent men. Lancet 1985;8422:181–4.

[18] Kloner RA. Erectile dysfunction and cardiovascular risk factors. In: Kloner RA, editor. Contemporary cardiology: heart disease and erectile dysfunction. Totowa (NJ): Humana Press; 2004. p. 39–49.

[19] Kloner RA, Mullin SH, Shook T, et al. Erectile dysfunction in the cardiac patient: how common and should we treat? J Urol 2003;170:S46–50.

[20] Katz SD, Balidemaj K, Homma S, et al. Acute type 5 phosphodiesterase inhibition with sildenafil enhances flow-mediated vasodilation in patients with chronic heart failure. J Am Coll Cardiol 2000;36: 845–51.

[21] Halcox JPJ, Nour KRA, Zulos G, et al. The effect of sildenafil on human vascular function, platelet activation, and myocardial ischemia. J Am Coll Cardiol 2002;40:1231–40.

[22] Gori T, Sicuro S, Dragoni S, et al. Sildenafil prevents endothelial dysfunction induced by ischemia and reperfusion via opening of adenosine triphosphate sensitive potassium channels. A human in vivo study. Circulation 2005;111:742–6.

[23] Desouza C, Parulkar A, Lumpkin D, et al. Acute and prolonged effects of sildenafil on brachial artery flow mediated dilatation in type 2 diabetes. Diabetes Care 2002;25:1336–9.

[24] Rosano GMC, Aversa A, Vitale C, et al. Chronic treatment with tadalafil improves endothelial function in men with increased cardiovascular risk. Eur Urol 2005;47:214–22.

[25] Kloner RA. Cardiovascular effects of the 3 phosphodiesterase 5 inhibitors approved for the treatment of erectile dysfunction. Circulation 2004;110:3149–55.

ELSEVIER
SAUNDERS

Urol Clin N Am 32 (2005) 403–417

UROLOGIC
CLINICS
of North America

Epidemiology of Erectile Dysfunction: the Role of Medical Comorbidities and Lifestyle Factors

Raymond C. Rosen, PhD[a],*, Rena Wing, PhD[b],
Stephen Schneider, MD[c], Noel Gendrano III, MPH[a]

[a]Department of Psychiatry, Robert Wood Johnson Medical School, 671 Hoes Lane, Piscataway, NJ 08854, USA
[b]Department of Psychiatry & Human Behavior, Brown University School of Medicine, Box G-BH,
Providence, RI 02912, USA
[c]Department of Medicine, Robert Wood Johnson Medical School, Clinical Academic Building,
Suite 5100A, 125 Paterson Street, New Brunswick, NJ 08901-1977, USA

Erectile dysfunction (ED) is a common male disability associated with aging that significantly impacts quality of life and interpersonal well-being [1–6]. Recent epidemiologic studies have highlighted the association between ED and broader indices of cardiovascular health and psychologic well-being, suggesting that ED may be an early marker for cardiovascular and other disease states [7–12]. At the same time, the availability of safe and effective oral therapies has led to a dramatic increase in the number of men seeking treatment. It is estimated that 25 to 30 million men worldwide are taking phosphodiesterase-5 (PDE-5) inhibitors, and that an additional 50 million or more are potential candidates for treatment [11,13,14].

Evidence from worldwide epidemiologic studies supports several observations:

- ED is highly prevalent in aging men, affecting approximately 50% of men older than 60 years of age. For many men, ED manifests in the 40s and 50s, increasing in frequency and severity after 60 years of age [1,10, 15,16].
- The degree of bother associated with ED is related inversely to aging; men older than 70 years of age typically report a lesser degree of bother than their younger counterparts.

Consequently, distress and treatment-seeking is usually higher in younger and middle-aged men [13,17,18].

- The prevalence and incidence of ED are correlated highly with the presence of known risk factors and comorbidities. In particular, cardiovascular comorbidities (eg, hypertension, hypercholesterolemia), diabetes mellitus, and metabolic syndrome have been associated with ED in multiple cross-sectional and longitudinal studies [7,17,19,20]. Most recently, depression and lower urinary tract symptoms (LUTS) have been added to the list of significant medical comorbidities and risk factors [21–24].
- Lifestyle factors, including smoking, obesity, and exercise, are also significant predictors of ED [19,25,26]. Moreover, intensive lifestyle modification improved erectile function and associated cardiovascular and inflammatory markers in a randomized, prospective controlled trial [27].

What factors account for early onset and progression of ED in some men, but not others? Despite the overall association with aging, some older men in their eighth and ninth decades continue to enjoy sexual activity and adequate penile erections [28–30]. This article considers the role of medical comorbidities (eg, hypertension, diabetes mellitus, LUTS) and lifestyle factors (eg, obesity, sedentary lifestyle) as key determinants of ED. By assessing the impact of specific

This article was supported by grant DK060438.
* Corresponding author.
E-mail address: Rosen@umdnj.edu (R.C. Rosen).

risk factors and comorbidities, the authors aim to identify suitable targets for future treatment and prevention. Current medical or surgical therapies for ED may be viewed as symptomatic or palliative treatments [13], which fail to address the underlying pathophysiologic mechanisms involved [9,31]. Findings from population-based studies should be used to guide clinical prevention or education efforts. These should be directed to the patient groups or individuals most likely to benefit from early intervention (eg, men without major illnesses or comorbidities) [26].

Conceptual and methodological issues need to be addressed. First, the definition and measurement of ED varies from study to study. All definitions of ED, however, are based on patients' self-report, which typically is assessed by single-item scales or questionnaire measures [4,14, 32–34]. Some differences are evident among these scales, although studies show overall concordance in the prevalence rates and association with well-known comorbidities and risk factors. Early landmark studies, such as the Massachusetts Male Aging Study (MMAS) and the National Health and Social Life Survey (NHSLS), used single-item scales, which assessed erection difficulties over several months or in the past year [32,33]. Subsequent studies used five- or 15-item versions of the International Index of Erectile Function (IIEF), a multidimensional, self-report scale that assesses male sexual function over a 4-week period [14]. Single-item instruments have the advantage of high completion rates and low patient burden. On the other hand, multidimensional scales provide broader and more complete assessment of disease severity. Despite such differences, similar results have been obtained across studies using these different measures.

A second, and potentially more challenging issue concerns the complex and often bidirectional interactions between variables. For example, depression may be a cause or a consequence of ED in many studies [12,24,35,36]. These studies support a direct association between ED and mood. In other studies, the causal relationships among the major risk factors for ED are less evident. Biomedical, psychosocial, and lifestyle factors may interact in complex ways. Separating the effects of one risk factor or comorbidity from another and determining the direction of causality among these factors can be difficult or impossible to ascertain in cross-sectional studies alone [28, 30,34,37]. More research is needed to elucidate these associations.

Prevalence and incidence of erectile dysfunction

The first large-scale, community-based studies of ED were reported in the early 1990s in the United States (Table 1). These studies included MMAS [1,7,15,33], the Olmstead County Study of Urinary Symptoms and Health Status [30,38], and NHSLS [4,39]. These well-known studies laid the foundation for current epidemiologic concepts and findings in this area. All three studies observed a strong effect of aging on ED using different measurement and sampling approaches. The presence of medical comorbidities, particularly cardiovascular disease, was identified as predictive of ED in each study.

The MMAS [1,7] was conducted between 1987 and 1989. A total of 1290 men living in the Boston, Massachusetts area were interviewed concerning sexual function and other aspects of health and lifestyle. Results showed that most men were sexually active, although the rates of ED ranged from approximately 20% of men 40 to 45 years of age, to approximately 50% of men 65 or more years of age. Diabetes mellitus, hypertension, and heart disease were significant predictors of ED in this study, as was depression. Among a battery of hormonal measures included, only dehydroepiandrosterone sulfate (DHEA-S) was associated significantly with ED [1]. Surprisingly, smoking was not a significant predictor and the amount of alcohol consumption was correlated only weakly with ED.

A similar association between aging and ED was reported in the Olmsted County Study [38]. In this observational study of 2115 men 40 to 79 years of age, a similar effect of aging on ED was observed that was correlated with the frequency of sexual behavior and overall sexual satisfaction. Only 18% of men over 70 years of age reported always or usually being able to maintain erections. Conversely, 25% of men over 70 years of age reported never being able to achieve an erection. The Olmsted County prevalence data were compared with a sample of Japanese men [40]. A similar age-related decline in erectile function was seen in both samples, although the overall rates of decline were slightly higher in the Japanese men compared with their American counterparts. The investigators suggest that cultural and perceptual factors might account for these differences.

The NHSLS [4,39] included in-depth, sexual behavior interviews with a nationally representative sample of men and women (N = 1749 women, 1410 men) 18 to 59 years of age in the United

Table 1
Erectile dysfunction (ED) prevalence by age and country (percentage[a] and risk ratio[b])

Reference	Study	Country	n	Age	Prevalence (%)	Risk ratio
Feldman et al. [1,7,33]	Massachusetts Male Aging Study (MMAS)	US	1,290	40–49	23	—
Johannes et al. [15]				50–59	32	—
				60–69	40	—
				70+	49	—
Panser et al. [38]	The Olmsted County Study	US	2,115	40–49	12.6	—
				50–59	13.3	—
				60–69	20.4	—
				70–79	25.2	—
Masumori et al. [40]	Shimamaki-Mura Study	Japan	289	40–49	14.9	—
				50–59	15.6	—
				60–69	13.4	—
				70–79	23.5	—
Laumann et al. [4,39]	National Health and Social Life Survey (NHSLS)	US	1,410	18–29	7	Referent
				30–39	9	1.46 (0.84–2.57)
				40–49	11	1.84 (0.97–3.47)
				50–59	18	3.59 (1.84–7.00)
Braun et al. [17]	Cologne Male Survey	Germany	4,489	30–39	2.3 (1.5–3.4)	—
				40–49	9.5 (7.6–11.7)	—
				50–59	15.7 (13.4–18.1)	—
				60–69	34.4 (31.6–37.3)	—
				70–80	53.4 (48.4–58.3)	—
Blanker et al. [21,46]	Krimpen Study	Netherlands	1,688	50–54	3	—
				55–59	5	—
				60–64	11	—
				65–69	18	—
				70–78	26	—
Bacon et al. [19]	Health Professionals Follow-up Study	US	31,742	Overall	33	—
				≤59	22	Referent
				60–69	44	2.9 (2.6–3.3)
				70–79	66	5.9 (5.2–6.7)
				≥80	69	9.9 (6.7–14.6)
Nicolosi et al. [42]	Cross National Study on the Epidemiology of Erectile Dysfunction	Brazil	2,513	40–44	9	—
		Italy		45–49	12	—
		Japan		50–54	18	—
		Malaysia		55–59	29	—
				60–64	38	—
				65–70	54	—

(continued on next page)

Table 1 (*continued*)

Reference	Study	Country	n	Age	Prevalence (%)	Risk ratio
Rosen et al. [22]	Multinational Survey of the Aging Male (MSAM-7)	US	1,915	Overall	54.9	—
		Europe	10,900	Overall	45.3	—
		All Countries	12,815	50–59	30.8	Referent
				60–69	55.1	2.67 (2.41–2.96)
				70–80	76.0	6.86 (6.02–7.82)
Fung et al. [8]	Rancho Bernardo Study	US	1,810	30–39	10	—
Barret-Connor et al. [41]				40–49	30	—
				50–59	45	—
				60–69	65	—
Rosen et al. [30]	Men's Attitudes of Life Events and Sexuality (MALES I) (MALES II)	Europe	10,729	20–29	8	—
Fisher et al. [13]		N. America	9,284	30–39	11	—
		S. America	7,826	40–49	15	—
				50–59	22	—
				60–69	30	—
				70–99	37	—
Laumann et al. [28]	Global Study of Sexual Attitudes and Behaviors (GSSAB)	N. Europe	1,402	40–49	—	Referent
				50–59	—	2.0 (1.0–4.1)
				60–69	—	3.9 (1.9–8.1)
				70-80	—	2.7 (1.0–7.1)
		S. Europe	1,879	40–49	—	Referent
				50–59	—	4.2 (2.1–8.5)
				60–69	—	6.5 (3.2–13.3)
				70–80	—	6.9 (3.1–15.4)
		Non-Europe West	1,447	40–49	—	Referent
				50–59	—	1.5 (0.9–2.4)
				60–69	—	3.7 (2.2–6.3)
				70–80	—	4.7 (2.5–9.0)
		Central/South America	520	40–49	—	Referent
				50–59	—	0.4 (0.1–1.0)
				60–69	—	0.4 (0.1–1.2)
				70–80	—	0.5 (0.1–2.1)
		Middle East	705	40–49	—	Referent
				50–59	—	1.3 (0.4–4.4)
				60–69	—	2.7 (0.7–10.4)
				70–80	—	6.8 (1.4–34.5)
		East Asia	1,101	40–49	—	Referent
				50–59	—	1.9 (1.0–3.7)
				60–69	—	4.3 (2.3–8.3)
				70–80	—	6.6 (3.2–13.6)

(*continued on next page*)

Table 1 (*continued*)

Reference	Study	Country	n	Age	Prevalence (%)	Risk ratio
		Southeast Asia	566	40–49	—	Referent
				50–59	—	1.1 (0.5–2.1)
				60–69	—	1.1 (0.5–2.3)
				70–80	—	1.2 1.9 (1.0–3.5)
Nicolosi et al. [29]	Global Study of Sexual Attitudes and Behaviors (GSSAB)	China	250	55 ± 10	20 (15–25)	—
		Hong Kong	250	55 ± 11	8 (3–13)	—
		Taiwan	250	52 ± 11	9 (5–13)	—
		South Korea	600	53 ± 11	18 (14–21)	—
		Japan	750	57 ± 11	13 (11–16)	—
		Thailand	250	53 ± 11	29 (21–38)	—
		Singapore	250	50 + 8	2 (0–4)	—
		Malaysia	250	52 ± 10	28 (20–36)	—
		Indonesia	250	55 + 8	11 (7–15)	—
		Philippines	250	59 ±11	33 (26–41)	—
Holden et al. [18]	Men in Australia Telephone Survey (MATeS)	Australia	5,990	Overall	21.3	—
				40–49	3.8	—
				50–59	10.7	—
				60–69	31.0	—
				70+	67.4	—

[a] The percentage of ED in each study is based on single-item or multiple-item self-report measures. See text for further details.

[b] Risk ratios are calculated as either odds ratios or relative risks for ED using 95% confidence intervals.

States. One question was used to evaluate the presence or absence of sexual problems ("Which of the following problems have you had for several months or more during the past year…"). ED was defined as difficulty achieving or maintaining erection, and ranged from 7% of men under 30 years of age to 18% of men more than 50 years of age. ED was related significantly to overall health, and was associated strongly with emotional stress and a history of urinary symptoms (eg, LUTS). Unfortunately, the absence of men older than 60 years of age in the sample limits the assessment of aging effects and related comorbidities.

Further evidence for the age association, prevalence, and risk factors for ED comes from the Health Professionals Follow-Up Study [19] and the Rancho Bernardo Study [8,41]. The Health Professionals Study [19] is based on the largest United States sample to date in which ED was addressed specifically (31,742 health professionals aged 53 to 90 years). Men with prostate cancer were excluded from the analysis of ED to reduce the potential impact of this risk factor. A highly significant effect of aging was observed,

with a 40-fold higher risk of ED in the oldest compared with the youngest age group. The overall, age-standardized prevalence of ED in the Health Professional Study was 33%. Negative lifestyle behaviors, particularly sedentary behavior, overweight, and smoking, were significant predictors of ED in this landmark study.

Other large-scale, multinational surveys have confirmed the strong age association observed in the early United States studies. These latter studies have provided interesting cross-national investigations into prevalence and risk factors in different populations of men. The Global Survey of Sexual Attitudes and Behavior (GSSAB) [28] included a detailed survey of sexual behavior in highly diverse samples (N = 27,500). This study provides global estimates of the prevalence of ED and other sexual problems in adult men and women aged 40 to 80 years in 29 countries. Major strengths of the study include the large sample size and wide geographic and cultural diversity. Sampling methods ranged from random-digit dialing, computer-assisted telephone interviewing methodology in North America, Brazil, Europe, Australia, and New Zealand to door-to-door interviewing in the Middle East, and intercept sampling in East Asia. A single-item question similar to the original NHSLS question was used to ascertain the prevalence of each sexual dysfunction, along with a second question to assess the relative frequency of the problem (often, sometimes, never). Only those who reported "sometimes" or "often" in response to the frequency of dysfunction question were included in the analysis of responders. The average participation rates for the study ranged from 8% to 55%, although the authors have shown that the sampling method had little effect overall on prevalence rates or patterns of predictors. Moreover, prevalence rates in this study are comparable to those seen in other large-scale epidemiologic studies, and may represent a conservative estimate of the prevalence because many subjects did not acknowledge the presence of sexual problems and may have had a negative reporting bias.

In addition to ED, the GSSAB investigated the prevalence and predictors of premature ejaculation (PE), lack of orgasm (anorgasmia), and low sexual desire in women. The rates for the pattern of risk factors and comorbidities for each of these problems are presented by age, health status, and region of the world. The results are informative in showing a more consistent age association for ED compared with other male and female sexual problems. Moreover, the prevalence of ED and other male sexual problems was highest in the East Asian countries (eg, China, Korea, Japan, Malaysia, Indonesia, the Philippines). Regarding ED in the GSSAB study, presence or absence of vascular disease (hypertension, diabetes mellitus, stroke, and peripheral vascular disease), LUTS, and depression were major comorbidities observed. Education was a negative predictor (higher education predicted fewer problems) for some problems (eg, PE), but not for ED per se.

In subsequent analysis from the GSSAB, Nicolosi and colleagues [26,29,42] compared the prevalence rates and correlates of ED in four countries in the GSSAB: Japan, Italy, Brazil, and Malaysia. According to the definition above, the age-adjusted prevalence of moderate to severe ED was 34% in Japan, 22% in Malaysia, 17% in Italy, and 15% in Brazil. Overall, the prevalence of ED was higher in the two Asian countries compared with Italy and Brazil. Despite differences in the prevalence rates, similarities were observed in the pattern of comorbidities and risk factors. In particular, increased risk for ED was associated with presence of diabetes mellitus, heart disease,

LUTS, and depression in all four countries. Conversely, higher education and increased physical activity levels were correlated inversely with ED across all countries. In a secondary analysis of the data [26], the investigators analyzed the role of lifestyle factors in subjects in the four regions without comorbid illnesses or chronic diseases (see later discussion on lifestyle factors).

Prevalence rates for ED were somewhat lower in the recent MALES study [13,30]. This difference is likely a result of a younger sample of men in this study, as was the case in the earlier NHSLS study [4,39], and use of a more indirect method of ED assessment. Subjects were not informed specifically about the purpose of the study, and a single question about erection problems was embedded in a list of men's health conditions. ED prevalence rates in this study were highest in the United States (as in other studies), and lowest in Spain and Latin American countries (Mexico, Brazil). Other European countries (Germany, France, United Kingdom) had prevalence rates of approximately 15% for all age groups combined. The prevalence of ED was correlated with the presence of cardiovascular disease, diabetes mellitus, and depression. Approximately 50% of men in the MALES study who had ED had sought professional help for their ED, although less then half were treated actively at the time of study. Most of those who received prescription ED medication from their doctors had discontinued its use. This study is notable for the detailed assessment of help-seeking and treatment satisfaction [13], and for the involvement of female partners. This latter aspect is unique among recent epidemiologic studies.

Additional data on prevalence and risk factors for ED come from a recent large-scale, community-based study of Australian men (Men in Australia Telephone Survey, or MATeS) [18]. This national study made use of a computer-assisted, random-dialing methodology for assessing ED and other reproductive health problems in a large, representative sample of approximately 6000 men aged 40 or more years. ED as measured by the single-item, MMAS measure [32] was found in 21% of the sample. For purposes of the study, ED reporters were defined as only men reporting moderate to severe ED. As in the previous studies, a strong age correlation was observed, with the prevalence of ED rising sharply from 10.7% in those 50 to 59 years of age, to 31% in those 60 to 69 years of age, and 67.5% of those 70 or more years of age. Of note, the rate of severe ED (complete inability to achieve erection) increased at approximately the same or higher rate, from less than 1% of those younger than 50 years of age, to 39.5% of men 70 or more years of age. This study provided important data on help-seeking for ED in comparison to other reproductive health problems (eg, prostate disease, hypogonadism). Despite high rates of moderate and severe ED in the study, less than 30% of affected men sought medical help for their problem. This was significantly lower, for example, than the number of men who received digital-rectal examinations (47.8%) or prostate-specific antigen testing (48.5%) for suspected prostate disease. The percentage of men who had ED who sought medical help was highest in the group 50 to 59 years of age (50.9%), and lowest in the group of men more than 70 years of age (17.1%). This study was also notable for the high response rate obtained (78.5%) and representativeness of the sample.

The above studies offer consistent support for the age-association and prevalence of ED, as well as its association with specific comorbidities and risk factors. The next sections examine the associations between ED and its major comorbidities and risk factors, particularly cardiovascular disease and LUTS. Finally, the authors consider the role of lifestyle factors, including obesity, smoking, and exercise, on ED.

The role of comorbidities and chronic illnesses

Epidemiologic studies of ED usually are conducted in large, community-based cohorts of men 40 to 80 years of age [10,16–19,22,28,40]. Men interviewed in these studies typically report a wide range of comorbidities, including LUTS, hypertension, hypercholesterolemia, obesity, diabetes mellitus, heart disease, and depression. Some studies have included men who have a history of prostate cancer, whereas others have specifically excluded men who have this condition [19,26]. Most studies reported in this section are based on samples of men who have one or more of the major comorbidities, such as diabetes mellitus, hypertension, depression, and LUTS (Table 2). Only one study has investigated separately the association of major risk factors in relatively healthy men without overt evidence of cardiovascular disease or diabetes mellitus [26].

The normal physiology of erection depends on adequate vasodilation and smooth muscle relaxation of the penile corpora [6,31,42]. These vascular mechanisms depend, in turn, on adequate neural innervation and release of nonadrenergic, noncholinergic neurotransmitters, notably nitric oxide, in the gap junctions and endothelial lining of the penile corpora [6,43]. Spinal and supra-spinal mechanisms are involved in the control of erection, which also depends on the presence of adequate levels of androgen. Given the interactive role of vascular, neurologic, and hormonal mechanisms, it is not surprising that diseases (eg, diabetes mellitus) or drugs (eg, alpha-blockers) that affect these processes may affect erectile function significantly. Recently, studies also have observed a strong association between ED and benign prostatic hyperplasia (BPH) or LUTS, although the specific mechanisms for this association are unclear [23].

Assessing comorbid disease and cardiovascular risk factors in men who have ED is clinically important given the strong links between ED and diabetes mellitus, heart disease, and hypertension. Accordingly, ED commonly is considered an early-warning sentinel or harbinger for coronary heart disease, just as cardiovascular disease is seen as a major risk factor for ED [9,31,44]. In particular, ED shares underlying mechanisms and risk factors with vascular disease, and it has been suggested that subclinical arterial insufficiency may be manifested as ED [31,44,45]. In the MMAS cross-sectional study [1], the age-adjusted probability of severe ED was 28% in treated diabetes mellitus, 39% in treated heart disease, and 15% in treated hypertension, compared with an overall prevalence of 9.5% in the entire MMAS sample [7].

Longitudinal studies similarly have shown a significant association between cardiovascular risk factors and ED [7,8,19,41]. In the MMAS longitudinal study, incident ED over a 9-year interval from 1989 to 1997 was predicted by the composite cardiovascular risk source at baseline, in addition to the degree of obesity [7]. The Rancho Bernardo study with a longer follow-up period (25 years) and fewer men (N = 570) also assessed the predictors of ED [8,41]. This well-known study observed that age, overweight (body mass index [BMI] > 28), and hyperlipidemia were major risk factors for the development of incident ED. The odds of developing ED in this study also were predicted by the number of cardiovascular risk factors; men with three or more risk factors had an odds ratio of 2.2 for developing ED, compared with men without any risk factors. In the Health Professionals Follow-Up Study [19], smoking

Table 2
Erectile dysfunction (ED) prevalence by co-morbidity and associated illness (percentage[a] and risk ratios[b])

Reference	Age	Diabetes	HTN	LUTS	Cancer	CVD	Hyper-cholesterolemia	Stroke	Depression
Feldman et al. [1]	40–69	Overall ED: 9.6% 28%	Overall ED: 9.6% 15%	—	—	Overall ED: 9.6% 39%	—	—	—
Braun et al. [17]	Overall	20.2%	32.0%	72.2%	—	—	—	—	—
	30–39	0.0%	11.5%	38.5%					
	40–49	11.1%	17.3%	43.2%					
	50–59	22.8%	37.6%	71.8%					
	60–69	22.1%	33.3%	79.5%					
	70–80	20.8%	33.9%	74.7%					
Feldman et al. [7]	40–69	—	1.79 (0.98–3.28)	—	—	—	—	—	0.88 (0.37–2.11)
Johannes et al. [15]	40–69	1.83 (1.23–2.73)	1.52 (1.11–2.07)	—	—	1.96 (1.32–2.91)	—	—	—
Blanker et al. [21,46]	50–78	2.4 (1.2–4.5)	2.1 (1.5–2.9)	Mild: 2.4 (1.0–5.6) Mod: 6.0 (2.6–14.2) Sev: 9.9 (3.5–27.9)	—	3.1 (1.9–5.0)	—	—	—
Bacon et al. [19]	≤59 to ≥80	1.5 (1.5–1.6)	1.3 (1.3–1.3)	—	1.1 (1.1–1.2)	1.3 (1.3–1.3)	1.2 (1.2–1.2)	1.3 (1.2–1.4)	—
Nicolosi et al. [26]	40–70	—	—	Mod: 2.15 (1.32–3.48) Sev: 4.23 (1.49–12.06)	—	—	—	—	2.11 (1.48–3.02)
Rosen et al. [22]	50–80	2.36 (2.02–2.76)	1.49 (1.35–1.66)	Mild: 1.98 (1.67–2.34) Mod: 3.76 (3.14–4.50) Sev: 7.67 (5.87–10.02)	—	1.61 (1.41–1.84)	1.19 (1.06–1.33)	—	—
Fung et al. [8]	4.56 ± 10.2	—	Overall: 33.0%	—	—	—	1.54 (1.05–2.26)	—	—
Barret-Connor et al. [41]	1.07 (1.04–1.09)	—	ED: 11.2%	—	—	—	—	—	—

Rosen et al. [30]	20–70+	No ED: 4.0% ED: 14.0%	No ED: 19.0% ED: 36.0%	No ED: 7.0% ED: 17.0%	No ED: 16.0% ED: 29.0%	No ED: 13.0% ED: 25.0%
Laumann et al. [28]	40–80	N. Europe 1.6 (1.0–2.7) S. Europe 2.2 (1.5–3.4) Non-Europe West 1.4 (1.0–2.1) Central/South America 4.1 (1.7–10.1) Middle East 4.4 (1.8–10.7) East Asia 2.5 (1.6–3.8) Southeast Asia 2.0 (1.1–3.6) [Vascular Diseases]	N. Europe 1.8 (0.8–3.7) S. Europe 2.0 (1.1–3.6) Non-Europe West 1.5 (0.8–2.9) Central/South America 1.9 (0.7–5.6) Middle East 2.2 (0.5–9.6) East Asia 1.3 (0.7–2.5) Southeast Asia 1.8 (0.4–8.9) [Prostate Diseases]	—	—	—
Holden et al. [18]	>40	2.4 (1.8–3.1)	1.3 (1.1–1.5)	—	—	1.7 (1.4–2.1) 1.8 (1.4–2.3)

[a] The percentage of ED in each study is based on single-item or multiple-item self-report measures. See text for details.

[b] Risk ratios are calculated as either odds ratios or relative risks for ED using 95% confidence intervals.

and physical activity added to the risk for ED beyond the effects of aging and cardiovascular health status.

Other community-based studies provide support for the role of cardiovascular risk factors in ED. For example, the Cologne Survey observed a high comorbidity of hypertension and diabetes mellitus in a large sample of German men who had ED [17]. Subjects who had ED in the Dutch community study [21,46] were more likely to have comorbidities such as diabetes mellitus, hypertension, and hyperlipidemia. In the GSSAB study [28], two medical comorbidities were evident across all countries and age groups: a history of vascular conditions (eg, hypertension, diabetes mellitus) and prostate problems (eg, prostate cancer, LUTS). Most recently, cardiovascular disease, hypertension, and diabetes mellitus were associated significantly with ED in the MATeS study [18]. Patients who had diabetes mellitus in this study had a 2.4× higher rate of ED, and patients who had cardiovascular disease had a 1.7× higher odds ratio for developing ED. Depression was associated in this study with a significant increase in the risk for ED, as in previous studies. In these cross-sectional studies, the direction of causality is not necessarily evident.

Less widely recognized as a major risk factor for ED, BPH and LUTS have been associated with ED in an increasing number of well-controlled, community-based studies. LUTS is an independent risk factor for ED in each of these studies. In the Cologne Survey [17], the prevalence of LUTS was 72% in men who had ED compared with 38% of those who did not have ED. Based on multivariate analyses in this study, LUTS was an independent predictor for ED, beyond the effects of age, diabetes mellitus, hypertension, and pelvic surgery. Similarly, results of a community-based study of 1688 men in the Netherlands showed that the prevalence of severe ED increased from 3% in men 50 to 54 years of age to 26% in those 70 to 78 years of age [21,46]. Age, LUTS, obesity, cardiovascular disease, chronic obstructive pulmonary disease, and smoking were independent risk factors for ED in this study [21].

The Cross-National Study assessed the prevalence of ED in relatively healthy men (ie, those without significant comorbidity) in four countries (Brazil, Italy, Japan, and Malaysia) [26]. The prevalence of moderate or complete ED in these otherwise healthy men was 16%, approximately one half the 32% prevalence reported in 1077 men in the same study who reported one or more concomitant medical conditions. In these relatively healthy men, multivariate logistic regression analysis indicated that moderate (odds ratio 2.2, 95% confidence interval [CI]: 1.2–3.9) and severe (odds ratio 4.9, 95% CI: 1.4–16.7) ED were age-related. The presence of urinary symptoms or BPH/LUTS diagnosis was the most significant predictor, overall, in this study for ED. This study provides strong confirmation of the significance of BPH/LUTS as a key risk factor for ED, particularly in the absence of other major illnesses or comorbidities.

The role of LUTS in ED and related ejaculatory disorders in aging men was investigated systematically in the MSAM-7 Study [22]. This large, multinational study evaluated comorbidities and risk factors for male sexual dysfunction, including ED and ejaculatory dysfunction. The MSAM-7 survey included 12,815 men 50 to 80 years of age in the United States and six European countries [22]. Overall, results strongly confirmed the negative association between LUTS and sexual function in aging men, independent of the effects of other comorbidities and lifestyle factors. In the MSAM-7 [22], the overall prevalence of ED was 49%, with 10% reporting complete absence of erection. The prevalence of ED in this study was higher in American men (55%) compared with European men (45%). The prevalence of ED was age-dependent, with rates of 31%, 55%, and 76% in men 50 to 59 years, 60 to 69 years, and 70 to 80 years of age, respectively. Logistic regression analysis, which controlled for the effects of age, medical comorbidities, tobacco use, and alcohol consumption, showed that age and the severity of LUTS were independent risk factors for ED. Furthermore, age and LUTS were stronger risk factors for ED than were diabetes mellitus, hypertension, heart disease, or hyperlipidemia in this study. The mechanism for this association has been reviewed recently [23].

Finally, depression has been implicated as an important risk factor or comorbidity in several studies [12,18,30,35,36,46]. Data from the MMAS were analyzed to examine the association between ED and depression, as measured by the Center for Epidemiological Studies—Depression (CES-D) scale [35]. In this analysis, an overall significant relationship (odds ratio 1.82; CI = 1.21–2.73) was observed between depression and ED, after controlling for the effects of aging and other risk factors. The risk for ED was approximately doubled (13% versus 25%) in men who had depression in the MALES study, compared with their age-matched counterparts without ED [30]. The direction of causality is unclear, however, given the cross-sectional nature of the study designs. Results of recent randomized, prospective trials have shown that pharmacologic treatment of ED with sildenafil or vardenafil results in significant improvements in measures of mood and depression, suggesting that ED may be a significant risk factor for depression [26,47,48].

Taken together with the data on cardiovascular disease and diabetes mellitus, the relationship between ED and its important comorbidities has been investigated comprehensively. These studies provide evidence of a clear and robust association with these medical comorbidities and risk factors, and support the concept of ED as an early marker of medical and psychiatric illnesses, particular cardiovascular disease, LUTS, diabetes mellitus, and depression.

The role of lifestyle factors

The role of lifestyle factors in ED has been investigated in cross-sectional and longitudinal studies. Despite methodologic difficulties in assessing behaviors such as diet and exercise in large-scale, observational studies, as well as variations in the sampling design and assessment methodology from one study to another, some interesting trends can be observed across studies (Table 3). In particular, obesity and sedentary lifestyle have been shown consistently to be risk factors for ED in men who have comorbid illnesses such as hypertension and diabetes mellitus, and especially in men without overt cardiovascular disease [26]. Other lifestyle factors, such as smoking and alcohol consumption, have been implicated in some studies. Intervening on cardiovascular and lifestyle factors may have broader benefits beyond restoration of erectile function. This important concept should be evaluated further because recent studies have implicated the role of the metabolic syndrome, obesity, insulin resistance, and lack of exercise as independent risk factors for ED and cardiovascular disease [7,20,31,44,45].

Obesity long has been considered a risk factor for ED, and several epidemiologic studies have considered body weight and diet in the assessment of risk. In the original MMAS study, the prevalence of ED was not affected directly by BMI or waist-to-hip ratio [1]. Subsequent longitudinal data from the same study [7,25], however, showed that baseline obesity (BMI $\geq$ 28) significantly

Table 3
Lifestyle Factors and erectile dysfunction (ED) (percentages[a] & risk ratios[b])

Reference	Age	Country	BMI	Sedentary/Active Lifestyle	Alcohol consumption	Smoking
Feldman et al. [33]	40–69	US	—	—	—	1.17 (0.87–1.58)
Feldman et al. [7]	40–69	US	Over: 1.96 (1.17–3.28)	Active: 0.71 (0.42–1.22)	Low: 0.95 (0.54–1.67) High: 0.87 (0.41–1.86)	1.97 (1.07–3.63)
Blanker et al. [46]	50–78	Netherlands	Over: 1.4 (1.0–2.0) Obese: 2.3 (1.4–3.8)	—	Low: 0.7 (0.5–1.0) High: 0.7 (0.4–1.1)	1.3 (0.9–1.8)
Bacon et al. [19]	53–90	US	Over: 1.1 (1.1–1.2) Obese: 1.4 (1.3–1.5)	Low: 0.9 (0.8–0.9) High: 0.7 (0.6–0.7)	1.0 (1.0–1.1)	1.3 (1.2–1.4)
Nicolosi et al. [26]	40–70	Brazil	Quartile 1: Referent	<Avg. Activity: Referent	None: Referent	Light: 1.23 (0.91–1.67) Heavy: 2.59 (1.46–4.61)
		Italy	Quartile 2: 0.73 (0.49–1.09)	Avg. Activity: 0.46 (0.27–0.76)	Low: 0.89 (0.62–1.29)	
		Japan	Quartile 3: 0.69 (0.46–1.03)	>Avg. Activity: 0.35 (0.22–0.54)	High: 1.11 (0.70–1.75)	
		Malaysia	Quartile 4: 0.57 (0.37–0.86)			
Rosen et al. [22]	50–80	US Europe	—	—	—	1.22 (1.09–1.36)
Fung et al. [8] Barret-Connor et al. [41]	45.6 +(10.2)	US	Obese: 1.93 (1.18–3.17)	—	—	16.5%
Laumann et al. [28]	40–80	N. Europe	—	1.1 (0.6–1.9)	—	1.1 (0.6–2.0)
		S. Europe		1.0 (0.6–1.7)	—	1.1 (0.6–1.7)
		Non-Europe West		2.1 (1.2–3.6)	—	1.5 (0.9–2.5)
		Central/South America		0.4 (0.1–1.4)	—	1.4 (0.6–3.4)
		Middle East		3.0 (0.8–11.4)	—	0.4 (0.2–1.1)
		East Asia		1.6 (0.9–3.0)	—	1.1 (0.7–1.9)
		Southeast Asia		1.8 (0.8–3.9)	—	1.0 (0.5–2.0)
Holden et al. [18]	≥40	Australia	Under: 2.4 (1.3–4.3) Over: 1.1 (0.9–1.3) Obese: 1.8 (1.4–2.2)	1.5 (1.3–1.8)	Low: 0.7 (0.6–0.9) High: 1.1 (0.8–1.6)	1.2 (1.0–1.4)

[a] The percentage of ED in each study is based on single-item or multiple-item self-report measures. See text for further details.
[b] Risk ratios are calculated as either odds ratios or relative risks for ED using 95% confidence intervals.

predicted the development of ED over an 8-year follow-up period [7], and that overweight subjects at baseline remained at higher risk for ED even in the event of follow-up weight loss. Subjects who ate a diet rich in cholesterol and unsaturated fats were also more likely to develop ED in the follow-up period than those with a more balanced diet [7].

The role of obesity in ED has been confirmed in large-scale cross-sectional and longitudinal studies [19,46,21,18]. In the study in the Netherlands, for example, 1700 Dutch men between 50 and 75 years of age were evaluated for the presence of ED and other health conditions [21]. BMI was a significant predictor of ED as a single factor and in combination with other risk factors (eg, LUTS, hypertension, diabetes mellitus). A linear association between BMI and ED was observed in this study; the odds ratio for ED increased from 1.5 for a BMI of 25 to 30 (relative to BMI < 25), and to 3.0 for BMI greater than 30. Similar findings were reported in the Health Professionals Follow-Up Study in the United States [19], and in the recent MATeS study in Australia [18]. In both large-scale, observational studies described above, obesity was a significant, independent risk factor for ED. Recently, obesity also was shown to be a significant risk factor for male and female sexual dysfunction [20], although the mechanisms for this association are complex and not well understood.

Physical activity is another lifestyle factor that has been linked strongly to the occurrence of ED in aging men. In the Health Professionals Follow-Up Study [19], for example, ED was associated strongly with BMI and level of physical activity. Participants were categorized according to their level of exercise or physical activity. Higher levels of sedentary behavior (less physical activity) were a strong, independent predictor of ED in this study. A linear, negative association was observed between the amount of exercise engaged in per week (metabolic equivalents [MET] h/wk) and the likelihood of ED. For example, men with exercise levels greater than 16 MET h/wk had an odds ratio of 0.7 (CI = 0.6, 0.8) for ED, compared with sedentary men (0–2.7 MET h/wk). Frequent vigorous exercise, according to the investigators, was associated with an approximately 30% reduction in the risk for ED. This effect was more evident in men under 60 years of age. Similar results for the effects of exercise were reported in the GSSAB study [28]. In this large multinational study, the United States and other western, non-

European countries (eg, Canada, Mexico) showed a significant negative association between the level of physical activity and probability of ED (odds ratio = 2.1; CI = 1.2, 3.6). Similar trends were observed in other geographic regions, although the level of association between exercise and ED was less clear in the European and Asian samples.

Other studies have shown that exercise impacts the prevalence and incidence of new cases of ED. Derby and colleagues [25] prospectively evaluated whether changes in sedentary activity and other lifestyle factors such as obesity, smoking, and alcohol consumption were associated with changes in erectile function in the MMAS sample. Among this sample, 593 men without ED at baseline who also did not have prostate cancer and were not being treated for heart disease or diabetes mellitus were followed closely for 8 years. In examining the probability of new-onset ED during the follow-up period, two significant findings were reported. First, the lowest risk for ED was among individuals who were initially sedentary, and then became physically active during the study. The highest risk for ED was among men who were sedentary at baseline and follow-up. Reductions in smoking, obesity, and amount of alcohol consumption were associated with lower incidence of ED, although not as consistently as the level of physical activity. The MMAS longitudinal study provides strong evidence for the association between ED and the presence or absence of regular exercise [25]. When subjects were stratified according to their level of exercise, ED was highest among men with sedentary lifestyles and lowest among those who were active or who initiated physical activity or exercise regimens over the course of the study [25].

In the cross-national sample from the GSSAB study, Nicolosi and colleagues [26] examined the association between lifestyle factors and ED in men without major medical comorbidities (eg, prostate cancer, diabetes mellitus). In this sample, 1335 men who had ED and no diagnosis of cardiovascular or prostate diseases, diabetes mellitus, ulcer, or depression were evaluated. The goal of this analysis was to determine the significance of lifestyle factors in determining ED in men without major medical illnesses or comorbidities. The associations between erectile function and lifestyle factors, particularly obesity and sedentary behavior, were most clearly evident in this study. Specifically, the investigators found that 31.8% of men who reported below-average levels of physical activity had ED, compared with 13.9% of those who exercised more than average. In other words, lack of exercise increased the risk for ED by approximately 2.5×. The protective effects of exercise and low BMI were apparent in this study, perhaps because other major comorbidities (eg, diabetes mellitus, heart disease) were not obscuring the association.

The effects of weight loss and exercise were examined further in a recent randomized intervention trial of lifestyle modification in men who had obesity-related ED [27]. This study compared 2 years of exercise and weight loss with an educational control in 110 obese men (mean BMI = 36.4) who had moderate to severe ED. As in the cross-national study [26], men who had overt diabetes mellitus or other cardiovascular diseases were excluded from the trial. Patients in the weight loss and exercise group lost more weight than the controls (5.7 versus 0.7 kg) and increased their amount of exercise weekly (150 versus 33 min/wk). These changes were associated with significant decreases in cholesterol, C-reactive protein, and interleukin levels in the intervention group compared with the controls. Improved erectile function was correlated with the amount of weight loss and increased activity levels. Approximately one third of men in the intervention group achieved normal levels of erectile function following treatment. Overall, this study confirmed in a prospective, randomized design the association of BMI and physical activity levels with erectile function.

The role of other lifestyle factors, such as cigarette smoking and alcohol consumption, is less clear. Cigarette smoking long has been linked with ED, is associated with increased cardiovascular risk, and represents a potentially modifiable risk factor for the occurrence of ED. In the baseline MMAS data, current tobacco use was not an independent risk factor for ED, but it amplified the links between other risk factors [1]. For example, complete ED was found in 56% of subjects who had heart disease and were also smokers, compared with 21% in nonsmokers who had heart disease. In hypertensive men, smoking more than doubled the probability of complete ED. Longitudinal data from MMAS showed that smoking at baseline almost doubles the likelihood of moderate or complete ED 8 years later (24% for smokers versus 14% for nonsmokers) [5]. Surprisingly, the longitudinal MMAS study on modifiable risk factors conducted over the same period [25] found that quitting smoking in midlife may not be sufficient to reverse or prevent progression to ED. The investigators suggest that irreversible,

vascular effects in penile arteries and smooth muscle may have occurred in men with a long history of tobacco use [25].

Smoking increased the risk for ED moderately (odds ratio = 1.3) in the Health Professionals Follow-Up Study [19] and in the Krimpen Study [21] (odds ratio = 1.6; smokers versus nonsmokers). Other large-scale studies have observed positive, albeit nonsignificant associations between smoking and ED (MATeS, MSAM-7, GSBB) [18,22,28]. In contrast, smoking was highly predictive of ED in the cross-sectional study of men without significant medical comorbidities [26]. In this latter study, heavy smokers (> 30 cigarettes per day) had an odds ratio of 2.31 for ED, compared with an odds ratio of 1.26 for men who smoked fewer than 30 cigarettes per day. Again, the role of smoking may be obscured partially in earlier studies of men who had ED and multiple comorbidities. This important hypothesis warrants investigation in future studies.

Alcohol consumption is another potentially modifiable risk factor for ED that has been investigated in several epidemiologic studies. In the cross-sectional MMAS data, for example, excessive alcohol consumption (> 600 mL/wk) modestly increased the likelihood of ED from 17% to 29% [1]. This association was not confirmed in the longitudinal data [15], however, or in the evaluation of lifestyle change in the MMAS cohort [25]. No consistent effects of alcohol consumption were observed in the Health Professionals Follow-Up Study [19] or the Krimpen Study [21,46]. Both of these large-scale studies evaluated the amount of alcohol consumption in their samples, and found no evidence of an association with ED. Based on these results, it has been suggested that alcohol consumption may not be predictive of ED in men with moderate or low levels of alcohol consumption. It may be a significant factor in men with high levels of alcohol use, however, who are less likely to participate in epidemiologic studies of ED.

Overall, lifestyle factors seem to play a significant role in the development or maintenance of ED. Obesity and lack of exercise, in particular, have been implicated strongly in a number of cross-sectional and longitudinal studies. Based on results of the recent study by Esposito and colleagues [27] in Naples, Italy, lifestyle intervention can effectively restore erectile function in many men who have obesity-related ED, at least among those without significant medical comorbidities. Two essential questions remain to be addressed. First, is there a specific mechanism by which lifestyle modification changes lead to improved sexual function? For example, the study by Esposito and colleagues [27] suggests that changes in endothelial function may underlie the observed improvements in ED and more general cardiovascular health. This important hypothesis warrants further investigation [20,31,44]. Second, given the high rate of success of PDE-5 inhibitor drugs, is lifestyle modification a viable treatment option, either alone or in combination with pharmacologic therapy? No studies have investigated this question.

Summary

ED is a highly prevalent disorder associated with a significant burden of illness. The prevalence and incidence of ED are strongly age-related, affecting more than half of men older than 60 years. Results of recent multinational studies have shown that the condition is worldwide, although North American and Asian men report somewhat higher rates in most studies than their European and South American counterparts. ED is an early symptom or harbinger of cardiovascular disease, perhaps as a result of changes in endothelial function and nitrergic innovation in the penile corpora. The major comorbidities include diabetes mellitus, hypertension, hyperlipidemia, and heart disease. More recently, LUTS and depression have been linked to ED, although the mechanisms for these latter associations are not established clearly. Lifestyle factors, particularly obesity and lack of exercise, are significant predictors of ED in several studies, particularly in men without comorbid medical illnesses. The evidence for smoking and alcohol consumption is less clear. Further research is needed to evaluate the effects of intervention on these potentially modifiable risk factors.

References

[1] Feldman HA, Goldstein I, Hatzichristou DG, et al. Impotence and its medical and psychosocial correlates: results of the Massachusetts Male Aging Study. J Urol 1994;151:54–61.

[2] Fugl-Meyer AR, Lodnert G, Branholm IB, et al. On life satisfaction in male erectile dysfunction. Int J Impot Res 1997;9:141–8.

[3] Guest JF, Das Gupta R. Health-related quality of life in a UK-based population of men with erectile dysfunction. Pharmacoeconomics 2002;20:109–17.

[4] Laumann EO, Paik A, Rosen RC. The epidemiology of erectile dysfunction: results from the National Health and Social Life Survey. Int J Impot Res 1999;11(Suppl 1):S60–4.

[5] Litwin MS, Nied RJ, Dhanani N. Health-related quality of life in men with erectile dysfunction. J Gen Intern Med 1998;13:159–66.

[6] Lue TF. Erectile dysfunction. N Engl J Med 2000; 342(24):1802–13.

[7] Feldman HA, Johannes CB, Derby CA, et al. Erectile dysfunction and coronary risk factors: prospective results from the Massachusetts Male Aging Study. Prev Med 2000;30(4):328–38.

[8] Fung MM, Bettencourt R, Barrett-Connor E. Heart disease risk factors predict erectile dysfunction 25 years later. The Rancho Bernardo Study. J Am Coll Cardiol 2004;43:1405–11.

[9] Jackson G. Erectile dysfunction and cardiovascular disease. Int J Clin Pract 1999;53:363–8.

[10] Martin-Morales A, Sanchez-Cruz JJ, Saenz de Tejada I, et al. Prevalence and independent risk factors for erectile dysfunction in Spain: results of the Epidemiologia de la Disfuncion Erectil Masculina Study. J Urol 2001;166(2):569–74.

[11] McKinlay JB. The worldwide prevalence and epidemiology of erectile dysfunction. Int J Impot Res 2000;12(Suppl 4):S6–11.

[12] Shabsigh R, Klein LT, Seidman S, et al. Increased incidence of depressive symptoms in men with erectile dysfunction. Urology 1998;52:848–52.

[13] Fisher W, Rosen RC, Eardley I, et al. The multinational men's attitudes to life events and sexuality (MALES) study phase II: understanding PDE5 inhibitor treatment seeking patterns among men with erectile dysfunction. J Sex Med 2004;1:150–60.

[14] Rosen RC, Riley A, Wagner G, et al. The International Index of Erectile Function (IIEF): a multidimensional scale for assessment of erectile dysfunction. Urology 1997;49:822–30.

[15] Johannes CB, Araujo AB, Feldman HA, et al. Incidence of erectile dysfunction in men 40 to 69 years old: longitudinal results from the Massachusetts male aging study. J Urol 2000;163(2):460–3.

[16] Pinnock CB, Stapleton AM, Marshall VR. Erectile dysfunction in the community: a prevalence study. Med J Aust 1999;171(7):353–7.

[17] Braun M, Wassmer G, Klotz T, et al. Epidemiology of erectile dysfunction: results of the Cologne Male Survey. Int J Impot Res 2000;12(6):305–11.

[18] Holden CA, McLachlan RI, Pitts M, et al. Men in Australia, Telephone Survey (MATeS) I: a national survey of the reproductive health and concerns of middle aged and older Australian men. Lancet 2005;366:218–24.

[19] Bacon CG, Mittleman MA, Kawachi I, et al. Sexual function in men older than 50 years of age: results from the Health Professionals Follow-Up Study. Ann Intern Med 2003;139:161–8.

[20] Esposito K, Giugliano D. Obesity, the metabolic syndrome and sexual dysfunction. Intl J Impot Res 2005;17:391–8

[21] Blanker MH, Bohnen AM, Groeneveld FP, et al. Correlates for erectile and ejaculatory dysfunction in older Dutch men: a community-based study. J Am Geriatr Soc 2001;49(4):436–42.

[22] Rosen R, Altwein J, Boyle P, et al. Lower urinary tract systems and male sexual dysfunction: the multinational survey of the aging male (MSAM-7). Eur Urol 2003;44(6):637–49.

[23] Rosen RC, Giuliano F, Carson CC. Sexual dysfunction and lower urinary tract symptoms (LUTS) associated with benign prostatic hyperplasia (BPH). Eur Urol 2005;47:824–37.

[24] Rosen R, Seidman S, Menza M, et al. Quality of life, mood, and sexual function: a path analytic model of treatment effects in men with erectile dysfunction and depressive symptoms. Int J Impot Res 2004;16:334–40.

[25] Derby CA, Mohr BA, Goldstein I, et al. Modifiable risk factors and erectile dysfunction: can lifestyle changes modify risk? Urology 2000;56:302–6.

[26] Nicolosi A, Glasser DB, Moreira ED, et al. Prevalence of erectile dysfunction and associated factors among men without concomitant diseases: a population study. Int J Impot Res 2003;15:253–7.

[27] Esposito K, Giugliano F, Di Palo C, et al. Effect of lifestyle changes on erectile dysfunction in obese men: a randomized controlled trial. JAMA 2004; 291:2978–84.

[28] Laumann EO, Nicolosi A, Glasser DB, et al. Sexual problems among women and men aged 40–80 years: prevalence and correlates identified in the Global Study of Sexual Attitudes and Behaviors. Int J Impot Res 2005;17:39–57.

[29] Nicolosi A, Glasser DB, Kim SC, et al. Sexual behavior and dysfunction and help-seeking patterns in adults aged 40–80 years in the urban population of Asian countries. BJU Int 2005;95:609–14.

[30] Rosen RC, Fisher W, Eardley I, et al. The multinational men's attitudes of life events and sexuality (MALES) study: prevalence of erectile dysfunction and related health concerns in the general population. Curr Med Res Opin 2004;20:607–17.

[31] Ganz P. Erectile dysfunction: pathophysiological mechanisms pointing to underlying cardiovascular disease. Am J Cardiol, in press.

[32] Derby CA, Araujo AB, Johannes CB, et al. Measurement of erectile dysfunction in population-based studies: the use of a single question self-assessment in the Massachusetts Male Aging Study. Int J Impot Res 2000;12(4):197–204.

[33] Feldman HA, Goldstein I, Hatzichristou DG, et al. Construction of a surrogate variable for impotence in the Massachusetts Male Aging Study. J Clin Epidemiol 1994;47(5):457–67.

[34] Prins J, Blanker MH, Bohnen AM, et al. Prevalence of erectile dysfunction: a systematic review of population-based studies. Int J Impot Res 2002;14:422–32.

[35] Araujo AB, Durante R, Feldman HA, et al. The relationship between depressive symptoms and male erectile dysfunction: cross-sectional results from the Massachusetts Male Aging Study. Psychosom Med 1998;60:458–65.

[36] Araujo AB, Johannes CB, Feldman HA, et al. Relation between psychosocial risk factors and incident erectile dysfunction: prospective results from the Massachusetts Male Aging Study. Am J Epidemiol 2000;152(6):533–41.

[37] Nicolosi A, Moreira ED, Shirai M, et al. Epidemiology of erectile dysfunction in four countries: cross-national study of the prevalence and correlates of erectile dysfunction. Urology 2003;61:201–6.

[38] Panser LA, Rhodes T, Girman CJ, et al. Sexual function of men ages 40 to 79 years: the Olmsted County Study of Urinary Symptoms and Health Status Among Men. J Am Geriatr Soc 1995;43(10): 1107–11.

[39] Laumann EO, Paik A, Rosen RC. Sexual dysfunction in the United States: prevalence and predictors. JAMA 1999;281(6):537–44.

[40] Masumori N, Tsukamoto T, Kumamoto Y, et al. Decline of sexual function with age in Japanese men compared with American man: results of 2 community-based studies. Urology 1999;54:335–44.

[41] Barrett-Connor E. Heart disease factors predict erectile dysfunction 25 years later: the Rancho Bernardo Study. Am J Cardiol, in press.

[42] Andersson KE, Wagner G. Physiology of penile erection. Physio Rev 1995;75:191–236.

[43] Rajfer J, Aronson WJ, Bush PA, et al. Nitric oxide as a mediator of relaxation of the corpus cavernosum in response to nonadrenergic, noncholinergic neurotransmission. N Engl J Med 1992;326:90–4.

[44] Solomon H, Man JW, Jackson G. Erectile dysfunction and the cardiovascular patient: endothelial dysfunction is the common denominator. Heart 2003; 89:251–3.

[45] Solomon H, Man JW, Wierzbicki AS, et al. Relation of erectile dysfunction to angiographic coronary artery disease. Am J Cardiol 2003;91:230–1.

[46] Blanker MH, Bosch JL, Groeneveld FP, et al. Erectile and ejaculatory dysfunction in a community-based sample of men 50 to 78 years old: prevalence, concerns and relation to sexual activity. Urology 2001;57(4):763–8.

[47] Rosen R, Shabsigh R, Berber M, et al. Efficacy and tolerability of vardenafil in men with mild major depressive disorder and erectile dysfunction. Am J Psychiatry, in press.

[48] Seidman SN, Roose SP, Menza MA, et al. Treatment of erectile dysfunction in men with depressive symptoms: results of a placebo-controlled trial with sildenafil citrate. Am J Psychiatry 2001; 158(10):1623–30.

ELSEVIER
SAUNDERS

Urol Clin N Am 32 (2005) 419–429

UROLOGIC
CLINICS
of North America

Phosphodiesterase-5 Inhibition: the Molecular Biology of Erectile Function and Dysfunction

Sharron H. Francis, PhD*, Jackie D. Corbin, PhD

Department of Molecular Physiology and Biophysics, Light Hall, Room 702,
Vanderbilt University School of Medicine, Nashville, TN 37232-0615, USA

The ability of male mammals to achieve and maintain an engorgement of penile tissues that is sufficient for sexual intercourse is a biologic imperative for continuation of the species. The erectile response of the penis is a highly complex and physiologically coordinated neurovascular process, and appropriate relaxation of penile vascular smooth muscle is key to achieving penile erection [1–5]. Impairment of any aspect of this specialized process can alter the changes that normally occur in blood flow to the penis following sexual arousal, the capacity for accumulation of blood within the sinusoids of the penis, and the rate of venous outflow. The resulting diminution in penile tumescence results in erectile dysfunction (ED). Other maladies, such as priapism, are associated with impaired regulation of penile rigidity and are understood poorly.

Advances in treatment of ED using oral pharmacotherapies have refocused efforts of the medical and pharmaceutical communities to understand more fully the physiology of the erectile response and the pathophysiology that results in ED. Although the vasculature of the penis is specialized in function, most basic molecular mechanisms that regulate penile blood flow and capacitance are shared with the systemic and pulmonary vascular beds. As a result, insights gained in studies of erectile function and dysfunction provide promise for advances in treating other vascular malfunctions [6–9].

Origins of ED vary; it may result from vascular, hormonal, neurogenic, iatrogenic, or psychogenic causes, or some combination thereof. ED is comorbid with other health problems and more advanced age. Approximately one half of men over 40 years of age are affected to some extent by ED [10–18]. ED is substantially more common in men who have diabetes mellitus, hypercholesterolemia, depression, renal disease, hypogonadism, hypertension, and cardiovascular disorders secondary to endothelial dysfunction [19–24]. Lifestyle factors such as smoking, obesity, stress, and sedentary living also increase the incidence and severity of ED. Physical trauma such as that associated with spinal cord injury, radical prostatectomy, or radiation therapy can produce or exacerbate ED by compromising innervation of penile tissues, thereby diminishing penile blood supply [20,25–29].

The signaling pathway that provides for penile erection

The first step in the male erectile response involves activation of specific neurologic pathways by sexually arousing stimuli; these can be either cerebral or physical in origin. Regulation of penile erection involves precise coordination of output from parasympathetic, sympathetic, and somatosensory neural pathways that results in vasodilation of penile arteries, increased blood flow to the penis, and increased volume capacity within penile vascular structures (Fig. 1). This vasodilation is the end result of a shift in the balance between the activity of procontractile and prodilatory pathways. Most vasodilatory effects associated with sexual arousal are mediated by nitric

This work was supported by National Institutes of Health grants DK40029 and 58277.

* Corresponding author.

E-mail address: sharron.francis@vanderbilt.edu (S.H. Francis).

oxide, a small gaseous signaling molecule [1,15,30]. Erogenous stimuli elicit increased production and release of nitric oxide, as a neurotransmitter, from penile nonadrenergic, noncholinergic nerve terminals. Nitric oxide also is produced and released by a thin layer of luminal endothelial cells that abut the smooth muscle cells embedded in the wall of penile arteries and line the sinusoids of the penile corpora cavernosa [1,4,30,31]. Both sources of nitric oxide are important in penile erection (see Fig. 1). Evidence suggests that in the initial phases of the erectile response nitric oxide is released from nerve terminals in relatively short bursts followed by a more sustained release from endothelial cells throughout the duration of the erection. Studies in mice indicate that deficiency in nitric oxide production from either source may not abolish capacity for achieving an erection. It generally is accepted, however, that impaired nitric-oxide release from nerves (eg, as a result of neuropathies or trauma) or from endothelium caused by endothelial damage or deterioration can cause or exacerbate the severity of ED in men.

Nitric oxide is a short-lived, small molecule comprised of one nitrogen and one oxygen atom (Fig. 2). It is produced in nerve terminals throughout the body, including those of the penis, and in endothelial cells throughout the vasculature by the catalytic action of a family of nitric oxide synthases (NOS) that convert the precursor amino acid, L-arginine, to nitric oxide and L-citrulline (see Fig. 2) [32–34]. Neuronal and endothelial cells contain closely related, but different, forms of NOS: neural NOS (nNOS) and endothelial NOS (eNOS), respectively. Both enzymes are expressed constitutively, exhibit low basal activity, and are stimulated by Ca^{2+}/calmodulin binding (see Fig. 2). Both forms of NOS are believed to produce nitric oxide in the absence of external stimuli: sexual arousal produces an influx of Ca^{2+} into these cells that in turn binds to calmodulin; the Ca^{2+}/calmodulin complex substantially increases the activity of both forms of NOS. In addition to regulation by Ca^{2+}/calmodulin, other mechanisms that modulate activities of these enzymes include phosphorylation/dephosphorylation of

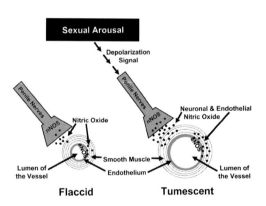

Fig. 1. Penile vascular dilatation in response to sexual arousal. Nitric oxide (*black dots*) is produced by nitric oxide synthases (NOS) located in penile nerve terminals (neuronal NOS [nNOS]) and endothelial cells (endothelial NOS [eNOS]). Gray band surrounding the vessel lumen represents the endothelial cell layer; concentric circles represent the smooth muscle encircling either penile arteries or sinusoids of the corpora cavernosa. Sexual arousal produces a depolarization signal in penile nerves that activates nNOS, resulting in increased nitric oxide production and release that elicits the initial phase of increased blood flow into the penile vasculature. Increased blood flow, acetylcholine release, and shear stress on the endothelium increase Ca^{2+} entry into the cell, activate eNOS, and increase nitric oxide production and vasodilatation.

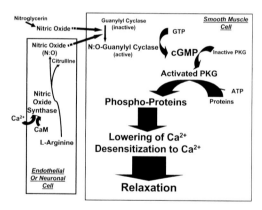

Fig. 2. Cascade of steps associated with nitric oxide–induced activation of the cyclic GMP (cGMP)-signaling pathway, amplification of the signal, and relaxation of penile vascular smooth muscle. Nitric oxide (N:O) is synthesized from L-arginine in neuronal and endothelial cells by NOS that are activated when cellular Ca^{2+} increases and the Ca^{2+}/calmodulin complex binds. Nitric oxide diffuses from the endothelial or neuronal cell into the extracellular space and vascular smooth muscle cell, where it activates guanylyl cyclase to synthesize cGMP. Increase in cGMP level activates cGMP-dependent protein kinase (PKG) and the cellular cGMP-signaling pathway that is amplified at each step (*increasingly larger arrows and text*). The result of the signaling cascade is relaxation of penile vascular smooth muscle.

several sites, interaction with cellular proteins, and cofactor/substrate availability [32,33,35,36].

Psychogenic and reflexogenic erogenous stimuli selectively increase production and release of nitric oxide from nNOS-containing nerve terminals in the penis. This is believed to result from depolarization of penile nerves in response to erogenous stimuli. Endothelial cells release nitric oxide in response to the mechanical sheer stress and viscous drag of blood coursing over the surface of these cells and to release of acetylcholine and perhaps other neurotransmitters; endothelial-derived nitric oxide acts as a paracrine factor on juxtaposed vascular smooth muscle cells. In the course of an erectile response, escalating blood flow into the penis following the initial release of nitric oxide from local nerve terminals provides increased sheer stress, activation of eNOS, and release of more nitric oxide from endothelial cells. The specific generation and release of nitric oxide within penile tissues provide an agonist drive that is highly localized and accounts for selective vasodilatation of penile vessels in response to sexual arousal (see Fig. 2).

Nitric oxide is also the active molecule released from nitrovasodilators such as nitroglycerin tablets commonly prescribed for treatment of chest pain known as *angina pectoris*. Nitric oxide that is produced naturally and that which is derived from medications such as nitroglycerin acts through the same mechanism to decrease tone in smooth muscle cells encircling blood vessels (see Fig. 2). When nitroglycerin is administered for relief of chest pain, the nitric oxide derived from the medication is distributed systemically and acts as an agonist to cause vasodilatory effects in the entire vascular bed. In contrast, nitric oxide produced in the nerves and endothelial cells of the penile vasculature following sexual arousal acts only on vascular smooth muscle cells in the penis.

The second step in the erectile response involves the rapid diffusion of nitric oxide across the plasma membrane of vascular smooth muscle cells and its interaction with its intracellular target, a heme group on guanylyl cyclase (GC) (see Fig. 2) [37–39]. This is not a trivial feat because nitric oxide is highly reactive and quickly declines in concentration because it can be bound covalently to certain amino acids on proteins, inactivated by chemical reducing factors in the cytosol such as glutathione, and complexes with protein heme groups. Nitric oxide binds tightly to the heme cofactor on GC resulting in activation of the enzyme; this GC is also known as *nitric oxide–*

activated GC or *soluble GC* (see Fig. 2). Unlike hemes in many proteins, the heme on GC discriminates strongly between nitric oxide and oxygen. Activated GC converts its substrate, GTP, to the second messenger, cyclic GMP (cGMP) (see Fig. 2). With increased sexual arousal, the nitric oxide provided to the smooth muscle cells of the penile vasculature is increased progressively, more GC is activated, cellular cGMP level rises, and the cGMP-signaling pathway is stimulated. The term *cGMP-signaling pathway* describes the biochemical processes by which elevation of cGMP brings about particular effects in a tissue, in this case vascular smooth muscle relaxation. In vascular smooth muscle, cGMP-dependent protein kinase (PKG) is the principal mediator of the cGMP-signaling pathway (see Fig. 2) [40].

Nitric oxide, the "first messenger" in the cGMP-signaling pathway, sets in motion a cascade of reactions in which the magnitude of each step is amplified enzymatically (ie, the number of molecules at each step increases). The progressively larger arrows and text for the different steps in Fig. 2 emphasize this. Stepwise amplification converts the effect initiated by a modest amount of nitric oxide into marked lowering of intracellular free Ca^{2+}, desensitization of contractile proteins to Ca^{2+}, and a decrease in the contractile state of the penile vascular smooth muscle (see Fig. 2). Nitric oxide and cGMP share the spotlight as linchpins in this signaling cascade; both are critical components in the physiologic pathway that promotes the vasodilatation leading to penile erection [1,30,31]. Even if sufficient nitric oxide is generated in penile tissues and GC is activated to synthesize more cGMP, impairment of proteins mediating subsequent steps in the cGMP-signaling pathway or an imbalance in the relative rates of cGMP synthesis and degradation can impair penile erection.

The third step leading to penile erection involves cellular biochemical effects elicited by the cGMP-signaling pathway (Fig. 3). cGMP binds to a limited number of target proteins in mammalian cells and alters their activities. In vascular smooth muscle cells such as those in the walls of penile arteries, cGMP mediates most of its effects through PKG [40–45]. cGMP binds to regulatory sites on PKG and causes a conformational change that activates catalysis. The extent of elevation of cGMP or activation of PKG required for optimum penile erection is uncertain; based on studies of these agents in other tissues, two- to threefold increases may be sufficient [46,47]. In the active state PKG transfers

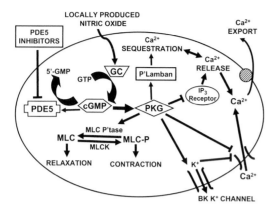

Fig. 3. Biochemical changes associated with nitric oxide–induced vasodilatation. cGMP content in vascular smooth muscle cells is determined by the balance between synthesis by the nitric oxide–activated GC and breakdown by phosphodiesterase-5 (PDE5). PDE5 inhibitors block PDE5 activity, thereby enhancing cGMP accumulation when synthesis is continuing. PKG is the main mediator of cGMP signaling in vascular smooth muscle cells; it phosphorylates and increases activity of (1) phospholamban (P'LAMBAN) to increase Ca^{2+} sequestration in the endoplasmic reticulum, (2) the BK K^+ channel resulting in increased K^+ efflux, increased hyperpolarization of the membrane and inhibition of Ca^{2+} influx through voltage-gated Ca^{2+} channels, (3) myosin light chain phosphatase (MLC P'TASE) to dephosphorylate myosin light chain (MLC) and (4) proteins that promote Ca^{2+} extrusion from the cell. PKG phosphorylation events have a negative effect on the function of (1) the inositol triphosphate (IP3) receptor, resulting in decreased sensitivity to IP3 and inhibition of Ca^{2+} release from intracellular stores, and (2) Ca^{2+} channels that mediate Ca^{2+} influx into the cell. PKG also phosphorylates PDE5 (not shown) and increases PDE5 catalytic activity and affinity for PDE5 inhibitors.

phosphate from cellular ATP to serines or threonines in numerous cellular proteins, although the number of proteins phosphorylated by PKG and the mechanism by which PKG brings about smooth muscle relaxation are unknown. In vascular smooth muscle, PKG phosphorylates myosin light chain phosphatase (also known as *phosphoprotein phosphatase 1M*), which dephosphorylates myosin light chain (MLC) [48]. Dephospho-MLC has a weakened interaction with other contractile proteins in the cell, thereby promoting smooth muscle relaxation [49].

Many other proteins phosphorylated by PKG contribute to regulation of intracellular Ca^{2+} homeostasis, including: (1) phospholamban, which modulates sequestration of Ca^{2+} in the endoplasmic reticulum—phosphorylation by PKG enhances this function; (2) a regulatory protein associated with the inositol triphosphate receptor (IP3 receptor), which when phosphorylated by PKG inhibits IP3-induced release of Ca^{2+} from intracellular stores; (3) the BK K^+ channel that is activated by phosphorylation by PKG, providing for increased K^+ exit, hyperpolarization of the cell membrane potential, and inactivation of voltage-gated Ca^{2+} channels; and (4) plasma membrane Ca^{2+} pumps that extrude more Ca^{2+} following phosphorylation by PKG (see Fig. 3) [40,42,43,45]. Two thin filament/actin-binding proteins (vasodilatory stimulated phosphoprotein and a heat shock-related protein) also are phosphorylated by PKG and may be involved in relaxation of vascular smooth muscle. The roles of these proteins are unclear.

In summary, as cGMP increases in the smooth muscle cells lining penile arteries and sinusoids, more PKG will be activated, resulting in decreased intracellular Ca^{2+} levels, decreased tension in the contractile machinery of the cell, and increased vasodilatation. In the cardiovascular system, the cGMP-signaling pathway plays a prominent role in numerous processes other than modulation of smooth muscle tone; these include certain cardiac functions, regulation of smooth muscle proliferation, and inhibition of platelet aggregation [40,43,50].

Adequate functioning of the components described above is critical to achieve a degree of penile erection sufficient for sexual intercourse. Insufficiency in any step can lead to ED, including inadequate sexual arousal, nerve dysfunction resulting from neuropathies or injuries, vascular insufficiencies, or biochemical imbalances. In neuropathies associated with particular diseases or injuries that impair the nerve supply, the nitric oxide produced and released from nerves and endothelial cells may be insufficient to activate GC and the downstream cGMP-signaling pathway [51,52]. In individuals who have vascular deterioration, cellular components such as NOS, GC, or PKG that are required to mediate dilation of penile vascular smooth muscle may be deficient. Lastly, an imbalance among the activities of cellular proteins that determine cellular cGMP level can produce ED or other erectile malfunctions [53].

Modulation of cellular cyclic GMP level

Cellular cGMP level is dictated by the balance between the rates of synthesis by GC and breakdown by cyclic nucleotide (cN) phospho-diesterases (PDE) [54–58]. PDEs cleave the cyclic phosphate ring that is required for the action of cGMP or cyclic AMP (cAMP) in the respective signaling pathways (see Fig. 3; Fig. 4). PDE activities in mammalian cells provide the primary counterpoint to cAMP and cGMP synthesis and act to dampen or terminate a cN signal such as that of cGMP in the penis. Mammalian PDEs have been divided into 11 families based on their amino acid sequences, regulatory features, and pharmacologic properties. Some are highly specific for hydrolyzing either cGMP or cAMP, whereas others hydrolyze both cNs.

Most tissues contain multiple forms of PDEs, including members of several different PDE families, but in tissues including the penile corpus cavernosum, the profile of PDEs is limited. In smooth muscle cells of the penile vasculature, phosphodiesterase-5 (PDE5), a cGMP-specific PDE, is the major cGMP-hydrolyzing PDE [59–61]. This pattern dictates that PDE5 activity will play a major role in determining cGMP level in these cells. The balance between the activities of GC and PDE5 in these cells largely determines the intracellular cGMP level. The activities of GC and PDE5 are subject to complex and dynamic regulatory processes that impact the balance of these activities, thereby altering cGMP level and, consequently, vascular tone [1,4,62,63]. Insufficient cGMP synthesis by GC or increased hydrolysis by PDE5 could result in low cellular cGMP, weak action in the cGMP-signaling pathway,

inadequate vasodilation, and impaired erectile function. Alternatively, excessive cGMP synthesis by GC or decreased breakdown of cGMP by PDE5 could result in more prolonged activation of the cGMP-signaling pathway and vasodilatation of penile tissues, as occurs in patients who have priapism, a life-threatening ailment [53].

Mechanism by which phosphodiesterase-5 inhibitors enhance erectile function

The prominence of PDE5 as a cGMP-PDE in vascular smooth muscle garnered the attention of investigators interested in developing pharmaceuticals that would block its action [64,65]. It was predicted that inhibition of PDE5 would elevate cellular cGMP and decrease vascular tone. As a result, PDE5 was considered an excellent pharmacologic target for treatment of systemic hypertension because the cGMP-signaling pathway seems to feature prominently in regulating cGMP levels in most blood vessels [41–45].

The culmination of years of work by many investigators to improve the potency and specificity of chemicals that would block PDE5 activity came to fruition in the mid-1990s with the introduction of sildenafil [66,67]. In contrast to predictions and despite the abundance of PDE5 in the systemic vasculature, sildenafil produced only modest effects on systemic blood pressure, likely because of the myriad counter-regulatory mechanisms involved in blood pressure control [68]. Remarkably, however, sildenafil improved erectile function in many men who have ED.

Introduction of sildenafil, and more recently two other potent and selective PDE5 inhibitors, tadalafil and vardenafil (Fig. 5), into the commercial market revolutionized treatment of ED worldwide [11,12,15,69,70]. These medications are administered easily, act quickly, are readily affordable, and have proved highly effective in the management of ED in many patients. The relatively minor side effects of the medications vary slightly (headache, flushing, dyspepsia, rhinitis, visual perturbation, backache), are transient, have low incidence, and tend to wane with use of the medications. Although tachyphylaxis has been suggested in at least one report, there is little evidence that it is a significant problem in individuals using the inhibitors on-demand for long-term intervals [71,72]. Incidence of tachyphylaxis may be minimized by the intermittent use of the inhibitors, which avoids sustained and regular exposure to drug.

cGMP

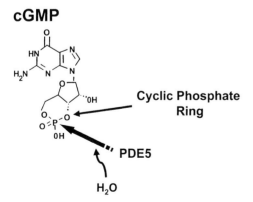

Fig. 4. Structure of cGMP and site of PDE5 action. cGMP is comprised of a guanine ring, a ribose ring, and a novel six-membered cyclic phosphate ring. PDE5 action breaks the cyclic phosphate ring by inserting a hydroxyl group from a solvent water molecule at the phosphorous atom (*thicker arrow*).

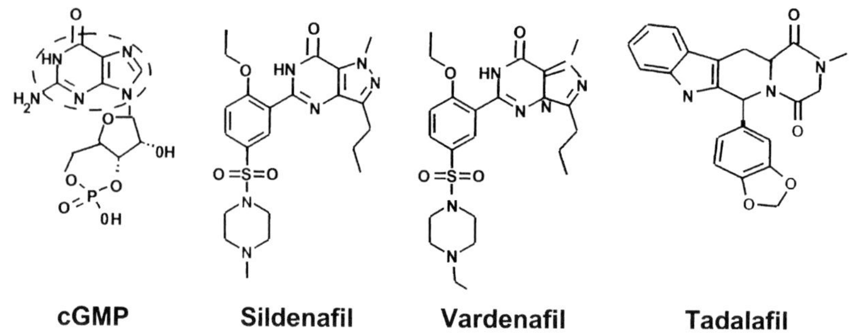

cGMP   **Sildenafil**   **Vardenafil**   **Tadalafil**

Fig. 5. Comparison of the molecular structures of cGMP, sildenafil, vardenafil, and tadalafil. Sildenafil, vardenafil, and tadalafil contain heterocyclic rings that in part mimic the guanine ring (*dashed circle*) of cGMP, but they lack the ribose and cyclic phosphate ring present in cGMP. Compared with cGMP, the three inhibitors have two to four additional rings that form contacts with amino acids in and around the PDE5 catalytic site and thereby increase their potency for binding to PDE5.

The molecular structures of all three inhibitors include a heterocyclic ring component that mimics the purine of the cGMP substrate of PDE5 (see Fig. 5); this similarity in structure between the inhibitors and cGMP provides for the action of these medications because the heterocyclic ring component in each of the inhibitors mimics the purine of cGMP (see Fig. 5) and binds into the catalytic site on PDE5 where cGMP binds and is degraded (Fig. 6). These medications compete directly with cGMP, the substrate, for access to the catalytic site [73,74]. If cGMP cannot gain access to the pocket on PDE5 containing the catalytic machinery, it cannot be inactivated by hydrolysis.

All three inhibitors have significant advantage over cGMP in interacting with the catalytic site of PDE5. First, unlike cGMP, the inhibitors are not degraded when they bind to the catalytic site, and second, the inhibitors have much higher affinity (1000- to 40,000-fold) than cGMP, as indicated by the relative thickness of the upper arrow in Fig. 6 [73,74]. The higher affinities are the result of multiple attractive forces made by the additional rings in the inhibitors that are absent in cGMP (see Fig. 5). These extra rings interact with amino acids in and around the catalytic site of PDE5 that cGMP does not contact. The number and types of attractive forces formed respectively by the three inhibitors account for vardenafil being 10 to 40 times more potent than sildenafil, and tadalafil being approximately twice as potent as sildenafil [73,75,76].

None of the inhibitors has been shown to interact significantly with other cellular proteins, although this possibility cannot be excluded. The high specificity and affinity of these inhibitors for PDE5 is consistent with the few side effects that have been reported and with the circulating concentration of each of the free inhibitors required for improvement of erectile function. The latter approximates the concentration of that inhibitor required to block PDE5 activity, and recommended range of doses for the inhibitors is in line with the varied potencies. Sildenafil, the

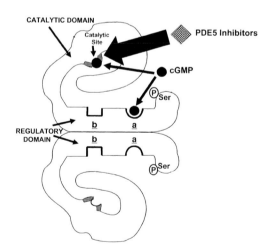

Fig. 6. Working model of PDE5 protein. PDE5 is a dimer comprised of identical subunits. cGMP (*black circle*) binds to the catalytic site in the catalytic domain and to allosteric sites in the regulatory domain. PDE5 inhibitors bind with much higher affinity than cGMP to the catalytic site, and, unlike cGMP, are not broken down by PDE5. PDE5 is phosphorylated (P) at a single serine (Ser). Phosphorylation and allosteric cGMP binding increase affinity of the catalytic site for inhibitors and for cGMP.

weakest of the three, is marketed in 25-, 50-, and 100-mg tablets compared with 5-, 10- and 20-mg tablets for vardenafil, the most potent of the three. Tadalafil may be marketed in relatively low recommended doses of 5-, 10-, and 20-mg in part because of a high bioavailability of this drug.

Impact of regulation of phosphodiesterase-5 on cyclic GMP signaling and inhibitor potency

PDE5 is highly regulated, and these regulatory mechanisms in part provide for negative feedback regulation of cGMP levels under normal physiologic conditions and for a feed-forward action to increase potency of pharmacologic inhibitors of PDE5 (see Fig. 6). First, by most estimates, the catalytic activity of PDE5 under basal physiologic conditions is relatively low because the cellular cGMP concentration is well below that required to saturate PDE5 and achieve the maximum hydrolytic rate (V_{max}). As cGMP synthesis increases in response to nitric oxide activation of GC, cellular cGMP begins to rise, and the activity of PDE5 increases linearly. Second, in addition to interaction of cGMP with the catalytic site, the nucleotide also binds to allosteric sites in the regulatory domain of PDE5 (see Fig. 6), and this binding is increased when the catalytic site is occupied; cGMP binding to the allosteric sites causes two effects: (1) increased affinity of the catalytic site for the cGMP substrate and (2) exposure of a single serine for phosphorylation by PKG. Ligand binding to the catalytic and allosteric sites induces a conformational change in PDE5 that converts the enzyme into a more active form.

These effects increase affinity of PDE5 catalytic site for cGMP, thereby increasing the degree of saturation of the site, resulting in increased cGMP hydrolysis. These molecular mechanisms provide for a classic negative feedback mechanism to dampen or terminate the magnitude of the cellular response to the cGMP signaling pathway. In individuals with normal erectile function, the increase in cGMP synthesis in response to sexual arousal is accompanied by countervailing activation of PDE5 to dampen or terminate cGMP signaling (see Figs. 3 and 6). Despite this delicate balance, in the normal erectile response cGMP level increases sufficiently to bring about the vasodilatation required for penile tumescence. Obviously, excess PDE5 activity compared with GC activity will produce ED. Pharmacologic blocking of PDE5 activity by sildenafil, vardenafil, or tadalafil shifts the balance to favor cGMP accumulation and improves the quality of the erectile response (see Figs. 3 and 6).

Activation of PDE5 by these mechanisms improves interaction of the PDE5 catalytic site with the three medications used for treatment of ED. Sildenafil, tadalafil, or vardenafil are most effective for relief of ED when taken 30 minutes to 2 hours before sexual activity. This allows sufficient time for the inhibitors to enter the vascular smooth muscle cells and bind to the catalytic site of PDE5. First, this binding produces a conformational change in PDE5 that transforms it into a higher-affinity binding partner for the inhibitors. Second, when cGMP begins to rise in the cells, it binds to the allosteric sites on PDE5, which further enhances affinity of the catalytic site for the inhibitors. Third, after binding cGMP at the allosteric sites, PDE5 becomes phosphorylated by PKG, a process that also enhances affinity of the catalytic site for the inhibitors. In this manner, the inhibitors increase their own potency and efficacy, a classic feed-forward regulation of function. In this instance, the inhibitors exploit a built-in natural negative feedback mechanism to accentuate their effects.

Cessation of inhibitor effects

The three commercially marketed PDE5 inhibitors are not metabolized in the smooth muscle cell where their primary actions take place. The inhibitors must dissociate from PDE5, successfully diffuse out of the cell, escape re-entry, and be transported to the liver where they are metabolized or inactivated by cytochromes CYP3A4, CYP2C9, CYP2C19, and CYO2D6 [77]. Certain metabolites of sildenafil, although less potent, account for part of its inhibition of PDE5. The high affinity with which sildenafil, vardenafil, and tadalafil bind to PDE5 is likely to slow reversal of the effects of these medications because even when the inhibitor dissociates from PDE5, it is likely to rebind quickly. This dynamic equilibrium will occur repeatedly before the drug diffuses through the plasma membrane into the extracellular space, enters the plasma, and is transported to the liver. Following sexual arousal, the affinity of PDE5 for the inhibitors would be greatest because of the regulatory mechanisms described above. Because PDE5 is the major cGMP-hydrolyzing PDE in corpus cavernosum, cGMP level will remain high until the inhibitor exits the cell. Several reports indicate that some individuals have improved erectile function after the time required for clearance of measurable drug from plasma [78,79]. Although the medication may have been cleared from plasma, it still may be present and blocking PDE5 in the vascular smooth muscle cells. A recent clinical study in men who already had used sildenafil successfully showed that efficacy declined only slightly from 1 (97%) to 12 hours (74%) after taking a 100-mg pill [79]. This observation is consistent with biochemical studies.

Tissues affected by action of phosphodiesterase-5 inhibitors

The perception of much of the medical and lay community is that PDE5 inhibitors act only in the penis. In fact, when any of the three inhibitors is ingested, the particular inhibitor will enter cells throughout the body, including vascular smooth muscle cells of the systemic and pulmonary beds, platelets, and heart; the inhibitors will block PDE5 action potently in all tissues containing PDE5. Box 1 summarizes factors that contribute to the selective action of these inhibitors to improve erectile function. These PDE5 inhibitors have a pronounced effect only in systems where there is significant cGMP synthesis. In the absence of sexual arousal, PDE5 inhibitors do not cause penile erection; nitric oxide release from the penile nerves and endothelium is required to increase cGMP production. Only under those conditions will the inhibitor's effect to block PDE5 hydrolysis of cGMP manifest as an erection.

The potential for broader action of the PDE5 inhibitors is evidenced by the slight (10–15 mm Hg) drop in systemic blood pressure experienced by many patients after taking these drugs [68,80,81]. Although the effect on blood pressure

is mild, it occurs because the endothelial cells that line the systemic vessels constantly produce and supply low levels of nitric oxide to the smooth muscle cells of these vessels. In some individuals, concomitant use of alpha-blockers, which decrease Ca^{2+} signaling and reduce contraction of vascular smooth muscle, and PDE5 inhibitors can cause significant hypotensive events; as a result, considerable caution should be used when administering PDE5 inhibitors to these patients [81].

All three manufacturers warn against concomitant use of the inhibitors and nitric oxide derived from nitrovasodilators, such as nitroglycerin, and certain recreational drugs [82,83]. In this case, the nitroglycerin medication provides a nitric oxide agonist drive to blood vessels throughout the body, and concomitant inhibition of PDE5 could produce a life-threatening or fatal hypotensive event. Recent reports indicate that sildenafil shows promise in treatment of other maladies associated with vascular dysfunction; this includes pulmonary hypertension where the nitric oxide agonist production in the affected vessels is robust and, therefore, the PDE5 inhibitors can act effectively to elevate cGMP [8,84–88]. Studies in animal models also suggest a role for sildenafil in improved recovery from stroke [89,90] and blunting or reversal of cardiac hypertrophy [91]. Sildenafil also seems to promote dilation of the lower esophageal sphincter in individuals who have idiopathic achalasia [92] and to relieve symptoms associated with Raynaud's phenomenon in some patients [93]. These examples demonstrate that PDE5 inhibitors act in tissues other than those of the penis. In all cases, active synthesis of cGMP is necessary for the effect of the PDE5 inhibitors to be manifest. This emphasizes that developing a clear understanding of the molecular basis of the action of these inhibitors is central to full exploitation of their potential.

Summary

Commercially marketed PDE5 inhibitors are highly specific for PDE5, and in the face of continuing cyclic GMP synthesis, elevate cellular cGMP. This elevation results from direct competitive inhibition of PDE5 and from blocking the negative feedback regulation of the enzyme. Elevation of cGMP activates PKG, which mediates the effects of the cGMP-signaling pathway to decrease smooth muscle tone and dilate penile vascular smooth muscle. By exploiting features of PDE5 regulatory mechanisms that modulate

---

Box 1. Factors that contribute to selective action of phosphodiesterase-5 inhibitors to improve erectile function

- Localized release of nitric oxide in penis
- Limited PDE5 tissue distribution
- High biochemical potency of inhibitors for PDE5
- Strong selectivity for PDE5 versus other PDEs
- Regulatory mechanisms of PDE5 that increase affinity for PDE5 inhibitors
- Pharmacokinetics of the inhibitors

PDE5 function, the inhibitors enhance their own potencies.

References

[1] Burnett AL, Lowenstein CJ, Bradt DS, et al. Nitric oxide in the penis: physiology and pathology. Science 1992;257:401–3.

[2] Andersson KE, Stief CG. Neurotransmission and the contraction and relaxation of penile erectile tissues. World J Urol 1997;15:14–20.

[3] Lincoln TM. Cyclic GMP and mechanisms of vasodilation. Pharmacol Ther 1989;41:479–502.

[4] Ignarro LJ, Cirino G, Casini A, et al. Nitric oxide as a signaling molecule in the vascular system: an overview. J Cardiovas Pharmacol 1999;34:879–86.

[5] Carvajal JA, Germain AM, Huidobro-Toro JP, et al. Molecular mechanism of cGMP-mediated smooth muscle relaxation. J Cell Physiol 2000;184: 409–20.

[6] Ghofrani HA, Wiedemann R, Rose F, et al. Sildenafil for treatment of lung fibrosis and pulmonary hypertension: a randomised controlled trial. Lancet 2002;360:895–900.

[7] Ghofrani HA, Rose F, Schermuly RT, et al. Oral sildenafil as long-term adjunct therapy to inhaled iloprost in severe pulmonary arterial hypertension. J Am Coll Cardiol 2003;42:158–64.

[8] Michelakis ED, Tymchak W, Noga M, et al. Long-term treatment with oral sildenafil is safe and improves functional capacity and hemodynamics in patients with pulmonary arterial hypertension. Circulation 2003;108:2066–9.

[9] Rosenkranz S, Diet F, Karasch T, et al. Sildenafil improved pulmonary hypertension and peripheral blood flow in a patient with scleroderma-associated lung fibrosis and the raynaud phenomenon. Ann Intern Med 2003;139:871–3.

[10] Feldman HA, Goldstein I, Hatzichristou DG, et al. Impotence and its medical and psychosocial correlates: results of the Massachusetts Male Aging Study. J Urol 1994;151:54–61.

[11] Goldstein I, Lue TF, Padma-Nathan H, et al. Oral sildenafil in the treatment of erectile dysfunction. J Urol 1998;167:1197–203.

[12] Burnett AL. The impact of sildenafil on molecular science and sexual health. Eur Urol 2004;46:9–14.

[13] Padma-Nathan H, Steers WD, Wicker PA. Efficacy and safety of oral sildenafil in the treatment of erectile dysfunction: a double-blind, placebo-controlled study of 329 patients. Sildenafil Study Group. Int J Clin Pract 1998;52:375–9.

[14] Lue TF. Neurogenic erectile dysfunction. Clin Auton Res 2001;11:285–94.

[15] Lue TF. Erectile dysfunction. N Engl J Med 2000; 342:1802–13.

[16] Rotella DP. Phosphodiesterase 5 inhibitors: current status and potential applications. Nat Rev Drug Discov 2002;1:674–82.

[17] Montorsi F, Salonia A, Deho F, et al. Pharmacological management of erectile dysfunction. BJU Int 2003;91:446–54.

[18] Montorsi F, Salonia A, Deho F, et al. The ageing male and erectile dysfunction. World J Urol 2002; 20:28–35.

[19] Spollett GR. Assessment and management of erectile dysfunction in men with diabetes. Diabetes Educ 1999;25:65–73.

[20] Rendell MS, Rajfer J, Wicker PA, et al. Sildenafil for treatment of erectile dysfunction in men with diabetes: a randomized controlled trial. Sildenafil Diabetes Study Group. JAMA 1999;281:421–6.

[21] Stuckey BG, Jadzinsky MN, Murphy LJ, et al. Sildenafil citrate for treatment of erectile dysfunction in men with type 1 diabetes: results of a randomized controlled trial. Diabetes Care 2003;26: 279–84.

[22] Koppiker N, Boolell M, Price D. Recent advances in the treatment of erectile dysfunction in patients with diabetes mellitus. Endocr Pract 2003; 9:52–63.

[23] Basu A, Ryder RE. New treatment options for erectile dysfunction in patients with diabetes mellitus. Drugs 2004;64:2667–88.

[24] Salonia A, Briganti A, Deho F, et al. Pathophysiology of erectile dysfunction. Int J Androl 2003;26: 129–36.

[25] Raina R, Lakin MM, Agarwal A, et al. Long-term effect of sildenafil citrate on erectile dysfunction after radical prostatectomy: 3-year follow-up. Urology 2003;62:110–5.

[26] Montorsi F, Salonia A, Zanoni M, et al. Counseling the patient with prostate cancer about treatment-related erectile dysfunction. Curr Opin Urol 2001;11: 611–7.

[27] Ramos AS, Samso JV. Specific aspects of erectile dysfunction in spinal cord injury. Int J Impot Res 2004;16(Suppl 2):S42–5.

[28] Derry F, Hultling C, Seftel AD, et al. Efficacy and safety of sildenafil citrate (Viagra) in men with erectile dysfunction and spinal cord injury: a review. Urology 2002;60(Suppl 2):49–57.

[29] Raina R, Lakin MM, Agarwal A, et al. Efficacy and factors associated with successful outcome of sildenafil citrate use for erectile dysfunction after radical prostatectomy. Urology 2004;63:960–6.

[30] Ignarro LJ, Bush PA, Buga GM, et al. Nitric oxide and cyclic GMP formation upon electrical field stimulation cause relaxation of corpus cavernosum smooth muscle. Biochem Biophys Res Commun 1990;170:843–50.

[31] McDonald LJ, Murad F. Nitric oxide and cyclic GMP signaling. Proc Soc Exp Biol Med 1996;211: 1–6.

[32] Marletta MA. Another activation switch for endothelial nitric oxide synthase: why does it have to be so complicated? Trends Biochem Sci 2001;26: 519–21.

[33] Alderton WK, Cooper CE, Knowles RG. Nitric oxide synthases: structure, function and inhibition. Biochem J 2001;357:593–615.

[34] Hemmens B, Mayer B. Enzymology of nitric oxide synthases. Methods Mol Biol 1998;100:1–32.

[35] Butt E, Bernhardt M, Smolenski A, et al. Endothelial nitric-oxide synthase (type III) is activated and becomes calcium independent upon phosphorylation by cyclic nucleotide-dependent protein kinases. J Biol Chem 2000;275:5179–87.

[36] Fleming I, Busse R. Molecular mechanisms involved in the regulation of the endothelial nitric oxide synthase. Am J Physiol Regul Integr Comp Physiol 2003;284:R1–12.

[37] Foster DC, Wedel BJ, Robinson SW, et al. Mechanisms of regulation and functions of guanylyl cyclases. Rev Physiol Biochem Pharmacol 1999;135:1–39.

[38] Lucas KA, Pitari GM, Kazerounian S, et al. Guanylyl cyclases and signaling by cyclic GMP. Pharmacol Rev 2000;52:375–414.

[39] Bellamy TC, Garthwaite J. The receptor-like properties of nitric oxide-activated soluble guanylyl cyclase in intact cells. Mol Cell Biochem 2002;230:165–76.

[40] Feil R, Lohmann SM, de Jonge H, et al. Cyclic GMP-dependent protein kinases and the cardiovascular system: insights from genetically modified mice. Circ Res 2003;93:907–16.

[41] Smolenski A, Burkhardt AM, Eigenthaler M, et al. Functional analysis of cGMP-dependent protein kinases I and II as mediators of NO/cGMP effects. Naunyn Schmiedebergs Arch Pharmacol 1998;358:134–9.

[42] Francis SH, Corbin JD. Cyclic nucleotide-dependent protein kinases: intracellular receptors for cAMP and cGMP action. Crit Rev Clin Lab Sci 1999;36:275–328.

[43] Lincoln TM, Dey N, Sellak H. Invited review: cGMP-dependent protein kinase signaling mechanisms in smooth muscle: from the regulation of tone to gene expression. J Appl Physiol 2001;91:1421–30.

[44] Schlossmann J, Feil R, Hofmann F. Insights into cGMP signaling derived from cGMP kinase knockout mice. Front Biosci 2005;10:1279–89.

[45] Hofmann F. The biology of cyclic GMP-dependent protein kinases. J Biol Chem 2005;280:1–4.

[46] Francis SH, Noblett BD, Todd BW, et al. Relaxation of vascular and tracheal smooth muscle by cyclic nucleotide analogs that preferentially activate purified cGMP-dependent protein kinase. Mol Pharmacol 1988;34:506–17.

[47] Jiang H, Colbran JL, Francis SH, et al. Direct evidence for cross-activation of cGMP-dependent protein kinase by cAMP in pig coronary arteries. J Biol Chem 1992;267:1015–9.

[48] Surks HK, Mochizuki N, Kasai Y, et al. Regulation of myosin phosphatase by a specific interaction with cGMP-dependent protein kinase Ialpha. Science 1999;286:1583–7.

[49] Chuang AT, Strauss JD, Steers WD, et al. cGMP mediates corpus cavernosum smooth muscle relaxation with altered cross-bridge function. Life Sci 1998;63:185–94.

[50] Li Z, Xi X, Gu M, et al. A stimulatory role for cGMP-dependent protein kinase in platelet activation. Cell 2003;112:77–86.

[51] Celermajer DS, Cullen S, Deanfield JE. Impairment of endothelium-dependent pulmonary artery relaxation in children with congenital heart disease and abnormal pulmonary hemodynamics. Circulation 1993;87:440–6.

[52] Kugiyama K, Yasue H, Okumura K, et al. Nitric oxide activity is deficient in spasm arteries of patients with coronary spastic angina. Circulation 1996;94:266–71.

[53] Champion HC, Bivalacqua TJ, Takimoto E, et al. Phosphodiesterase-5A dysregulation in penile erectile tissue is a mechanism of priapism. Proc Natl Acad Sci USA 2005;102:1661–6.

[54] Beavo JA. Cyclic nucleotide phosphodiesterases: functional implications of multiple isoforms. Physiol Rev 1995;75:725–48.

[55] Burns F, Zhao AZ, Beavo JA. Cyclic nucleotide phosphodiesterases: gene complexity, regulation by phosphorylation, and physiological implications. Adv Pharmacol 1996;36:29–48.

[56] Degerman E, Belfrage P, Manganiello VC. Structure, localization, and regulation of cGMP-inhibited phosphodiesterase (PDE3). J Biol Chem 1997;272:6823–6.

[57] Francis SH, Turko IV, Corbin JD. Cyclic nucleotide phosphodiesterases: relating structure and function. Prog Nucleic Acid Res Mol Biol 2001;65:1–52.

[58] Houslay MD, Adams DR. PDE4 cAMP phosphodiesterases: modular enzymes that orchestrate signalling cross-talk, desensitization and compartmentalization. Biochem J 2003;370:1–18.

[59] Taher A, Meyer M, Stief CG, et al. Cyclic nucleotide phosphodiesterase in human cavernous smooth muscle. World J Urol 1997;15:32–5.

[60] Wallis RM, Corbin JD, Francis SH, et al. Tissue distribution of phosphodiesterase families and the effects of sildenafil on tissue cyclic nucleotides, platelet function, and the contractile responses of trabeculae carneae and aortic rings in vitro. Am J Cardiol 1999;83:3–12.

[61] Gopal VK, Francis SH, Corbin JD. Allosteric sites of phosphodiesterase-5 (PDE5). A potential role in negative feedback regulation of cGMP signaling in corpus cavernosum. Eur J Biochem 2001;268:3304–12.

[62] Schmidt HH, Walter U. NO at work. Cell 1994;78:919–25.

[63] Corbin JD, Francis SH. Cyclic GMP phosphodiesterase 5: target for sildenafil. J Biol Chem 1999;274:13729–32.

[64] Lugnier C, Schoeffter P, Le Bec A, et al. Selective inhibition of cyclic nucleotide phosphodiesterases of human, bovine and rat aorta. Biochem Pharmacol 1986;35:1743–51.

[65] Wyatt TA, Naftilan AJ, Francis SH, et al. ANF elicits phosphorylation of the cGMP phosphodiesterase in vascular smooth muscle cells. Am J Physiol 1998; 274:H448–55.

[66] Boolell M, Allen MJ, Ballard SA, et al. Sildenafil: an orally active type 5 cyclic GMP-specific phosphodiesterase inhibitor for the treatment of penile erectile dysfunction. Int J Impot Res 1996;8:47–52.

[67] Ballard SA, Gingell CJ, Tang K, et al. Effects of sildenafil on the relaxation of human corpus cavernosum tissue in vitro and on the activities of cyclic nucleotide phosphodiesterase isozymes. J Urol 1998;159:2164–71.

[68] Jackson G, Benjamin N, Jackson N, et al. Effects of sildenafil citrate on human hemodynamics. Am J Cardiol 1999;83:13C–20C.

[69] Montorsi F, Briganti A, Salonia A, et al. The use of phosphodiesterase type 5 inhibitors for erectile dysfunction. Curr Opin Urol 2004;14:357–9.

[70] Sadovsky R, Miller T, Moskowitz M, et al. Three-year update of sildenafil citrate (Viagra) efficacy and safety. Int J Clin Pract 2001;55:115–28.

[71] El-Galley R, Rutland H, Talic R, et al. Long-term efficacy of sildenafil and tachyphylaxis effect. J Urol 2001;166:927–31.

[72] Steers W, Guay AT, Leriche A, et al. Assessment of the efficacy and safety of Viagra (sildenafil citrate) in men with erectile dysfunction during long-term treatment. Int J Impot Res 2001;13:261–7.

[73] Corbin JD, Francis SH. Pharmacology of phosphodiesterase-5 inhibitors. Int J Clin Pract 2002;56: 453–9.

[74] Corbin JD, Francis SH. Molecular biology and pharmacology of PDE-5-inhibitor therapy for erectile dysfunction. J Androl 2003;24:S38–41.

[75] Saenz de Tejada I, Angulo J, Cuevas P, et al. The phosphodiesterase inhibitory selectivity and the in vitro and in vivo potency of the new PDE5 inhibitor vardenafil. Int J Impot Res 2001;13:282–90.

[76] Sung BJ, Hwang KY, Jeon YH, et al. Structure of the catalytic domain of human phosphodiesterase 5 with bound drug molecules. Nature 2003;425: 98–102.

[77] Warrington JS, Shader RI, von Moltke LL, et al. In vitro biotransformation of sildenafil (Viagra): identification of human cytochromes and potential drug interactions. Drug Metab Dispos 2000;28:392–7.

[78] Porst H, Padma-Nathan H, Giuliano F, et al. Efficacy of tadalafil for the treatment of erectile dysfunction at 24 and 36 hours after dosing: a randomized controlled trial. Urology 2003;62:121–5 [discussion 125–6].

[79] Moncada I, Jara J, Subira D, et al. Efficacy of sildenafil citrate at 12 hours after dosing: re-exploring the therapeutic window. Eur Urol 2004;46:357–60.

[80] Zusman RM, Morales A, Glasser DB, et al. Overall cardiovascular profile of sildenafil citrate. Am J Cardiol 1999;83:35C–44C.

[81] Kloner RA. Cardiovascular effects of the 3 phosphodiesterase-5 inhibitors approved for the treatment of erectile dysfunction. Circulation 2004;110: 3149–55.

[82] Crosby R, Mettey A. A descriptive analysis of HIV risk behavior among men having sex with men attending a large sex resort. J Acquir Immune Defic Syndr 2004;37:1496–9.

[83] Smith KM, Romanelli F. Recreational use and misuse of phosphodiesterase 5 inhibitors. J Am Pharm Assoc 2005;45:63–72.

[84] Zhao L, Mason NA, Morrell NW, et al. Sildenafil inhibits hypoxia-induced pulmonary hypertension. Circulation 2001;104:424–8.

[85] Michelakis E, Tymchak W, Lien D, et al. Oral sildenafil is an effective and specific pulmonary vasodilator in patients with pulmonary arterial hypertension: comparison with inhaled nitric oxide. Circulation 2002;105:2398–403.

[86] Lepore JJ, Maroo A, Pereira NL, et al. Effect of sildenafil on the acute pulmonary vasodilator response to inhaled nitric oxide in adults with primary pulmonary hypertension. Am J Cardiol 2002;90:677–80.

[87] Kleinsasser A, Loeckinger A. Sildenafil for lung fibrosis and pulmonary hypertension. Lancet 2003; 361:262–3.

[88] Ghofrani HA, Wiedemann R, Rose F, et al. Combination therapy with oral sildenafil and inhaled iloprost for severe pulmonary hypertension. Ann Intern Med 2002;136:515–22.

[89] Zhang R, Wang Y, Zhang L, et al. Sildenafil (Viagra) induces neurogenesis and promotes functional recovery after stroke in rats. Stroke 2002;33: 2675–80.

[90] Zhang L, Zhang RL, Wang Y, et al. Functional recovery in aged and young rats after embolic stroke. Treatment with a phosphodiesterase type 5 inhibitor. Stroke 2005;36(4):847–52.

[91] Takimoto E, Champion HC, Li M, et al. Chronic inhibition of cyclic GMP phosphodiesterase 5A prevents and reverses cardiac hypertrophy. Nat Med 2005;11:214–22.

[92] Bortolotti M, Mari C, Lopilato C, et al. Effects of sildenafil on esophageal motility of patients with idiopathic achalasia. Gastroenterology 2000;118:253–7.

[93] Rosenkranz S, Caglayan E, Diet F, et al. Long-term effects of sildenafil in a patient with scleroderma-associated pulmonary hypertension and Raynaud's syndrome. Dtsch Med Wochenschr 2004;129: 1736–40.

ELSEVIER
SAUNDERS

Urol Clin N Am 32 (2005) 431–445

UROLOGIC
CLINICS
of North America

Psychosocial Evaluation and Combination Treatment of Men with Erectile Dysfunction

Michael A. Perelman, PhD

The New York Presbyterian Hospital, Weill Medical College of Cornell University, 70 East 77th Street, Suite 1C, New York, NY 10021, USA

From the perspective of the new millennium, it is clear that both organic and psychosocial factors play a role in the etiology of sexual function and dysfunction (SD), and consequently in the diagnosis and treatment of erectile dysfunction (ED). There are omnipresent psychogenic components existing in most potency problems regardless of the degree of organicity. Clinical experience demonstrates that anxiety can severely complicate the presenting picture of even a mild organic deficit, quickly escalating it into a complete and seemingly total dysfunction. The degree of manifest dysfunction frequently exceeds the degree of organic impairment even in "organically impotent" men. Despite the existence of organic pathogenesis, ED has always had a psychogenic component—even if the ED was initially the result of constitution, illness, surgery, or other treatment [1]. Yet our treatments for ED are overwhelmingly medical.

Approximately 90% of men who seek assistance for ED are treated with phosphodiesterase-5s (PDE-5s) [2]. Generally, PDE-5 inhibitors are safe and highly effective, restoring erections in approximately 70% of men. Yet there is a growing body of evidence suggesting that the frequently quoted 20% to 50% dropout rate for medical treatments is true for PDE-5 treatment as well [2]. Why? The adverse event profile is excellent for all three Food & Drug Administration (FDA)-approved PDE-5s, with few patients terminating treatment because of them. Some tried the medications out of curiosity and never intended to continue using a PDE-5. Others will discontinue PDE-5 use, because of the severity of their ED. For these individuals, the pharmaceuticals simply do not work. Regardless of the mode of administration, a certain percentage of the population will not experience restored capacity, because the degree of organicity is so profound as to overwhelm the salutary effects of the drug. In particular, some diabetics and radical prostatectomy survivors may need more powerful medical or surgical treatments, per the level two and three recommendations of the Process of Care Guidelines [3].

Significantly, primary care physicians (PCPs) have now become the principal health care providers for men with a primary complaint of ED, with urologists typically seeing the more recalcitrant cases. Unfortunately, the history obtained by PCPs and urologists is frequently limited to an end-organ focus, and fails to reveal significant psychosocial barriers to successful restoration of sexual health. These obstacles or "resistance" represent an important cause of nonresponse and discontinuation of treatment [4]. These barriers manifest themselves in varying levels of complexity, which individually and/or collectively must be understood and managed for pharmaceutical treatment to be optimized [2,5,6].

Only recently have clinicians begun incorporating sex therapy concepts, and recognized that resistance to lovemaking is often emotional. Clearly, medical and surgical treatments alone are often insufficient in helping couples resume a satisfying sexual life. There are a variety of biopsychosocial obstacles to recovery that contribute to treatment complexity. All of these variables impact compliance and sex lives substantially [5]. There are multiple sources of patient

E-mail address: perelman@earthlink.net

and partner psychologic resistance that may converge to sabotage treatment. Most of these barriers to success can be managed as part of the treatment, yet too few clinicians are trained to do so [5,7]. This article will focus on identifying psychosocial issues relevant to the diagnosis and management of ED.

Combining sexual pharmaceuticals and sex therapy is the "oral therapy" of choice to optimize treatment for all SD, including men with ED. Less medication is required when you modify immediate causes while appreciating other psychologic obstacles [5]. However, combination treatment (CT) is by no means a new idea, and sexual medicine is not the first specialty using a broad-spectrum approach to increase efficacy and satisfaction. Today, mainstream psychiatry is characterized by a CT with an emerging literature demonstrating the benefit of combining both pharmacologic and psychologic treatments for a number of conditions [8–10]. In urology and many medical specialties, CT usually referred to a two or more drug regimen, such as those described in the 2003, American Urological Association guidelines for benign prostatic hyperplasia [11].

There already is a history of using CT in sexual medicine. In the 1990s, sex therapists worked with urologists combining either intracavernosal injection, intraurethral insertion, or vacuum tumescence therapy [12–16]. Multiple case reports have summarized the benefits of combining sexual pharmaceuticals with cognitive or behavioral treatments for ED [17–21]. Later articles strengthened the recommendation for a combination of medical and psychologic approaches to the treatment of erectile dysfunction [2,5,6,16,22,23].

We know clinically that many PDE-5 nonresponders can be restored to sexual health through a CT, integrating sex therapy and sexual

pharmaceuticals. Yet how do we conceptualize such a model so that standard treatment algorithms could be stretched to incorporate this concept? The answer is a schema, which captures both organic and psychosocial factors, integrated into a treatment model.

The Sexual Tipping Point™ and combination treatment

The mind and body both inhibit and excite sexual response [24], creating a unique dynamic balance, which Perelman named the Sexual Tipping Point™ (STP) [25–27]. The STP is the characteristic threshold for the expression of a sexual response for any individual, which may vary dynamically within and between individuals and any given sexual experience. There is a variable expression of this response that may be inhibited or facilitated due to a mixture of both psychogenic and organic factors. The specific threshold for the sexual response is determined by multiple factors for any given moment or circumstance, with one factor or another dominating, while others recede in importance. This concept provides the basis of a model, which provides a fuller understanding of the interface between psychosocial factors and the medical and surgical treatment of ED (Fig. 1).

Clinicians can easily apply the STP model to conceptualize CT where sex coaching and sexual pharmaceuticals are integrated into diagnosis and an efficacious treatment, which addresses physiology, psychology, and culture. At any moment in the intervention process, the clinician determines the most elegant solution, which focuses the majority of effort on fixing the predominant factor while not ignoring the others. Clinicians using the STP model can fully conceptualize ED by understanding the predisposing, precipitating, and maintaining psychosocial aspects of their patient's

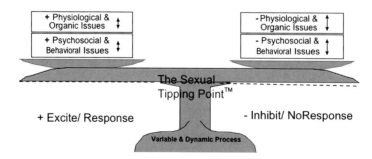

Fig. 1. The multifactorial etiology of sexual function and dysfunction. Copyright © Michael A. Perelman, PhD. All rights reserved; with permission.

diagnosis and management, as well as organic causes and risk factors.

Medicine and surgery today emphasize evidence-based research. There is a seeming inherent tension between this concept and the qualitative "art and science" of psychotherapy. This author will attempt to bridge that gap by discussing the STP and CT for erectile dysfunction, where sex-coaching strategies are integrated with sexual pharmaceuticals. Sex coaching integrates sex therapy and other psychologic techniques into office practice, improving effectiveness in treating ED. In this manner the clinician becomes informed about the psychologic forces of patient and partner resistance, which impact patient compliance and sex lives beyond organic illness and mere performance anxiety.

There is a synergy to this approach, which is not yet supported by adequate empirical evidence, but is rapidly gaining adherents, who, over time, will document its successful benefits. An excellent summary of the existing evidence for combination treatments, primarily for ED, with a few female sexual dysfunction studies, can be found in Table 10 of the WHO 2nd Consultation on Erectile and Sexual Dysfunction, Psychological and Interpersonal Dimensions of Sexual Function and Dysfunction Committee report [28]. There is a growing consensus that CT will be the treatment of choice for all SD, as new pharmaceuticals are developed for desire, arousal, and orgasm problems in both men and women [6].

This article will discuss the diagnosis and case management of ED from the perspective of the following key areas of CT: (1) nosology; (2) etiology; (3) a focused sex history using a "sex status exam"; (4) partner/couple's issues; (5) patient expectations, pharmaceutical preference, and sexual script issues; (6) follow-up strategies and the use of sexual pharmaceuticals as a "therapeutic probe" illuminating causes of failure or nonresponse; (7) "weaning" and relapse prevention; (8) referral.

Nosology and definition

The sexual response cycle can be conceptualized as having four interactive, nonlinear phases: desire, arousal, orgasm, and resolution [4,29–31]. Sexual dysfunctions are disruptions of any of these phases including the sexual pain and muscle spasm disorders [32]. Although defined independently, each SD may overlap another. ED is defined as the inability to achieve or maintain an erection adequate for satisfactory sexual performance [33]. Psychogenic ED is defined as the persistent inability to achieve or maintain an erection satisfactory for sexual performance owing predominantly or exclusively to psychologic or interpersonal factors. Epidemiologic studies have highlighted the prevalence of psychosocial factors in the etiology of erectile dysfunction, with special emphasis on self-reported depressive symptoms. In addition to the clinical subtypes of generalized versus situational, psychogenic erectile dysfunction can be characterized as life-long (primary) or acquired (secondary) [34].

Etiology

Psychogenic

Our current perspective, which emphasizes the importance of *both* organic and psychosocial factors in the etiology of ED, was not always the predominant view. For nearly a half of the twentieth century, the etiology of ED was primarily attributed to a variety of psychogenic causes. Early in the century, Freud highlighted deep-seated anxiety and internal conflict as the root of sexual problems. Then, psychodynamic theorists postulated multiple psychosocial explanations for ED, with unconscious aggression and unexpressed anger recurring as themes. Although historically suggested, there is no evidence that specific psychologic traits or styles are clearly associated with ED, although depression and anxiety disorders may manifest as sexual dysfunction. Relationship problems and other psychosocial events/stresses frequently contribute to, result from, or sometimes cause ED, and especially should be considered for men with acquired or situational ED. Specifically, pregnancy fears should be explored when the reason for professional referral was related to the female partner's wish to conceive.

By mid-century, Masters and Johnson [29,31] and then Kaplan [4] designated limited sexual knowledge, predisposing negative sexual experiences, and anxiety as the primary culprits; while providing a nod to organic factors. They catalyzed the emergence of sex therapy, which relied on cognitive and behavioral prescriptions to improve patient functioning. They and later sex therapists viewed interpersonal and relationship factors as both a cause and a consequence of ED for many couples. For the next 2 decades, a psychologic sensibility dominated discussions of the causes and cures of SD.

Many psychologic theories included anxiety as an important component, and anxiety does play a definite role in ED. Bancroft described a delicate balance between central excitatory and inhibiting mechanisms adding greater understanding of the role of anxiety and other psychogenic factors in ED [24]. Several investigators and clinicians have described how anxiety's role in initiating or maintaining sexual arousal difficulties are frequently mediated by cognition. Alterations in perceptual and attentional processes can directly result in erectile variation [34,35]. In addition, performance anxiety may lead a man to engage in behaviors such as "spectatoring" during intercourse, which focuses attention away from arousing stimulus and instead on negative cognitions, and consequently has a dampening effect on erectile capacity and response [31].

Organic

Despite the large literature suggesting a variety of psychogenic etiologies, there is also significant evidence of organic determinants of variability in male erectile response. During the late 1980s, along with increased diagnostic sophistication, there was a progressive shift toward surgical and predominantly pharmaceutical treatments for ED. By the 1990s, urologists had established hegemony with the successful marketing of various penile prostheses, as well as intracavernosal injection and intraurethral insertion systems. The monumentally successful 1998 Sildenafil launch (Pfizer, New York, New York) and its subsequent publicity at the end of the twentieth century, symbolized the apex of biologic determinism. Most clinicians and most of the general public saw ED and its treatment solely in organic terms.

Mixed

The new millennium finds us embracing a more enlightened and sophisticated "mixed" paradigm where the importance of both organic and psychogenic factors are appreciated for their role in predisposing, precipitating, maintaining, and reversing SD. This rebalancing of perspective reflected a growing consensus of thought, catalyzed by mental health professionals (MHPs) [5,17,36,37]. These MHPs have successfully advanced the obvious concept once again: psychosocial factors are also critical to the understanding of sexual function and dysfunction. Sexual pharmaceuticals are highly efficacious, and can very frequently restore sexual capacity, but rewarding sexual function is only experienced when psychosocial factors also support restored sexual activity.

ED, like other sexual dysfunctions, is best understood as being caused by an interaction of organic and psychogenic factors. There is a strong likelihood of biologic variability in the arousal threshold. Although the exact nature of a biologic predisposition is not known, it is reasonable to conclude that the "threshold" for erectile onset and latency may have a distribution curve like numerous other human variables. This view is similar to theories regarding biologically predisposed thresholds for ejaculation described by Perelman [19] and Waldinger [38,39]. Determining whether the exact physiologic mechanism(s) of such a "threshold" are central, peripheral, or some combination, requires further research. However, this pattern of susceptibility presumably interacts with a variety of sexual circumstances and intra- and interpersonal dynamics, in addition to environmental and medical risk factors, resulting in a manifest dysfunction. One can easily hypothesize that normal variation in the function of the nervous systems could result in a somatically determined variation in both men and women's desire, arousal, and orgasm response, in terms of onset, latency, capacity, and so on.

Finally, a biologic set point for erectile latency is affected by multiple organic and psychogenic factors in varying combinations over the course of a man's life cycle. The assessment process required to appreciate each of these factors determines the endpoint dysfunction for a particular individual, at a particular moment in time, as illustrated by using the STP model. Each man has a variably expressed erectile threshold or erectile tipping point (ETP). It is presumed that the ETP may be inhibited or facilitated due to a mixture of both psychosocial and organic factors. The specific threshold for erection is determined by multiple factors for any given moment or circumstance, with one factor or another dominating, as others become less important. We then have a useful heuristic device to describe the variety of vectors impacting both normal erections and ED. Here again, the ETP model can be used to illustrate CT, where sex coaching and sexual pharmaceuticals are integrated together to provide the most elegant solution for the treatment of ED (Fig. 2).

Evaluation and diagnosis

History taking

Obviously, the clinician must determine whether the patient has an illness or is taking a drug that

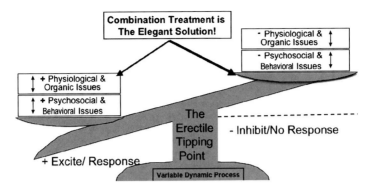

Fig. 2. Combination treatment optimizes response: integrating sex therapy and sex pharmaceuticals. Copyright © Michael A. Perelman, PhD. All rights reserved; with permission.

could be causing the symptom. However, this article presumes the necessary assessment steps and procedures, including physical examination, as well as laboratory tests, have been conducted in a manner consistent with the parameters recommended elsewhere in this volume. Here, the focus is on the psychosocial balance to the equation. However, the clinician should not arbitrarily separate the psychosocial/sexual history from the medical history. An integrated medical and sexual history yields a significant amount of information regarding all aspects of a man's sexual health and relationships.

A focused sex history or "sex status" rapidly identifies the numerous maintaining causes of sexual dysfunction (eg, insufficient stimulation, depression) and points toward predisposing and precipitating factors. It provides a broad understanding of the current sexual experience within the context of a man's life. The ideal history is an integrated, fluid assessment, where the patient's response is continuously reevaluated during follow-up. Assessing response to the initial pharmaceutical and behavioral prescriptions, which function as a therapeutic probe, is a critical component of the psychosocial evaluation process.

The successful treatment of ED requires a specific data set that provides answers to three key questions regarding diagnosis, etiology, and treatment:

a) Does the patient really have a sexual disorder, and what is the differential diagnosis?
b) What are the underlying organic or psychosocial factors?

1. What are the organic factors?
2. What are the "immediate" maintaining psychosocial causes (eg, current cognitions, emotions, and behaviors)?
3. What are potential "deeper" psychosocial causes (predisposing, precipitating)?

c) Should the patient be treated or not? Does the severity of the underlying organic and psychosocial factors require direct treatment, or can treatment of these factors be bypassed or concurrent? These decisions are dynamic, and should be consistently reevaluated as treatment proceeds [40].

The methodology used to answer these questions is a focused sexual history. Once this method is mastered, all initial necessary data can be captured in <10 minutes, even if additional consultations or a later referral is required. The clinician should obtain the necessary information to answer the above three questions in a manner that does not sabotage the relationship with the patient. Treatment for the ED should be started as soon as possible, with reevaluations of the patient's responses occurring as treatment proceeds. A fuller comprehension of psychosocial issues optimizes patient response and minimizes relapse potential.

This method suggests a rapid assessment of the immediate and remote causes of sexual dysfunction, using the previously mentioned four-phase model of human sexual response (ie, desire, excitement, orgasm, and resolution). The primary goal of the evaluation visit is to obtain the necessary information to assess the nature of the ED and to begin developing a treatment plan. However, empathy and rapport with the patient must never be sacrificed in the service of obtaining the critical details. Rapport is strengthened if the patient is asked direct questions in a comfortable, reassuring, empathic manner. Both patient and clinician will obtain an understanding of the problem resulting in a mutually derived treatment plan. The therapeutic context works best when it is humanistic, emphasizing good communication and mutual respect.

Numerous continuing medical education programs have addressed the problem of encouraging clinicians to both initiate and discuss sexual issues by emphasizing the importance of sexual dysfunction as a biologic marker of disease, among other reasons. Clinicians must use a direct approach with the inquiry initiated in a neutral manner, using nonjudgmental screening questions. Inquire directly about any change in the patient's sexual experience and his beliefs regarding the cause of those changes [41,42]. His story should be allowed to unfold in the available time. He should be carefully guided with a short list of predetermined questions, yet the clinician must be mindful about interrupting in the middle of the patient's explanation.

Although most patients are eager to "tell their story" to an accessible knowledgeable clinician, others may be ambivalent about discussing details. This anxiety must be appreciated even as the clinician proceeds. Reciprocally, the interviewing must be conducted at the clinician's comfort level. While pursuing an analysis of sexual behavior, it is essential that the clinician monitor their own comfort, to instill confidence and facilitate openness on the patient's part.

The format for both evaluation and treatment may vary, as patients may be single or coupled. Whether single or coupled, most patients visiting a clinician are likely to be seen alone [5]. When time permits, the clinician should encourage partner attendance with committed couples, allowing assessment and counseling for both. However, the issue should not be forced. Treatment format is a therapeutic issue, and rapport should never be sabotaged. Although conjoint consultation is a good policy, it is not always the right choice or a practical one. A man in a new dating relationship is probably better off seeing the clinician alone, than stressing a new relationship by insisting on a conjoint visit. The reality and cost/benefit of partner participation is a legitimate issue for both the couple and the clinician, and not always a manifestation of resistance. Furthermore, sometimes there is no partner; sometimes the current sexual partner is not the spouse, raising legal, social, and moral sequelae.

Finally, the patient's desire for his partner's attendance may be mitigated by a variety of intrapsychic and interpersonal factors, which, *at least initially, should be respected and heeded.*

The clinician's challenge is not necessarily requiring an office visit with the partner, as many continuing medical education programs have advocated. Although important information can be obtained from the partner's perception of the problem, partner cooperation is more important than partner attendance in the evaluation and treatment of ED [5,43]. Sex pharmaceuticals plus sex counseling and education work for many people, if the partner was cooperative in the first place. Importantly, many women were cooperating with their partners, or facilitating sexual activity even independently of their knowledge of the use of a sexual aid or pharmaceutical. In other words, serendipitous matching of sexual pharmaceutical and previous sexual script equaled success: "we did, what we used to do, and it worked" [5,6]. This important issue of treatment format is reexamined during the discussion of follow-up.

The sexual status examination or "sex status" examination

The sex status examination is the single most important diagnostic tool at the clinician's disposal, and is most consistent with the "review of systems" common to all aspects of medicine [5,32]. A focused sex status critically assists in understanding and identifying the immediate cause of the ED (ie, the actual behavior or cognition causing or contributing to the sexual disorder). The sex status focuses on finding potential physical and specific psychosocial factors relating to the disorder. A description of the sexual symptom, the history of the sexual symptom, must all be pursued in detail. All patients who are being evaluated for sexual difficulties should be briefly screened for psychopathology. However, this does not need to be pursued in depth unless there is evidence of a significant emotional disorder.

The clinician should obtain a clear and detailed description of the patient's sexual symptoms, as well as information about the onset and progression of symptoms. The details of the physical and emotional circumstances surrounding the onset of a difficulty are important for the assessment of both physical and psychologic causes. The clinician must elicit these details, if not spontaneously offered. Both sex therapists and clinicians juxtapose detailed questions about the patient's current and past sexual history, unveiling an understanding of the causes of dysfunction and noncompliance.

A detailed description of the patient's current sexual experience and an analysis of his sexual behavior and of the couple's erotic interaction can help rule out organic causes. Furthermore, the sexual information evoked in history-taking will help anticipate noncompliance with medical and surgical interventions. Modifying immediate psychologic factors may result in less medication being needed, regardless of the specific SD. In general, clinicians will intervene with pharmacotherapy and brief sex coaching, which address immediate causes (eg, insufficient stimulation) directly and intermediate issues (eg, partner issues) indirectly, and will rarely focus on deeper issues (eg, sex abuse). In fact, when deeper psychosocial issues are the primary obstacles, it is usually time for referral [6].

It is particularly useful for the clinician when initiating the discussion of sex with the patient to obtain a description of a recent experience which incorporates the sexual symptom. One question that will help pin down many of the immediate and remote causes is, "Tell me about your last sexual experience." Common immediate causes of ED will be quickly evoked by the patient's response. There are several frequently identified contributors to ED, including insufficient stimulation (eg, a lack of adequate friction), a lack of subjective feelings of arousal, fatigue, and negative thinking [44]. Sex is fantasy and friction, mediated by frequency [5]. To function sexually, men need sexy thoughts, not only adequate friction. Although fatigue is a common cause of SD in our culture, negative thinking/antifantasy, whether a reflection of performance anxiety or partner anger, is also a significant contributor.

Usually the clinician obtains the last sexual experience within the context of assessing, if this is a typical experience. What are the differences between this experience and those with other partners is a question that can be asked of almost any man. He may be conservative and presume the clinician is referencing only premarital comparisons; while for many single and some married men a current comparison will be made, which will inform the clinician of numerous etiologic issues. Although sex therapists assess the pattern and quality of the man's romantic relationships, urologists will typically obtain only a brief status of the current relationship.

The clinician follows up with focused, open-ended questions to obtain a mental "video picture." Inquiries are made about desire, fantasy, frequency of sex, and effects of drugs and alcohol. Did arousal vary during manual, oral, and coital stimulation? What is the masturbation style, technique, and frequency? Idiosyncratic masturbation is a frequent hidden cause of ED, as well as retarded ejaculation [45–47]. When possible, the clinician should ascertain the patient's thoughts during various types of sexual behavior. The following questions can be helpful: When does antisexual thinking emerge? Is the patient anxious about sexual failure early in the day before sex is even on the horizon? Does he worry that he "getting too soft" and "pull out" even though he has not "fallen out." What is the content of his negative thinking? Is there a fear of negative partner reaction and worry over what his partner thinks. Is he judging himself negatively? The mind is capable of derailing normal sexual arousal as well as interfering with the restorative benefit of current and future sexual pharmaceuticals. Understanding cognition can be key to facilitating sexual recovery and satisfaction. Although usually not pursued in depth by urologists, discovering why a man has intrusive thoughts that interfere with his sexual functioning is an issue of great interest to sex therapists.

Which psychosocial factors are currently maintaining the psychic structure that results in the distracted thoughts and implicitly/explicitly reduces sexual arousal? It is interesting to understand what predisposed the patient to have that type of distressing thought and to know his full psychosocial history. However, it is only critical to know and understand the current psychosocial obstacles (PSOs) that are maintaining the dysfunctional process. Often, listening will provide answers to these questions before they even need to be asked out loud. When not spontaneously articulated by the patient, inquiries should be made, guided by clinical judgment and sensitivity.

Exploring other psychosocial issues

It is not necessary to do an exhaustive sexual and family history for most evaluations. The investigation of these issues should be selective so that the interview does not become unnecessarily lengthy. The patient's description will probably indicate whether he experiences the difficulty at all times or only under certain circumstances. However, a fluctuating pattern does not necessarily discriminate between psychogenic and organic etiology. In cases of a secondary problem, the clinician will hear of an important change from function to dysfunction. Was the change preceded by, or concurrent with, major life stress, (eg, loss of a job)? The patient may guide the clinician to the specific cause, or the clinician may need to examine the time period of the sexual change for clues to causation. The clinician should examine any of the areas known to possibly alter sexual function from the point of view of psychosocial stress, including, but not limited to, health, family, and work. Again, all does not have to be accomplished in the first visit.

Sometimes the patient will be able to tell the clinician the cause of change. The guideline is frequently, "interview the crisis." The clinician should not only get a clear picture of the current situation, but also obtain a full understanding of exactly what occurred and the patient's response to the change. Yet, it is also informative to assess if the ED was slowly progressing with age, rather than an acute shift in capacity. It is equally important to ascertain why the patient is seeking assistance at that moment in time.

Sometimes the patient will provide too much detail regarding background information, which is tangentially relevant, but not primary. In this situation the clinician should gently interrupt, acknowledging the potential importance of the patient's statement, and move the interview forward. For instance, the clinician could say, "That's very interesting, but I wonder if we might postpone those details. I'd like to come back to that, but today I need a broader understanding of your problem." Alternatively, "That's helpful, but what happened next"? The goal should be to establish and maintain rapport while gathering the relevant details.

Previous treatment approaches

Depending on the particular patient, the discussion of last sexual experience and an elaboration on current functioning will inevitably evoke information about what previous approaches the patient has attempted. The results of earlier treatments for this condition, including herbal therapies, folk therapies, and earlier professional treatments should be assessed. Additionally, past treatment for psychiatric issues (eg, depression), early sexual experiences, developmental issues, substance use or abuse, and partner issues may be mentioned by the patient. The clinician should decide which material seems most important to

understand the sexual disorder's etiology, following the pattern that emerges naturally from the patient's description.

Psychiatric considerations

The clinician should briefly screen all patients for obvious psychopathology that would significantly interfere with the initiation of treatment for the ED. Yet, the clinician will also want to know whether psychiatric symptoms, if present, are the cause or the consequence of the sexual disorder. There is a statistically significant increase in depression for men with ED. If the patient is depressed, the severity of his depression should be clarified. Furthermore, all patients who experience major depression should be queried about suicide risk. Treatment of ED may improve mild reactive depression, while depressive symptoms might alter response to therapy of ED [48]. A clinician's history-taking must parse out the question of whether the ED is causing depression or whether the depression and its treatment (eg, selective serotonin reuptake inhibitors) is causing the ED. For a detailed discussion of pharmacology and sex, the reader is recommended to the "WHO" Sexual Medicine text [28].

When a patient with a variety of psychopathologic states (eg, stress, phobias, personality disorders) is evaluated for sexual complaints, the clinician must consider whether that patient's emotional conflicts are too severe for a focused treatment of the sexual problem, and whether such treatment should either be safely postponed for another time or occur concurrently with treatment for the emotional distress. With more severe situations the modal choice is likely to be a simultaneous initiation of the sexual dysfunction treatment along with a referral to a mental health practitioner to facilitate patient management. Yet, a person who is currently addicted to drugs or alcohol is not a suitable candidate for treatment until he has been detoxified and is off the drug. There are situations when it is appropriate to postpone treating the patient for the ED until psychotherapeutic consultation is able to assist the individual in developing a more reality-based view. Although sometimes this can be done simultaneously, other times treatment for ED must wait. More subtle personality factors, such as fragile self-esteem, anxiety, and fear of being negatively evaluated by others, are frequently prevalent in men with sexual concerns. Yet, usually this would not result in postponing treatment for the sex problem [30,40].

Family and early psychosexual history

A psychosexual and family history may provide insight into the deeper causes of the patient's problem, and may reveal cultural or neurotic origins of the problem. Significant factors from the past might include losses, traumas, negative past sexual relationships, and negative past interpersonal relationships. They may also include cultural and religious restrictions. However, unless dissuaded by the evaluation otherwise, the urologist may usually proceed with level 1 treatments [3] with confidence that rapport will preserve an opportunity for further exploration should that prove to be necessary.

Partner/relationship issues

Although sex therapists assess the pattern and quality of the man's romantic relationships, urologists typically obtain a brief status of the current relationship. For all men, clinicians should assess marital status as well as living and dating arrangements. Contextual factors, including difficulties with the current interpersonal relationship and whether the partner has a sexual dysfunction, should be clarified. The clinician may grasp the couple's interactions from the first interview's sex status. It remains to be determined if deeper difficulties in the couple's relationship determine the patient's sexual problem. Numerous partner-related nonsexual issues may also adversely impact outcome. These issues can be screened through inquiry. A reassuring, "No one's relationship is perfect; what do you both argue about"? can be helpful. Additionally, monitor the degree of acrimony when the patient describes his complaints. For example, is the anger, resentment, hurt, or sadness a maintaining or precipitating factor, or are the emotions more mild manifestations of the frustrations of daily life?

Previous sexual scripts also need assessment [49]. Several questions should be asked, including whether sexual relations were ever good with the current partner, what changed, and what the patient's view of causation is. For all men, whether or not the problem is partner-specific needs to be determined. If the problem is partner-specific, the clinician must ascertain which of several categories are etiologically relevant: inadequate sexual technique, poor communication, incompatible sexual script or fantasies, no physical attraction. Power struggles, transferences, partner psychopathology, and commitment/intimacy issues are elusive, and may have implications for the sexual

problem. Initially, all that is required is to decide if the degree of relationship strife is too severe to initiate the ED treatment. Otherwise, concurrent relationship treatment is provided or a referral is made and ED treatment is postponed. However, it will be the bias of many to err on the side of giving the relationship and ED treatment every possible chance.

The single patient

The single patient with a psychosexual dysfunction must be assessed in the same manner as if the patient was in a relationship. The patient's sexual symptom may or may not relate to difficulties in his relationships. Clinician time constraints and competencies, along with patient predilections, will determine whether the patient's single status becomes a therapeutic focus. This issue must be managed with sensitivity. Needless to say, sexual orientation issues, for both single and coupled men, require the same, if not even greater sensitivity on the clinician's part. Several treatment interventions have been described for single males with chronic erectile difficulties. Treatment strategies include sexual attitude change, assertiveness training, masturbation exercises, and social skill development, in addition to sexual pharmaceuticals and surgery all per Process of Care Guidelines [3,34].

Questionnaires

Questionnaires can be used in both training and research. In training, questionnaires provide students with a range of potentially relevant material of interest in the diagnosis and treatment of ED. In research, questionnaires allow for a standardization of both diagnostic data collection, and provide recognized consistent endpoints. A complete review of this topic may be found in the WHO Sexual Medicine text [28]. Additionally, some clinicians may choose to use current or future instruments to facilitate the history-taking process. Such instruments must be incorporated in a manner that does not interfere with rapport.

Treatment

Treatment proceeds from evaluation, but remains a dynamic process that requires constant reassessment. The sex status methodology described in the previous section is continuously used and reapplied during the treatment process. The treatments themselves will frequently be pharmaceutical with a progressive escalation regarding degree of intrusiveness, including potential surgical intervention as dictated by "Process of Care" guidelines [3] .However, there must be a continuous awareness of the intra- and interpersonal forces that may interfere or be used to enhance response to these same medical and surgical treatments. It is the essence of sex coaching to optimize pharmaceutical efficacy.

In cases of primarily psychogenic ED, Rosen [37]. summarized the following approaches as used by sex therapists: (a) anxiety reduction and desensitization, (b) cognitive-behavioral interventions, (c) increased sexual stimulation, and (d) interpersonal assertiveness and couples' communication training. Yet today, most physicians will initiate treatment with a PDE-5 regardless of etiology. This is usually the case even if the ED is primarily psychogenic in origin, given the extremely high PDE-5 efficacy rate with that population [50]. Currently, there are three highly efficacious PDE-5, FDA-approved treatments for ED: Sildenafil, Vardenafil, Tadalafil. All three PDE-5s are used worldwide. All have good success rates! Simple cases do respond well to oral agents, with proper advice on pill use, expectation management, and a cooperative sex partner. However, clinicians should offer patients choices, especially those who are pharmaceutically naïve. Providing an unbiased, fair-balanced description of treatment options, including pharmaceutical benefits based on the pharmacokinetics, efficacy studies, and the clinician's own patients' experience; will result in the patient attributing greater importance to the clinician's opinion. Incorporating patient preference provides important guidance, and will enhance healer/patient relations, minimize PSOs, and improve compliance. Anecdotal data has suggested patient preferences reflected key marketing messages of the respective pharmaceutical companies. Prescribing clinicians might take advantage of that hypothesis to increase efficacy. If safety and long-term side effects are the primary concern, Sildenafil has the oldest/longest database [51]. If, pressed by questions regarding hardness of erection; in vitro selectivity may or may not translate to clinical reality, yet some patients believe Vardenafil provides, the best quality erection with the least side effect [52]. Tadalafil will provide the longest duration of action [53]. What is the clinician's experience with their own patients?

The focused sexual history creates awareness of the patient's sexual script and expectations, leading to more precise and improved recommendations and management [5]. For instance, a clinician would improve outcome by briefly clarifying whether a patient was better off practicing with masturbation, or reintroducing sex with a partner. A recently divorced man, who was using condoms for the first time in years, was probably better off masturbating with a condom rather than attempting sex with his partner, the first time he tried a new sex pharmaceutical.

Knowledge of pharmacokinetics (onset, duration of action, and so on) plus sexual script analysis helps optimize treatment, by improving probability of initially selecting the right prescription. Understanding the couples "sexual script" can help the clinician fine tune pharmaceutical selection, leading to better orgasm and sexual satisfaction, not merely improved erection [6]. Sexual script in this situation refers to style and process of the couple's premorbid sex life [49]. For those fortunate enough to have had a good premorbid sex life, dosing instructions should focus on returning to previously successful sexual scripts—as if medication was not a necessary part of the process. This maximizes patient likelihood of getting adequate stimulation in a manner likely to be comfortable and conducive to partner sensitivities. Awareness of within individual differences improves the quality of recommendations made for that person or couple's sexual recovery. Between individual differences in sexual style (sex script analysis), can determine which medication might be used by a couple effectively, with less change required in their "normal" sexual interactions. For instance, some couples mutually presume that the man is "in charge," and that he should initiate and seduce. Because he is planning the sexual encounter, Sildenafil or Vardenafil might be good choices. However, predosing with Tadalafil might be preferable if a response to an externally evoked situation (partner) over an extended time is desired. Fitting the right medication based on pharmacokinetics to the individual/couple will increase efficacy, satisfaction, compliance, and improve continuation rates. Rather than changing the couples' sexual style to fit the treatment, try to fit the right medication to the couple [6].

Follow-up and therapeutic probe

Discussions of follow-up most vividly illustrate the importance of integrating sex therapy and pharmacotherapy. Urologists Barada and

Hatzichristou improved Sildenafil nonresponders by emphasizing patient education (eg, food/alcohol effect), repeat dosing, partner involvement and follow-up [54,55]. Patient education about the proper use of sildenafil was crucial to treatment effectiveness. Clinicians can increase their success by scheduling follow-up the day they first prescribe. As with any therapy, follow-up is essential to ensure an optimal treatment outcome. Initial failures examined at follow-up reveal critical information. The pharmaceutical acts as a therapeutic probe, illuminating the causes of failure or nonresponse [2,4–6].

Retaking a quick current "sex status" provides a convenient model for managing follow-up. Other components of the follow-up visit include monitoring side effects, assessing success, and considering whether an alteration in dose or treatment is needed. Future comparator trials will help determine which drug works best, for which person(s), under which context. Until then, clinicians will likely trust their own judgment and experience. However, clinicians must provide ongoing education to patients and their partners, as well as involving them in treatment decisions whenever possible. Because nonerotic thoughts are such a frequent cause of nonresponse, encouraging immersion in the sexual experience through fantasy is helpful to eroticize both the experience and the partner. However, fantasy could be about anything erotic; masturbatory fantasies are usually quite effective. Fantasy of an earlier time with the current partner may be especially helpful for those who feel guilty about fantasizing in their own partner's presence.

A continuing dialog with patients is critical to facilitate success and prevent relapse. The numerous psychosocial issues previously discussed, may evoke noncompliance. These are important issues in differentiating treatment nonresponders from "biochemical failures," in order to enhance success rates. Early failures can be reframed into learning experiences and eventual success.

Partner cooperation must be anticipated pretreatment, and follow-up provides opportunity to confirm whether or not such cooperation is present. If cooperation is not present, the recognition of a need for contact with the partner should increase. If the partner's support for successful resolution of the ED is not present, then active steps must be taken to evoke it. When evaluation or follow-up reveals significant relationship issues, counseling the individual alone may help, but interacting with the partner will

often increase success rates. If the partner refuses to attend, or the patient is unwilling or reluctant to encourage them, seek contact with the partner by telephone. Ask to be called, or for permission to call the partner. Most partners find it difficult to resist speaking "just once," about "potential goals" or "what's wrong with their spouse." The contact provides opportunity for empathy and potential engagement in the treatment process, which may minimize resistance and improve outcome further. This effective approach could be modified depending on the clinician's interest and time constraints. Clinicians should counsel partners when necessary and possible. Although some partners will require direct professional intervention, many others could benefit from obtaining critical information from the ED patient or multiple media formats both private and public. Other times a referral for adjunctive treatment to a sex therapist for the partner may be required. It is likely that the more problematic the relationship, the less likely that patient–partner sex education will be able to successfully augment treatment in and of itself. Inevitably, a mental health referral would be required, albeit not necessarily accepted [5,6,25].

Weaning and relapse prevention

In general, the concept of relapse prevention has not been incorporated into sexual medicine. Yet ED is recognized as a progressive disease in terms of underlying organic pathology, which may play a role in altering threshold for response and potential reemergence of dysfunction. Both McCarthy and Perelman have recommended that the clinician schedule "booster" or follow-up sessions to help the patient stay the course and provide opportunity for additional treatment when necessary [5,6,56]. These concepts are derivative of an "addiction" treatment model where intermittent, but continuous care is the treatment of choice. Additionally, using sex therapy concepts in combination with sexual pharmaceuticals offers potential for minimizing dose and temporary or permanent weaning from medication depending on severity of organic and psychosocial factors. SDs are frequently progressive diseases, but this is especially true for ED. Over time the progressive exacerbation of either organic factors (endothelial disease, and so on) or PSOs may adversely impact a previously successful treatment regimen. Furthermore, although there is no current evidence for tachyphylaxis, neither are there extensive studies beyond 10 years indicating long-term efficacy of PDE-5s. No doubt escalating dose and providing alternative medications would be most clinicians' initial response of choice. However, both these processes may be modulated and mediated by sexual counseling and education. Sex therapy and other cognitive behavioral techniques and strategies could be extremely important in facilitating long-term medication maintenance, and helping to ensure continuing medication success [6].

Combination therapy: who, and when?

There are two alternative models for combination therapy: both will likely be adopted within the framework of sexual medicine, by different clinicians. First, working alone, PCPs and urologists will integrate sex counseling with their sexual pharmaceutical armamentarium to treat sexual dysfunction. In a second model, the above clinicians will collaborate with sex therapists through a coordinated multidisciplinary team approach to treatment. The clinical combinations will vary according to the presenting symptoms, as well as the varying expertise of these health care providers. The use of these two different models will require three steps. (1) The clinician first consulted by the patient will consider his/her interest, training, and competence. (2) The biopsychosocial severity and complexity of the sexual dysfunction, as a manifestation of both psychosocial and organic factors will be evaluated. (3) The clinician in consideration of the two previous criteria, together with patient preference, will determine who initiates treatment, as well as how and when to refer. The guidelines for managing the dysfunction will essentially be expanded (depending on severity), but continue to match the type of treatment algorithm described in "The Process of Care" and other step-change approaches [3].

Whether or not a clinician works alone, as in the first model, or as part of a multidisciplinary team, as in the second, will be partially determined by the psychosocial complexity of the case [2,6,28]. The treating clinician would diagnose the patient(s) as suffering from mild, moderate, or severe PSOs to successful restoration of sexual function and satisfaction. These three PSO categories would be defined as follows: (1) mild PSOs: no significant or mild obstacles to successful medical treatment; (2) moderate PSOs: some significant obstacles to successful medical treatment; (3) severe PSOs: substantial to overwhelming obstacles to successful medical treatment [6]. This characterization would be based on an assessment of all the available information obtained during the evaluation. This would be a dynamic diagnosis, continuously reevaluated as treatment progressed. The consulted clinician would continue treatment or make referrals based on progress obtained. The matrix determining who might treat is presented in Table 1.

Clearly, a multidisciplinary team including multiple medical specialists and a sex therapist could attempt to treat almost every case. However, a team is a very labor-intensive approach and frequently unrealistic, both economically and geographically in terms of available expertise and manpower. However, in the first two cells, which reflect common scenarios in clinical practice, a clinician who first evaluates a patient suffering from ED could integrate sex counseling with their sexual pharmaceuticals, often resulting in a successful outcome. Clinician difficulty with either moderate or severe psychosocial complexity would lead to appropriate referral and presumably the use of the multidisciplinary team model [6].

Referral

The clinician's "time crunch" can be managed, when coaching combined with a sexual pharmaceutical is sufficient for treatment success. If the partner's support for successful resolution of the ED is not present, then active steps must be taken to evoke it. Sometimes a conjoint referral for adjunctive treatment to a sex therapist for the partner may also be required [5]. Of course, the more problematic the relationship, the more profound the marital strife, the less likely that patient–partner sex education will be able to successfully augment treatment in and of itself. Inevitably, a referral to a MHP would be required,

Table 1
ED management guidelines based on PSO severity

	Mild PSOs	Moderate PSOs	Severe PSOs
Clinician sex coach	Frequently	Sometimes	Rarely
Multidisciplinary team	Frequently	Frequently	Frequently

Abbreviation: PSOs, Psychosocial obstacles. Copyright © Michael A. Perelman, PhD; adapted with permission.

albeit not necessarily accepted successfully. Additionally, there are numerous organically determined reasons making referral to a multiplicity of medical specialists (gynecologists, neurologists, psychopharmacologists, endocrinologists, and so on) necessary and appropriate [6].

Does a multidimensional understanding of ED always require a multidisciplinary team approach? Clearly, the answer is no. What is needed by the clinician is a viewpoint consistent with the biopsychosocial consensus initially reflected by the "Process of Care Guidelines," and elaborated upon in the published Proceedings of the WHO 2nd International Consultation on Erectile and Sexual Dysfunction [3,28]. These publications are the result of multidisciplinary cooperation, with collaborative knowledge being appreciated, independent of specialty of origin. These consensus reports speak to the importance of integrating medical, surgical, and psychosocial treatments for ED [3,5,28].

Treatment may require a multidisciplinary team in cases of severe dysfunction, and yet be recalcitrant to success even under this circumstance. There are many models for working together. Team approaches and composition will vary according to clinician specialty training, interest, and geographic resources. Although some expert clinicians work alone, other PCPs, urologists, and gynecologists have set up "in-house" multidisciplinary teams where nurses, clinician associates, and master's level MHPs provide the sex counseling [57]. This approach has obvious advantages and disadvantages. In cases of more severe PSOs, the patient(s) will be "referred out" for psychopharmacology, cognitive-behavioral therapy, and marital therapy in various permutations, provided by doctoral level MHPs. However, typically a clinician refers within his or her own academic institution, or within their own professional referral network—a kind of "virtual" multidisciplinary team. Referrals for the patient or partner may be required, and would usually be readily available. Identifying psychologic factors does not necessarily mean all clinicians must treat them. Clinicians not inclined to counsel, or uncomfortable, should consider referring or working conjointly with a sex therapist. All clinicians should be encouraged to practice to their own comfort level. Indeed, some PCPs and urologists will not have the expertise to adequately diagnose PSOs, independent of their ability or willingness to treat these factors. Awareness of their own limitations will appropriately prompt these clinicians to refer their patients for adjunctive consultation. Some clinicians are uncomfortable discussing sex, and many important issues remain unexplored because of clinician anxiety and time constraints. Whether the referral is clinician or patient initiated, sex therapists are ready to effectively assist in educating the patient about maximizing their response to the sexual situation. Additionally, they can help patients adjust to "second- and third-line" interventions such as injection and penile prosthesis.

Summary

Sexuality is a complex interaction of biology, culture, developmental, and current intra- and interpersonal psychology. A biopsychosocial model of sexual dysfunction provides a compelling argument for a combination treatment that integrates sex therapy and sexual pharmaceuticals. Although more research is needed, it seems probable to this author that combination therapy will be the treatment of choice for all SD, as new pharmaceuticals are developed for desire, arousal, and orgasm problems in both men and women [5,6,40,45]. The sex status or focused sex history, and continuous reassessment based on follow-up are the foundations of this approach. Restoration of lasting and satisfying sexual function requires a multidimensional understanding of all of the forces that created the problem, whether a solo clinician or multidisciplinary team approach is used. Each clinician needs to carefully evaluate their own competence and interests when considering the treatment of a man's ED, so that regardless of the modality used, the patient receives optimized care. Frequently, neither sex therapy nor medical/surgical interventions alone are sufficient to facilitate lasting improvement and satisfaction for a patient or partner suffering from ED. This author is optimistic for a future that uses combination therapy, integrating sex therapy and new medical and surgical treatments to restore sexual function and satisfaction.

References

[1] Perelman MA. Rehabilitative sex therapy for organic impotence. In: Segraves T, Haeberle E, editors. Emerging dimensions of sexology. New York: Praeger Publications; 1984.

[2] Althof SE. Therapeutic weaving: the integration of treatment techniques. In: Levine SB, editor. Handbook of clinical sexuality for mental health professionals. New York: Brunner-Routledge; 2003. p. 359–76.

[3] Rosen RC, et al. The process of care model for evaluation and treatment of erectile dysfunction. The Process of Care Consensus Panel. Int J Impot Res 1999;11:59–70 [discussion 70–4].

[4] Kaplan HS. The new sex therapy. New York: Brunner/Mazel; 1974.

[5] Perelman MA. Sex coaching for physicians: combination treatment for patient and partner. Int J Impot Res 2003;15(Suppl 5):S67–74.

[6] Perelman MA. Combination therapy for sexual dysfunction: integrating sex therapy and pharmacotherapy. In: Balon R, Segraves RT, editors. Handbook of sexual dysfunction. London: Taylor & Francis; 2005. p. 13–41.

[7] Althof SE. When an erection alone is not enough: biopsychosocial obstacles to lovemaking. Int J Impot Res 2002;14(Suppl 1):S99–S104.

[8] Keller MB, McCullough JP, Klein DN, et al. A comparison of nefazodone, the cognitive behavioral-analysis system of psychotherapy, and their combination for the treatment of chronic depression. N Engl J Med 2000;342:1462–70.

[9] Seligman ME. The effectiveness of psychotherapy. The Consumer Reports study. Am Psychol 1995; 50:965–74.

[10] Nathan PE, Gorman JM. A guide to treatments that work. New York: Oxford University Press; 1998.

[11] Committee AUAPG. AUA guideline on management of benign prostate hyperplasia (2003). Chapter 1: diagnosis and treatment recommendations. J Urol 2003;170:530–47.

[12] Turner LA, Althof SE, Levine SB, et al. Self-injection of papaverine and phentolamine in the treatment of psychogenic impotence. J Sex Marital Ther 1989;15:163–76.

[13] Hartmann U, Langer D. Combination of psychosexual therapy and intra-penile injections in the treatment of erectile dysfunctions: rationale and predictors of outcome. J Sex Educ Ther 1993;19: 1–12.

[14] Colson MH. Intracavernous injections and overall treatment of erectile disorders: a retrospective study. Sexologies 1996;5:11–24.

[15] Lottman PE, Hendriks JC, Vruggink PA, et al. The impact of marital satisfaction and psychological counselling on the outcome of ICI-treatment in men with ED. Int J Impot Res 1998;10: 83–7.

[16] Wylie KR, Jones RH, Walters S. The potential benefit of vacuum devices augmenting psychosexual therapy for erectile dysfunction: a randomized controlled trial. J Sex Marital Ther 2003;29: 227–36.

[17] McCarthy BW. Integrating sildenafil into cognitive-behavioral couples sex therapy. J Sex Educ Ther 1998;23:302–8.

[18] Segraves RT. Two additional uses for sildenafil in psychiatric patients. J Sex Marital Ther 1999;25: 265–6.

[19] Perelman MA. Integrating sildenafil and sex therapy: unconsummated marriage secondary to ED and RE. J Sex Educ Ther 2001;26:13–21.

[20] Perelman MA. FSD partner issues: expanding sex therapy with sildenafil. J Sex Marital Ther 2002; 28(Suppl 1):195–204.

[21] Leiblum S, Pervin L, Cambell E. The treatment of vaginismus: success and failure. In: Leiblum SR, Rosen RC, editors. Principles and practice of sex therapy: update for the 1990s. New York: Guilford Press; 1989. p. 113–40.

[22] Hawton K. Integration of treatments for male erectile dysfunction. Lancet 1998;351:7–8.

[23] Rosen RC. Medical and psychological interventions for erectile dysfunction: toward a combined treatment approach. In: Leiblum SR, Rosen RC, editors. Principles and practice of sex therapy. New York: Guilford Press; 2000.

[24] Bancroft J. Central inhibition of sexual response in the male: a theoretical perspective. Neurosci Biobehav Rev 1999;23:763–84.

[25] Perelman MA. Integration of sex therapy and pharmacological therapy in FSD. Invited Presentation to the Female Sexual Dysfunction 2005: A Multidisciplinary Update on Female Sexual Dysfunction Conference, Columbia University Department of Urology. Columbia University Medical Center, New York, New York, April 23, 2005.

[26] Perelman MA. Prevalence, definition, etiology and diagnosis of premature ejaculation. Invited Presentation to the Male Sexual Dysfunction and Men's Health Conference, Columbia University Department of Urology, Columbia University Medical Center, New York, New York, June 4, 2005.

[27] Perelman MA. AUA Poster, Abstract 1254: Idiosyncratic masturbation patterns: a key unexplored variable in the treatment of retarded ejaculation by the practicing urologist. 2005. Available at: http://www.posters2view.com/aua/lookup_view.php?word=Perelman&where=authors&return=%2Faua%2Fauthorindex.php%3Fnum%3D15.

[28] Lue TF, Basson R, Rosen R, et al. Sexual medicine: sexual dysfunctions in men and women. Paris: Health Publications; 2004.

[29] Masters WH, Johnson VE. Human sexual response. Boston: Little, Brown & Co.; 1966.

[30] Kaplan HS. The evaluation of sexual disorders: psychologic and medical aspects. New York: Brunner/Mazel; 1995.

[31] Masters WH, Johnson VE. Human sexual inadequacy. Boston: Little, Brown, & Co.; 1970.

[32] Kaplan HS, Perelman MA. The physician and the treatment of sexual dysfunction. In: Usdin G, Lewis J, editors. Psychiatry in general medical practice. New York: McGraw-Hill; 1979.

[33] Consensus development conference statement. National Institutes of Health. Impotence. December 7–9, 1992. Int J Impot Res 1993;5:181–284.

[34] Rosen RC. Psychogenic erectile dysfunction: classification and management. In: Lue TF, editor. Urologic Clinics of North America: erectile dysfunction. Philadelphia: W.B. Saunders Company; 2001. p. 269–78.

[35] Zilbergeld B. The new male sexuality. New York: Bantam Books; 1992.

[36] Althof SE. New roles for mental health clinicians in the treatment of erectile dysfunction. J Sex Educ Ther 1998;23:229–31.

[37] Leiblum SR, Rosen RC. Couples therapy for erectile disorders: conceptual and clinical considerations. J Sex Marital Ther 1991;17:147–59.

[38] Waldinger MD. The neurobiological approach to premature ejaculation. J Urol 2002;168:2359–67.

[39] Waldinger MD, Zwinderman AH, Olivier B, et al. Proposal for a definition of lifelong premature ejaculation based on epidemiological stopwatch data. J Sex Med 2005;2:498–507.

[40] Perelman MA. Psychosocial history. In: Goldstein I, Meston C, Davis S, Traish A, editors. Women's sexual function and dysfunction: study, diagnosis and treatment. United Kingdom: Taylor and Francis; 2005.

[41] Warnock JK. Assessing FSD: taking the history. Prim Psychiatry 2001;8:60–4.

[42] Viera AJ. Managing hypoactive sexual desire in women. Med Aspects Hum Sex 2001;1:7–13.

[43] Perelman MA. Premature ejaculation. In: Leiblum S, Pervin L, editors. Principles and practice of sex therapy. New York: Guilford Press; 1980.

[44] Perelman MA. The urologist and cognitive behavioral sex therapy. Contemp Urol 1994;6:27–33.

[45] Perelman MA, McMahon C, Barada J. Evaluation and treatment of the ejaculatory disorders. In: Lue T, editor. Atlas of male sexual dysfunction. Philadelphia: Current Medicine, Inc.; 2004.

[46] Perelman MA. Retarded ejaculation. Curr Sex Health Rep 2004;1:95–101.

[47] Perelman MA. AUA Abstract 1254: idiosyncratic masturbation patterns: a key unexplored variable in the treatment of retarded ejaculation by the practicing urologist. J Urol 2005;173:340.

[48] Seidman SN, Roose SP, Menza MA, et al. Treatment of erectile dysfunction in men with depressive symptoms: results of a placebo-controlled trial with sildenafil citrate. Am J Psychiatry 2001;158: 1623–30.

[49] Gagnon JH, Rosen RC, Leiblum SR. Cognitive and social aspects of sexual dysfunction: sexual scripts in sex therapy. J Sex Marital Ther 1982; 8:44–56.

[50] Goldstein I, Lue TF, Padma-Nathan H, et al. Oral sildenafil in the treatment of erectile dysfunction. Sildenafil Study Group. N Engl J Med 1998;338: 1397–404.

[51] Carson CC, Burnett AL, Levine LA, et al. The efficacy of sildenafil citrate (Viagra) in clinical populations: an update. Urology 2002;60:12–27.

[52] Hellstrom WJ. Vardenafil: a new approach to the treatment of erectile dysfunction. Curr Urol Rep 2003;4:479–87.

[53] Lilly/ICOS. Tadalafil package insert. Indianapolis (IN): Author; 2005.

[54] Hatzichristou D, Moysidis K, Apostolidis A, et al. Sildenafil failures may be due to inadequate patient instructions and follow-up: a study on 100 non-responders. Eur Urol 2005;47:518–22 [discussion 522–3].

[55] Barada JA. Successful salvage of sildenafil (Viagra) failures: benefits of patient education and re-challenge with sildenafil. 4th Congress of the European Society for Sexual and Impotence Research; Rome, Italy. October 2, 2001.

[56] McCarthy BW. Relapse prevention strategies and techniques with erectile dysfunction. J Sex Marital Ther 2001;27:1–8.

[57] Albaugh J, Amargo I, Capelson R, et al. Health care clinicians in sexual health medicine: focus on erectile dysfunction. Urol Nurs 2002;22:217–31.

ELSEVIER
SAUNDERS

Urol Clin N Am 32 (2005) 447–455

UROLOGIC
CLINICS
of North America

Clinical Evaluation of Erectile Dysfunction in the Era of PDE-5 Inhibitors

John R. Lobo, MD, Ajay Nehra, MD*

Department of Urology, Mayo Clinic, 200 1st Street SW, Rochester, MN 55905, USA

Erectile dysfunction (ED) is a multifactorial disorder that is receiving greater attention from patients and their sexual partners, the medical community, industry, popular culture, and society at-large. ED is the consistent or recurrent inability to attain or maintain penile erection adequate for sexual intercourse [4]. The introduction of relatively safe and effective oral therapy in the form of selective phosphodiesterase-5 (PDE-5) inhibitors has heightened patient and physician interest in the evaluation and treatment of this disorder. The incidence of ED has been quantified by population-based cohort studies in the United States, Brazil, and Europe [1–3]. In the Massachusetts Male Aging Study (MMAS), a community-based survey of men between 40 and 70 years of age, 52% of all respondents reported some degree of ED: 17% mild, 25% moderate, and 10% complete [1]. The MMAS described a crude incidence rate of 25.9 cases per 1000 man-years (95% confidence interval 22.9–29.9) with a mean follow-up of 8.8 years. As expected, incidence rates (cases per 1000 man-years) increased with patient age, with an incidence of 12.4 for men aged 40 to 49 years, 29.8 for men aged 50 to 59 years, and 46.4 for men aged 60 to 69 years. Diabetes mellitus, coronary artery disease, hypertension, decreased high-density lipoprotein (HDL) levels, and lower education were factors that increased the age-adjusted risk for ED [1].

A 3-month minimum duration is accepted for establishment of the diagnosis, although in certain cases of trauma or surgically induced ED, a 3-month minimum may not be necessary. Although objective testing or partner reports may be used to support the diagnosis of ED, these cannot replace the patient's self-report in classifying the dysfunction or establishing the diagnosis [5].

Identification of risk factors

ED is recognized increasingly as an important presentation of various organic and psychiatric illnesses. The introduction of oral PDE-5 inhibitors seems to have resulted in patients presenting to their physicians in increasing numbers for evaluation and treatment [6]. Identification of organic and psychogenic risk factors is therefore of great importance. An accepted classification is that recommended by the International Society of Sexual Medicine (ISSM), which categorizes ED into three main groups: (1) psychogenic, (2) organic, and (3) mixed (organic and psychogenic), the most common type [4]. Identification of risk factors and classification of the patient who has ED into one of these three groups is the first goal of the clinical evaluation.

According to the ISSM classification, psychogenic ED may be generalized or situational. The generalized type usually relates to a primary lack of sexual arousability, aging-related decline in arousability, personality characteristics or a chronic disorder of sexual intimacy, and usually is not associated with a particular sexual partner, situation, or performance concern [5,7]. The situational type of psychogenic ED, however, is associated specifically with a specific partner, performance concerns, or adjustment-related issues. Partner-related issues may include lack of arousability in a specific relationship, sexual object preference, and partner conflict or threat [8]. Performance-related

* Corresponding author.

E-mail address: nehra.ajay@mayo.edu (A. Nehra).

issues may be associated with situational performance anxiety or with other sexual dysfunctions
such as premature ejaculation or disorders of orgasm [9,10]. Adjustment-related issues include
major life stress such as significant illness and death
of partner [10]. Depressive and anxiety disorders
have been associated with ED and adequate treatment of these disorders reduces the severity of and
possibly eliminates ED [11–14]. Identification of
the psychogenic component to ED is useful in
guiding the treatment plan. In such patients, psychologic counseling and behavioral therapy approaches may be used in conjunction with or as
alternatives to medical treatments [10,14–17].

Organic erectile dysfunction

If the clinical evaluation suggests an organic
etiology, the ISSM classification system identifies
six major subgroups: neurogenic, hormonal, arterial, cavernosal (venogenic), and drug-induced [4].
In addition, various disease states are identified as
potential causes of ED through unclear mechanisms (Box 1).

Neurologic

Various neurologic conditions affect erectile
function. In theory, any neurologic condition
affecting autonomic innervation of the corpora
cavernosa may impact the ability to have a normal
erection. Polyneuropathy, which commonly involves autonomic dysfunction, is a source of ED
[18]. Vardi and colleagues [19] reported a 38% coincidence of polyneuropathy and ED in diabetics
and a 10% coincidence of the two in nondiabetics.
Other neurologic conditions that may lead to male
sexual dysfunctions are Parkinson's disease, de-
mentia, multiple sclerosis, and other neurodegen-
erative diseases [17,20–24]. In these patients, ED
is believed to be secondary to a complex interplay
among altered erectile nerve function, generalized
sensorimotor impairment, cognitive decline, ill-
ness-related stress, and decreased interpersonal
interaction [20–22]. Epilepsy also has been associated with ED and reduced sexual interest and desire [20]. In the case of multiple sclerosis, the
incidence of ED is reportedly 40% to 80%, typically presenting 5 to 10 years after the onset of
progressive neurologic symptoms [23]. Stroke,
a common neurologic condition worldwide, is associated with loss of sexual interest and desire,
ejaculatory dysfunction, and ED in 50% to 65%
of patients [24–26]. In spinal cord injury, ED
and other related sexual dysfunctions are among

Box 1. Common conditions associated with erectile dysfunction

Cardiovascular
Coronary artery disease
Peripheral vascular disease
Cerebrovascular disease
Congestive heart failure
Aortic aneurysm
Hypertension

Psychiatric
Schizophrenia
Depression
Anxiety

Pulmonary
Chronic obstructive pulmonary disease

Endocrine
Diabetes mellitus
Hypogonadism
Hyperthyroidism
Hypothyroidism
Hyperprolactinemia
Adrenal disorders

Neurologic
Stroke
Epilepsy
Multiple sclerosis
Parkinson's disease
Spinal cord injury
Peripheral neuropathy
Central nervous system tumors
Alzheimer's disease

Gastrointestinal
Chronic liver disease

Renal
Chronic renal failure
Renal vascular disease

Urologic
Peyronie's disease
Prostate cancer
Penile trauma
Pelvic trauma
Perineal trauma
Congenital anomalies

Miscellaneous
Smoking
Obesity
Chemotherapy
Radiation
Pelvic surgery
Pelvic trauma
Perineal trauma
Vascular surgery
Scleroderma

the most pronounced problems for future quality of life [17,20].

Endocrine

Abnormalities of endocrine function affect sexual behavior, desire, and interest [27,28]. In addition, gonadal function in men is affected adversely in a progressive way as part of the normal aging process [29,30]. Although reduced testosterone level is the most widely recognized and investigated hormonal alteration associated with the aging process, the production of several hormones, including dehydroepiandrosterone, thyroxine, melatonin, prolactin, and growth hormone, also is affected profoundly by age and may have implications in erectile function [28]. The role of androgens in normal and abnormal erectile function remains controversial [31]. To what extent the changes in the hormonal milieu contribute to the development and persistence of ED remains speculative. Androgen-replacement therapy improves the results of nocturnal penile tumescence (NPT) testing as well as erotic stimulus-evoked erections in significantly hypogonadal men [31–33]. In the MMAS, of the 17 hormones measured, dehydroepiandrosterone sulfate levels seemed to affect erectile function [34]. Although the role of androgens in normal erectile function has been viewed traditionally as permissive, there is increasing evidence that androgens are fundamental, not just for sexual behavior, but also for various physiologic and signaling pathways regulating erection [35].

Vascular

Vascular disease is the most common cause of organic ED [36]. Reduction of inflow into the cavernosal arteries and veno-occlusive dysfunction secondary to atherosclerotic occlusive disease is the accepted pathophysiologic mechanism in most cases of organic ED [36]. Penile arterial occlusive disease therefore shares a etiologic pathway with other vascular disease states such as cerebrovascular disease, myocardial infarction, coronary artery disease, hypertension, hyperlipidemia, and peripheral vascular disease [37]. In one study, 64% of men surveyed during hospitalization for myocardial infarction had some degree of ED [38]. Another study reported an 18% prevalence of ED in men before experiencing a myocardial infarction compared with 45% after the event [39]. In the MMAS report, heart disease, hypertension, and low serum HDL levels were correlated significantly with ED [1]. In an analysis of

MMAS studies, it is suggested that ED and coronary artery disease share some behaviorally modifiable determinants [40].

Four other disease states are encountered commonly during the clinical evaluation of the patient who has ED: cigarette smoking, diabetes mellitus, chronic renal failure, and treated prostate cancer. Cigarette smoking deleteriously affects the arterial endothelium on a microvascular level and is a risk factor for various vascular disease states [41,42]. A meta-analysis of the available literature over the last 20 years revealed that 40% of men who had ED were smokers, compared with 28% of men in the general population [43]. A literature review focusing on global epidemiology also correlated cigarette smoking with ED [44].

ED has been reported to occur in at least 50% of men who have diabetes mellitus, with the onset of symptoms occurring at an earlier age than in those without diabetes mellitus [45]. A review of the literature suggests that 26% to 35% of diabetic men will develop ED, and in the MMAS, the age-adjusted probability of complete ED was three times higher in men who had treated diabetes mellitus than in nondiabetics [46]. Numerous mechanisms by which diabetes mellitus causes ED have been proposed, although diabetes-induced microvascular and atherosclerotic disease and diabetes-induced autonomic and somatic peripheral neuropathies likely are the most important [36].

Chronic renal failure (CRF) is a risk factor for ED, and is encountered during the urologic evaluation. Effective treatment of CRF with renal transplantation reduces the severity of ED in these patients [47]. A common patient population encountered by the urologist includes that treated for prostate cancer by radical prostatectomy, radiotherapy, hormonal therapy, and most recently, cryosurgery. A recent report indicates a 60% incidence of ED post–radical prostatectomy, regardless of whether a nerve-sparing procedure had been performed [48]. Other reports have shown that in younger males, bilateral nerve-sparing radical prostatectomy results in higher retention of erectile function compared with the non–nerve-sparing procedure [49,50]. External-beam prostate radiotherapy and interstitial prostate brachytherapy result in posttreatment ED [51]. Interstitial prostate cryosurgery is an emerging treatment modality for prostate cancer, but recent reports indicate a high likelihood of posttreatment ED [52]. Medical and surgical treatment of symptomatic benign prostate hyperplasia (BPH) generally is not injurious to the cavernosal nerves, and it has been reported that sexual functions usually remain stable after BPH treatments [53].

The Second International Consultation on Sexual Dysfunction has identified risk factors for men who have ED, some of which are discussed here [4]. Poor overall health, tobacco use, diabetes mellitus, hormonal disorders, cardiovascular disease, hypertension, CRF, lower urinary tract symptoms, chronic neurologic diseases, spinal cord injury, surgery and radiotherapy for prostate cancer, psychiatric conditions including anxiety disorders and depression, medications, and recreational drugs are among the well-studied risk factors for ED. Identification and screening for these risk factors is an important goal of the clinical evaluation of ED.

Clinical assessment of erectile dysfunction

ED is a presenting symptom and an established disease state that may be primary or secondary to various other disease states. As with all other medical evaluations, an ED evaluation should be systematic, focusing sequentially on (1) identification of the chief complaint, (2) a detailed history of the present and prior illnesses and surgical procedures, (3) physical examination, (4) basic laboratory testing, (5) identification of the need for specialized referrals, and (6) specialized evaluation and testing. Of primary importance is the establishment of a clinician-patient partnership and an atmosphere of trust and openness between clinician and patient [54].

Symptom scales

The complexity of human sexual dysfunction historically has defied attempts at scientific quantification. Nevertheless, the use of ED symptom scales and questionnaires is an invaluable resource in identifying risk factors and potential etiologies. Symptom scales have obvious benefits of providing validated and cost-efficient identification of the problem as well as preliminary assessment of current and past sexual functioning. Numerous validated sexual questionnaires are available (Table 1) [55]. According to Rosen and colleagues [54], "the symptom scale used should reflect a high-level of sensitivity and regard for the individual's unique ethnic, cultural and personal background."

Medical and sexual history

A detailed medical history is essential to the clinical evaluation of ED. The clinician must be aware that ED may be symptomatic of an underlying medical disorder (see Box 1). Effective screening for these underlying diseases may be performed by taking a careful and targeted history. A substantial proportion of ED in the United States is believed to be secondary to vascular occlusive disease, and ED shares a common pathophysiology with other vascular disease states such as heart disease, stroke, and peripheral vascular disease. In the era of PDE-5 inhibitors, an ED evaluation therefore may be the first presentation of systemic vascular occlusive disease. A cursory history of cardiovascular symptomatology, including exercise tolerance, presence of angina, dyspnea, claudication, transient ischemic attacks, smoking history, and family history of cardiovascular disease, may identify a patient with cardiac and vascular risk factors [56]. A targeted urologic history also should be obtained, including that of lower urinary tract symptoms, urologic trauma, urologic malignancies, urinary tract infections, and sexually transmitted infections. A complete list of the patient's medications, including herbal medicines, nutritional supplements, and other alternative

Table 1
Commonly used validated questionnaires and symptoms scales in the evaluation of erectile dysfunction

Instrument	Target population	Parameters evaluated	Modality
International Index of Erectile Function (IIEF)	Men	Desire and interest, erections, orgasm, overall satisfaction	Self-administered
Derogatis Interview for Sexual Functioning (DISF-SR)	Men and women	Arousal, orgasm, sexual behavior, cognitive assessment	Generally <15 min Self-administered and clinician-administered, <15 min
Changes in Sexual Functioning Questionnaire (CISF)	Men	Desire and interest, arousal, erections, overall satisfaction	Self-administered and clinician-administered, <15 min

therapies should be obtained, especially because numerous medications cause ED (Box 2).

A comprehensive sexual history is essential in confirming the patient's diagnosis and in evaluating the patient's sexual function. The pre-evaluation questionnaire may be used to identify specific patient concerns that may be elaborated on and investigated further. Sexual history taking may focus on patient concerns regarding arousal, libido, performance, ejaculation and orgasm, and overall satisfaction. A major goal of sexual history taking should be to differentiate between potential organic and psychogenic causes in the etiology of a patient's sexual problem, with recognition of the potentially significant overlap between organic and psychogenic etiologies.

Physical examination

The physical examination is essential to a complete ED evaluation. A general screening for medical risk factors and comorbidities associated with ED should be performed. This includes a focused cardiovascular and neurologic examination, as well

---

Box 2. Classes of medications associated with erectile dysfunction

Antihypertensives
Beta blockers
Diuretics
Calcium channel blockers
Centrally acting antihypertensives

Hormonal Agents
Leutinizing hormone–releasing
  hormone agonists
5-alpha reductase inhibitors
Estrogens/progesterones
Antiandrogens

Psychotropics
Antidepressants
Selective serotonin reuptake inhibitors
Monoamine oxidase inhibitors
Lithium
Antipsychotics
Amphetamines

Miscellaneous
Alcohol
Cimetidine
Metoclopramide
Antiepileptics

---

as examination of other organ systems as suggested by the medical history. Urologic examination should include an assessment of body habitus and proper development of secondary sexual characteristics, abdominal and inguinal examination, and scrotal examination with assessment of testicular size and consistency and any abnormal scrotal size. Examination of the penis should include an assessment of cutaneous sensation and screening for any cutaneous lesions, congenital anomalies, traumatic lesions, or plaques. A proper digital rectal examination with assessment of prostate size, consistency, and the presence or absence of masses, is an essential part of the ED evaluation in all men. Evaluation of cutaneous sensation in the perineum is useful in identifying potential neurogenic causes of ED [57].

Basic laboratory testing

The goal of basic laboratory testing is cost-efficient screening for common systemic disorders that may result in ED. The Second International Consultation on Sexual Dysfunction (2004) Committee on Sexual Dysfunction Assessment in Men has recommended that fasting blood glucose, fasting cholesterol and lipid panel, and testosterone levels be obtained routinely as part of a basic ED evaluation [54]. Optional diagnostic tests that may be indicated specifically by the medical history and physical examination include levels of prolactin, leuteinizing hormone, follicle-stimulating hormone, prostate-specific antigen (PSA), complete blood count, and a thyroid function panel.

Specialized evaluation of erectile dysfunction

The goal of specialized evaluation is to define further the cause of ED and offer effective treatments. In most cases of ED, a detailed medical and sexual history, general medical examination, a focused genitourinary examination, and thorough review of relevant comorbidities and medications can identify the likely etiology and allow formulation of a treatment plan. Generally accepted indications for specialized evaluation are failure of initial treatment, Peyronie's disease, primary ED, history of pelvic or perineal trauma, cases requiring vascular or neurosurgical intervention, complicated endocrinopathy, complicated psychiatric disorder, complex relationship problems, and medico-legal concerns [54].

Vascular evaluation

The goal of specialized vascular testing is the quantitative and qualitative assessment of penile arterial and veno-occlusive function. In practice, vascular ED is subclassified as: arterial, veno-occlusive, or mixed vascular insufficiency [36]. The quality of penile inflow has been related directly to common vascular comorbidities including age, diabetes mellitus, hypertension, atherosclerotic vascular diseases, hyperlipidemia, and cigarette smoking [36].

Many tests evaluate penile vascular inflow and veno-occlusive function: intracavernous injection (ICI) pharmacotesting, penile blood flow study (PBFS), dynamic infusion cavernosometry (DICC), and selective penile angiography [54]. An ICI pharmacotest is an easily performed office-based diagnostic test. Although many intracavernosal vasoactive agents have been described for pharmacotesting, prostaglandin-E1 (PGE1) is the most commonly used agent at a dosage of 10 to 20 mcg for initial injection. Following intracavernosal injection, a subjective assessment of response is used: visual rating of erection with the patient asked to compare the erection to the best erection at home. In this manner, a subjective assessment of an inadequate versus adequate erection can be made. An ICI pharmacotest has the advantages of being simple to perform, minimally invasive, and being done relatively quickly in the office. A normal ICI pharmacotest in a neurologically intact patient may imply psychogenic ED. According to Rosen and colleagues [54], "comparison to other hemodynamic tests suggests a normal ICI pharmacotest is associated with normal veno-occlusive function (flow to maintain rigidity values of 0.5-3 mL/min)" [54]. In cases where the response from ICI pharmacotesting is abnormal, however, it is impossible to distinguish arterial insufficiency from veno-occlusive dysfunction. In addition, it is impossible to know if the pharmacologic challenge was sufficient and whether visual or other erotic stimuli need to be added to replicate a real-life setting. Despite pharmacologic erection, there may be abnormal arterial inflow. In addition, patient anxiety during testing situations may prevent duplication of best home erection. A normal ICI pharmacotest is useful in guiding the clinician toward investigation of psychogenic etiologies; an abnormal ICI pharmacotest raises several diagnostic questions that require further testing. An ICI pharmacotest alone therefore is believed to be a misleading diagnostic

test to exclude vascular ED unless performed with penile Doppler ultrasonography [58].

The PBFS uses intracavernous injection and assessment of penile vascular flow by color duplex Doppler ultrasound. It is the most informative and least invasive means of evaluating vasculogenic ED [54]. A PBFS provides an objective measurement of penile hemodynamics, especially arterial inflow. It can distinguish high-flow from low-flow priapism, and identify Peyronie's plaques. Although an intracavernosal agent such as PGE-1 typically is used, the combination of oral sildenafil citrate and a visual erotic stimulation may be an effective noninvasive pharmacologic induction [59]. This additionally may be useful in predicting treatment success with PDE-5 inhibitors. The important vascular parameters assessed by PBFS include peak systolic arterial velocity (PSV), cavernous artery diameters, and cavernous artery end-diastolic arterial velocity. A PSV less than 25 cm/sec reflects insufficient cavernous arterial inflow; PSV less than 25 cm/sec following ICI pharmacotesting and erotic stimuli has a 100% sensitivity and 95% specificity in selecting patients with abnormal penile arteriography [54]. A PSV greater than 30 cm/sec is considered normal. An inadequate erection in the setting of a normal arterial inflow following ICI pharmacotesting suggests veno-occlusive dysfunction [60]. Although this study cannot diagnose ED conclusively secondary to veno-occlusive dysfunction, it can suggest the diagnosis and identify patients in need of further and more invasive diagnostic testing, including cavernosometry and cavernosography.

DICC was a commonly used test in the routine evaluation of ED. With the widespread availability of PBFS and its usefulness in identifying patients who have vasculogenic ED and ability to distinguish arterial, venous-leak, or mixed vascular ED, "DICC is now reserved for the rare patient who might have a site-specific venous leak, or a history of penile fracture or perineal and pelvic trauma," according to Rosen and colleagues [54]. The DICC is the most sensitive test to detect sites of venous leak. In current practice, DICC generally is used in young men who might be candidates for penile vascular surgery to correct a veno-occlusive leak secondary to congenital or posttraumatic etiologies, and at times in men who have Peyronie's disease with poor rigidity before penile reconstructive surgery. DICC is an invasive evaluation of intracavernosal hemodynamics, requiring a needle in each corporal body, one infusing and one recording, as well as intracavernosal injection of a vasoactive agent at higher doses than that required for PBFS. Saline solution is infused into the corporal bodies to maintain specified intracavernosal pressures, and the vasoactive agent is redosed until a linear relationship exists between the infusion rate and cavernosal pressure. The first parameter assessed during DICC is "flow to maintain" an intracavernosal pressure of 150 mm Hg. A "flow to maintain" value of more than 3 mL/min is diagnostic of veno-occlusive dysfunction. Once the saline infusion is stopped, intracavernosal pressure decline is measured over time. An intracavernosal pressure decay of more than 45 mm Hg in 30 seconds is indicative of veno-occlusive dysfunction. Cavernosography, which may be performed with direct infusion of a dilute isoosmotic contrast medium followed by a plain-film radiograph of the lower pelvis, also may be used to radiographically confirm a venous leak.

Pudendal angiography remains the most invasive diagnostic test for vasculogenic ED. This diagnostic modality is reserved for the few cases of young men with decreased cavernosal arterial inflow on PBFS and a history of pelvic or perineal trauma. The expected finding in these cases is a discrete focus of arterial occlusion that may be corrected with microvascular surgery. A prior history of pelvic or perineal trauma is common in such patients. Pudendal angiography is not indicated when operative revascularization is not an option.

Penile MRI is a new diagnostic technique with significant opportunities for application in the field of penile pathologies. Advantages of penile MRI include better definition of anatomic details and penile circulation [61]. It may be used to detect penile fractures and plaques. Signal intensity depends on the rate of blood flow in the intracavernosal spaces. At present, penile MRI is probably too expensive and time-consuming to render it a routine diagnostic test.

Neurologic evaluation

As with all ED evaluations, the medical history and physical examination form the basis for further neurologic evaluation. Specialized testing for neurogenic ED is generally unnecessary. Often, a patient who has presumed neurogenic ED will have been diagnosed previously with an acute or chronic neurologic condition. Young age at presentation, acute onset of ED, and a normal or excellent response on PBFS following ICI or oral PDE-5 inhibitor pharmacotesting may be consistent with neurogenic ED. Some available neurologic tests include nerve conduction velocity studies, biothesiometry, bulbocavernosus electromyography (EMG),and corpus cavernosus EMG. Based on available evidence, neurologic testing lacks adequate sensitivity and reliability for routine clinical diagnosis [54]. A recent study, however, has correlated strongly abnormal penile thermal sensory testing with the clinical diagnosis of neurogenic ED [62]. Further evaluations are necessary before this test may be brought into routine clinical practice.

Psychologic evaluation

Most evaluations for ED will identify psychologic risk factors, either independently or in coexistence with organic risk factors. The authors' practice is to refer all patients suspected to have a significant psychogenic component to clinical psychologists, psychiatrists, and behavioral therapists with specific expertise in sexual dysfunction.

Traditionally, NPT testing has been used to distinguish psychogenic ED from organic ED. The test is expensive and time-consuming, requiring a specifically equipped sleep center. Documentation of a normal erection during an NPT test suggests that the neurologic and vascular axes are generally intact, and that psychogenic ED is likely.

Summary

The introduction of PDE-5 inhibitors has broadened the scope of ED evaluations to include primary care providers, urologists, cardiovascular specialists, endocrinologists, neurologists, psychiatrists, psychologists, and other specialties. A truly multidisciplinary approach is beneficial to the patient seeking evaluation and treatment. An awareness of the numerous medical illnesses associated with ED is essential for proper diagnosis. A systematic approach to the evaluation of ED must include sexual problem identification through the appropriate use of questionnaires and symptom scales, a detailed medical and sexual history, physical examination, and basic laboratory testing. Most ED evaluations do not require specialist referrals and invasive tests, but the clinician must be familiar with the indications and identify the need for further evaluations and investigations.

References

[1] Johannes CB, Araujo AB, Feldman HA, et al. Incidence of erectile dysfunction in men 40–69 years old: longitudinal results from the Massachusetts Male Aging Study. J Urol 2000;163:460–3.

[2] Moreira ED, Lbo CF, Diament A, et al. Incidence of erectile dysfunction in men 40–69 years old: results from a population-based cohort study in Brazil. Urology 2003;61:431–6.

[3] Schouten BW, Bosch JL, Bernsen RM, et al. Incidence rates of erectile dysfunction in the Dutch general population: effects of definition, clinical relevance and duration of follow-up in the Krimpen Study. Int J Impot Res 2005;17(1):58–62.

[4] Lizza EF, Rosen RC. Definition and classification of erectile dysfunction: report of the nomenclature committee of the International Society of Impotence Research. Int J Imp Res 1999;11:141–3.

[5] Lewis RW, Fugl-Meyer KL, Bosch R, et al. Definitions, classification, and epidemiology of sexual dysfunction. In: Lue TF, Basson R, Rosen R, et al, editors. Sexual medicine: sexual dysfunctions in men and women. 2004 edition. Paris: Health Publications; 2004. p. 39–72.

[6] Gopalakrishnan M, Buckner SA, Wyllie MG. Directions in urological research and drug therapies. Drug News Perspect 2001;4(9):544–50.

[7] Mas M. The influence of personality traits on the erectile response to intracavernosal PGE-1 injections. Int J Impot Res 2002;14(Suppl.4):S3.

[8] Wiederman MW. The state of theory in sex therapy. J Sex Res 1998;35:88–99.

[9] Feil MG, Richter-Appelt H. Control beliefs and anxiety in heterosexual men with erectile disorder: an empirical study. Z Sexualforschung 2002;15:1–20.

[10] Levine S. Sexual life, a clinicians guide. New York: Plenum; 1992.

[11] Araujo AB, Durante R, Feldman HA. The relationship between depressive symptoms and male erectile dysfunction: cross-sectional results from the Massachusetts Male Aging Study. Psychosom Med 1998; 60:458–65.

[12] Barlow DH. Causes of sexual dysfunction: the role of anxiety and cognitive interference. J Consult Clin Psychol 1986;54:140–8.

[13] Althof S. When an erection alone is not enough: biopsychosocial obstacles to lovemaking. Int J Imp Res 2002;(Suppl 1):99–104.

[14] Wincze JP, Carey MP. Sexual dysfunction: a guide for assessment and treatment. 2nd edition. New York: Guilford Press; 2001.

[15] Wylie KR. Treatment outcome of brief couple therapy in psychogenic male erectile disorder. Arch Sex Behav 1997;26(5):527–45.

[16] Perelman MA. The impact of the new sexual pharmaceuticals on sex therapy. Curr Psychiatry Rep 2001;3:195–201.

[17] Nehra A, Moreland RB. Neurologic erectile dysfunction. Urol Clin North Am 2001;28(2):289–308.

[18] Low PA. Autonomic neuropathies. Curr Opin Neurol 2002;15(5):605–9.

[19] Vardi Y, Sprecher EK, Kanter Y, et al. Polyneuropathy in impotence. Int J Imp Res 1996;8:65–8.

[20] Lundberg PO, Brackett NL, Denys P, et al. Neurological disorders: erectile and ejaculatory dysfunction. In: Jardin A, Wagner G, Khoury S, et al, editors. Erectile dysfunction. London: Health Publication; 1999. p. 591–649.

[21] Kaufman JM, Hatzichristou DG, Mulhall JP, et al. Sexual function in Parkinson's disease. Clin Neuropharmacol 1990;13:461–3.

[22] Brown RG, Jahanshahi WT, Quinn N, et al. Sexual dysfunction in patients with Parkinson's disease and their partners. J Neurol Neurosurg Psychiatry 1990; 53(6):480–6.

[23] Litwiller SE, Frohman EM, Zimmern PE. Multiple sclerosis and the urologist. J Urol 1999;161:743–57.

[24] Monga TN, Lawson JS, Inglis J. Sexual dysfunction in stroke patients. Arch Phys Med Rehab 1986;67: 19–22.

[25] Sjogren K, Damber JE, Liliequist B. Sexuality after stroke. Aspects of sexual function. Scand J Rehab Med 1983;15:55–61.

[26] Hawton K. Sexual adjustment of men who have had strokes. J Psychosom Res 1984;28:243–9.

[27] Morales A. Androgens, sexual endocrinopathies and their treatment. In: Erectile dysfunction: issues in current pharmacotherapy. London: Martin-Dunitz; 1998. p. 141–55.

[28] Morales A, Buvat J, Gooren LJ, et al. Endocrine aspects of male sexual dysfunction. In: Lue TF, Basson R, Rosen R, et al, editors. Sexual medicine: sexual dysfunctions in men and women, edition 2004. Paris: Health Publications; 2004. p. 345–83.

[29] Vermeulen A. Andropause. Maturitas 2000;35: 5–15.

[30] Feldman HA, Longcope C, Derby CA. Age trends in the levels of serum testosterone and other hormones in middle-aged men: longitudinal results of the Massachusetts Male Aging Study. J Clin Endocrinol Metab 2002;87:589.

[31] Nehra A. Treatment of endocrinologic male sexual dysfunction. Mayo Clin Proc 2000;75(Suppl):S40–5.

[32] Bancroft J, Wu FW. Changes in erectile responsiveness during androgen replacement therapy. Arch Sex Behav 1983;12:59–66.

[33] Carani G, Granata AR, Bancroft J, et al. The effects of testosterone replacement on nocturnal penile tumescence testing, rigidity and erectile response to visual erotic stimuli in hypogonadal men. Psychoneuroendocrinology 1995;20:743–53.

[34] Gray A, Feldman HA, McKinley JB, et al. Age, disease and changing sex hormone levels in middle-aged men: Results of the Massachusetts Male Aging Study. J Clin Endo and Met 1991;73:1016–105.

[35] Wespes E. The ageing penis. World J Urol 2002; 20(1):36–9.

[36] Russell S, Nehra A. The physiology of erectile dysfunction. Herz 2003;28(4):277–83.

[37] Sullivan ME, Thompson CS, Dashwood MR, et al. Nitric oxide and penile erection: is erectile dysfunc-

tion another manifestation of vascular disease? Cardiovasc Res 1999;43:658–65.

[38] Wabrek AJ, Burchell RC. Male sexual dysfunction associated with coronary artery disease. Arch Sex Behav 1990;9:69–75.

[39] Sjogren K, Fugl-Meyer AR. Some factors influencing quality of sexual life after myocardial infarction. Int Rehabil Med 1983;5(4):197–201.

[40] Feldman HA, Johannes CB, Derby CA, et al. Erectile dysfunction and coronary risk factors: prospective results from the Massachusetts Male Aging Study. Prev Med 2000;30:328–38.

[41] Puranik R, Celermajer DS. Smoking and endothelial function. Prog Cardiovasc Dis 2003;45(6):443–58.

[42] Bazzano LA, He J, Muntner P, et al. Relationship between cigarette smoking and novel risk factors for cardiovascular disease in the United States. Ann Intern Med 2003;138(11):891–7.

[43] Tengs TO, Osgood ND. The link between smoking and impotence: two decades of evidence. Prev Med 2001;32:447–52.

[44] Nehra A, Kulaksizoglu H. Global perspectives and controversies in the epidemiology of male erectile dysfunction. Cur Opin Urol 2002;12:493–5.

[45] Benet AE, Melman A. The epidemiology of erectile dysfunction. Urol Clin North Am 1995;22(4):699–709.

[46] Feldman HA, Goldstein I, Hatzichristou DG, et al. Impotence and its medical and psychosocial correlates: results of the Massachusetts Male Aging Study. J Urol 1994;151:54–61.

[47] Abdel-Hamid I. Mechanisms of vasculogenic erectile dysfunction after kidney transplantation. BJU Int 2004;94(4):497–500.

[48] Stanford JL, Feng Z, Hamilton AS, et al. Urinary and sexual function after radical prostatectomy for clinically localized prostate cancer: the Prostate Cancer Outcomes Study. JAMA 2000;283:354–60.

[49] Rabbani F, Stapleton AMF, Kattan W, et al. Factors predicting recovery of erections after radical prostatectomy. J Urol 2000;164:1929–34.

[50] Nehra A. Medical and surgical advances in the radical prostatectomy patient. Int J Impot Res 2000;12(Suppl 4):S47–52.

[51] Goldstein I, Feldman MI, Deckers PJ, et al. Radiation associated impotence: a clinical study of its mechanism. JAMA 1984;251:903–10.

[52] Robinson JW, Donnelly BJ, Saliken JC, et al. Quality of life and sexuality of men with prostate cancer 3 years after cryosurgery. Urology 2002;60(2 Suppl. 1):12–18.

[53] Leliefeld HHJ, Stovelaar HJ, McDonnell JM. Sexual function after various treatments for symptomatic benign prostatic hyperplasia. BJU Int 2002;89:208–13.

[54] Rosen R, Hatzichristou D, Broderick G, et al. Clinical evaluation and symptom scales: sexual dysfunction assessment in men. In: Lue TF, Basson R, Rosen R, et al, editors. Sexual medicine: sexual dysfunctions in men and women, edition 2004. Paris: Health Publications; 2004. p. 175–206.

[55] Rosen R, Hatzichristou D, Broderick G, et al. Clinical evaluation and symptom scales: sexual dysfunction assessment in men [annex I]. In: Lue TF, Basson R, Rosen R, et al, editors. Sexual medicine: sexual dysfunctions in men and women, edition 2004. Paris: Health Publications; 2004. p. 207–20.

[56] Russell ST, Khandheria BK, Nehra A. Erectile dysfunction and cardiovascular disease. Mayo Clin Proc 2004;79(6):782–94.

[57] Klausner AP, Batra AK. Pudendal nerve somatosensory evoked potentials in patients with voiding and/or erectile dysfunction: correlating test results with clinical findings. J Urol 1996;156(4):1425–7.

[58] Aversa A, Isidori AM, Caprio M, et al. Penile pharmacotesting in diagnosing male erectile dysfunction: evidence for lack of accuracy and specificity. Int J Androl 2002;25(1):6–10.

[59] Speel TG, Bleumer I, Diemont WL, et al. The value of sildenafil as a mode of stimulation in pharmacopenile duplex ultrasonography. Int J Impot Res 2001;13(4):189–91.

[60] Teh HS, Lin MB, Tsou IY, et al. Color duplex ultrasonography as a screening tool for venogenic erectile dysfunction. Ann Acad Med Singapore 2002;31(2):165–9.

[61] Bellorofonte C, Dellacqua S, Mastromarino G, et al. Penile nuclear magnetic resonance. Arch Ital Urol Androl 1994;66(4):187–93.

[62] Lefaucheur KP, Yiou R, Colombel M, et al. Relationship between penile thermal sensory threshold-measurement and electrophysiologic tests to assess neurogenic impotence. Urology 2001;57(2):306–9.

**ELSEVIER
SAUNDERS**

Urol Clin N Am 32 (2005) 457–468

**UROLOGIC
CLINICS
of North America**

Androgen Deficiency in the Etiology and Treatment of Erectile Dysfunction

John L. Gore, MD[a],*, Ronald S. Swerdloff, MD[b], Jacob Rajfer, MD[c]

[a]*Department of Urology, David Geffen School of Medicine, University of California-Los Angeles,
CHS Rm 66-124, 10833 LeConte Avenue, Los Angeles, CA 90095-1738, USA*
[b]*Division of Endocrinology, Department of Medicine, Harbor-UCLA Medical Center and Los Angeles Biomedical
Research Institute, David Geffen School of Medicine, University of California-Los Angeles,
1000 West Carson Street, Torrance, CA 90509, USA*
[c]*Department of Urology, David Geffen School of Medicine, University of California-Los Angeles,
CHS Rm 66-131, 10833 LeConte Avenue, Los Angeles, CA 90095-1738, USA*

The last decade has witnessed a substantial paradigm shift in the management of erectile dysfunction (ED). The introduction of oral phosphodiesterase-5 (PDE-5) inhibitors in 1998 drastically altered algorithms previously used in the evaluation of ED as PDE-5 inhibitors have replaced other interventions as first-line ED management. As our understanding of the multifactorial mechanisms that combine to cause ED evolves and therapies directed at impotent men continue to improve, the assessment of men who have ED must be reevaluated continuously.

Testosterone supplementation has experienced a similar upsurge, especially in aging men, as the news media and other agencies have popularized the notion of a male menopause, or "andropause." Between 1993 and 2000, prescription sales of testosterone preparations increased by 500% [1]. Of those receiving prescriptions for testosterone, most were 45 or more years of age [2]. In 2002, 71% of prescriptions for testosterone were for patients in this age range, a rate not likely to decrease given the rapid growth in the number of Americans 65 or more years of age [2]. In 2000, Medicare-aged Americans accounted for 12.4% of the United States population [3]. By 2030, that figure is expected to rise to 19.6%, with a projected 71 million Americans 65 or more years of age. With an expanding elderly population and a growing interest in androgen deficiency and testosterone supplementation, annual testosterone product sales that currently total $400 million can be expected to increase [4].

Despite an exponential increase in the use of testosterone replacement therapy (TRT), the role of testosterone in erectile physiology remains unclear. Furthermore, the sexual and nonsexual benefits of TRT have not been proven definitively, prompting a recent Institute of Medicine (IOM) report mandating new randomized, controlled trials to establish the risks, benefits, and optimal routes of administration of TRT in men who have androgen deficiency [2]. Elderly men were targeted specifically in these recommendations. Until these trials are completed, the proper evaluation and management of ED related to androgen deficiency will continue to generate controversy.

Testosterone and erectile function

Between 1990 and 1992, investigators at UCLA elucidated the role of nitric oxide (NO) as the chemical mediator of penile erection [5]. Immediately thereafter, Burnett and colleagues [6] localized NO to the cavernosal nerve and suggested that NO was the neurotransmitter that initiated penile erection. More recently, animal studies have shown that nitric oxide synthase (NOS), the enzyme that synthesizes NO in the axons of the cavernosal nerve, is regulated by the testosterone metabolite dihydrotestosterone (DHT) [7]. Indeed, castration induces a reduction

---

* Corresponding author.
E-mail address: jgore@mednet.ucla.edu (J.L. Gore).

in the expression of NOS, which results in a decreased maximal intracavernosal pressure, whereas the administration of exogenous testosterone restores neuronal NOS expression and erectile function in this animal model [8]. Testosterone also may affect the ultrastructural and neuroeffector mechanisms involved in penile tumescence. In animal models castration results in smooth muscle apoptosis and increased collagen deposition within the corpora cavernosa [9]. Consequently, the maximal intracavernosal pressure that can be achieved with an electrically induced erection in this experimental setting is reduced, whereas the administration of exogenous testosterone reverses this process and restores the erectile response. Animal models designed to mimic the effects of aging on ED also have suggested that the erectile response is androgen-dependent. Androgen therapy in older rats significantly improved erectile quality as measured by mean intracavernosal arterial pressure independent of NO or NOS activity [10].

Although androgens may be crucial to erectile function in animal models, the androgen dependence of the human erectile response is less defined. Foresta and colleagues [11] performed nocturnal penile tumescence (NPT) and penile Doppler ultrasound studies on 15 men who had severe hypogonadism and compared this cohort with 20 eugonadal men who had psychogenic ED. The hypogonadal men demonstrated impaired NPT results, with a decreased peak systolic velocity (PSV) and resistive index (RI) on ultrasound studies compared with controls. Following a 6-month course of parenteral testosterone therapy, the neurophysiologic parameters normalized. Further evidence that testosterone modulates penile erection in humans derives from studies that correlate free testosterone levels with ultrasound-measured PSV and RI independent of subject age and comorbidity [12]. Low levels of bioavailable testosterone may induce smooth muscle apoptosis, as in the rat model, causing impaired cavernosal smooth muscle relaxation and decreased PSV and RI on ultrasound examination. Therefore, although definitive evidence supporting a causal relationship between testosterone and ED is lacking, testosterone likely influences erectile function through neurogenic and myogenic mechanisms.

Androgen deficiency in the aging male

Andropause describes a constellation of symptoms associated with the changing hormonal milieu in aging men. Defined as a male equivalent of menopause, the term *andropause* is a misnomer. Menopause defines a dramatic hormonal change associated with the sudden anovulatory state of the female. Conversely, the androgenic sequelae of aging in men constitute a slowly progressive process without a distinct transition point. The wide variability in the severity of androgen decline among men further discredits the term andropause [13]. The authors prefer the term *androgen deficiency in the aging male (ADAM)*, which more properly reflects the pathophysiology behind this common condition. ADAM produces sexual and nonsexual effects, including decreased lean muscle mass, increased body fat, osteoporosis, decreased libido, ED, and depression. These changes reflect alterations not only in the hypothalamic-pituitary-gonadal axis, but also decreased production of growth hormone, disordered melatonin release, impaired thyroxine production, and elevated levels of leptin [14]. The physical manifestations of ADAM reflect decreased production of insulin-like growth factor–I, under the influence of growth hormone. Sexual dysfunction seems to correlate with age-related changes in serum testosterone levels, although adrenal androgens may play a limited role [8].

Testosterone secretion follows a circadian pattern, with peak serum testosterone levels in the early morning and a nadir in the late afternoon [15]. Testosterone that circulates in free and albumin-bound forms comprises bioavailable testosterone. The remainder of the body's testosterone circulates in an inactive form bound to sex hormone–binding globulin (SHBG). The prevalence of testosterone deficiency varies with the definition, threshold cutoffs used, population studied, and assay measurements used to define androgen deficiency in the elderly population. Beyond 40 years of age, total serum testosterone declines at an average rate of 0.8% per year [16]. Conversely, levels of inactive testosterone bound to SHBG increase with age at a rate of 1.6% per year. Thus, a moderate decrease in total serum testosterone masks a more dramatic decrease in bioavailable testosterone (Fig. 1).

Although the fall in serum testosterone in men is gradual, the Baltimore Longitudinal Study of Aging demonstrated that by the eight decade of life, 30% and 50% of men have total and free testosterone levels, respectively, below the normal range for young healthy men [17]. Studies of African American men also confirmed an age-related decline in testosterone [18]. On multivariate

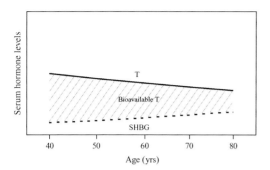

Fig. 1. Longitudinal trend of total and bioavailable testosterone levels with age. T, testosterone; SHBG, sex-hormone binding globulin.

analysis this association remains significant independent of other influential factors, including body mass index, comorbid disease, medications, cigarette smoking, and alcohol intake [17]. The time trend in serum testosterone levels parallels an age-related decline in the number of Leydig cells within the testes [19]. Further age-related changes include loss of the diurnal variation in testosterone secretion producing relatively constant blood levels throughout the day [20–23], resulting in a decrease in the morning concentrations of testosterone. Unlike younger patients who have primary gonadal failure, older testosterone-deficient men have regulatory dysfunction at the hypothalamic-pituitary and testicular levels. Thus, many older men with low serum testosterone levels have low or inappropriate serum leutinizing hormone (LH) concentrations.

In a population-based study of aging men, the prevalence of hypogonadism increases from 7% in men 40 to 60 years of age to 20% in men 60 to 80 years of age [24]. A secondary analysis of the same population revealed a significant increase in the prevalence of testosterone deficiency over the subsequent decade [25]. Defining androgen deficiency with low free testosterone, the prevalence of hypogonadism increased from 19.4% to 37.1% over this interval. Incorporating signs or symptoms of androgen deficiency into the definition, the prevalence of hypogonadism increased from 9.4% to 11.5% over the same interval. Likewise, the prevalence of ED increases with age, with approximately 50% of men 70 years of age affected [26]. Age also confers an increased risk for comorbid disease, further confounding delineation of a discrete etiology in elderly men who have ED. The rates of hypogonadism and ED are increased among men who have chronic comorbid

conditions, especially obesity and diabetes mellitus. Low serum testosterone levels in these patients may result from a decrease in production of SHBG, with little effect on bioavailable testosterone [27,28].

Evaluation of androgen deficiency

Questionnaires and physical examination findings thought to be pathognomonic of low testosterone fail to diagnosis hypogonadism with reasonable specificity. Although the ADAM questionnaire developed by Morley and colleagues [29] provides excellent sensitivity as a screening tool for men with low bioavailable testosterone levels, the specificity and reliability of the instrument are limited. Other screening questionnaires have similar constraints, although the ADAM questionnaires may be useful in following hypogonadal men on testosterone supplementation [29,30]. The combination of symptomatology and physical examination may reveal patients with low serum testosterone values. Classically, these patients endorse a history of decreased libido and demonstrate atrophic testes on physical examination. In the absence of a hormonal evaluation, history and physical examination rarely detect hypogonadism, however [31]. Symptomatology provides only 48% sensitivity and 66% specificity for diagnosing hypogonadism [32], and loss of sexual interest is a symptom common to several other conditions, including major depression. In a cohort of 1022 men reported by Buvat and colleagues [32], 32 of 533 men (6%) with normal sexual desire had subnormal levels of total testosterone. In the absence of a routine hormonal evaluation, 40% of the men in this cohort that responded to parenteral testosterone therapy never would have been diagnosed.

Overall, approximately 1 in 200 men have abnormally low levels of testosterone [33]. Based on routine screening of an elderly male population with assessments of bioavailable testosterone, a substantial proportion of elderly men are hypogonadal [34]. Among populations of men who have ED, as measured in several large retrospective reviews, the prevalence of hypogonadism ranges from 2.1% to 18.7% [32,35–38]. Combining these results, approximately 12.2% of patients who have ED may have low serum levels of testosterone.

The changing population of men seen in ED specialty clinics further justifies routine hormonal evaluation. Most patients referred to impotence specialists in the PDE-5 era already have failed PDE-5 inhibitors. In a cohort of diabetic men with impotence, Kalinchenko and colleagues [39] demonstrated that those who failed sildenafil had significantly lower total serum testosterone levels than controls. Combination therapy with oral testosterone undecanoate (not available in the United States) and sildenafil resulted in satisfactory erections in 84 of 120 (70%) men. Aversa and colleagues [40] demonstrated similar results in men with below-normal serum testosterone levels treated concomitantly with testosterone gel and a PDE-5 inhibitor.

The lack of specificity of questionnaires, history, and physical examination affirms the need for a biochemical assessment. A serum total testosterone drawn in the morning should be the first screening test for hypogonadism. In older men, the requirement for a morning blood draw is less strict because testosterone levels vary less throughout the day [20–23]. A finding of low total serum testosterone requires confirmation because free and total testosterone can exhibit marked week-to-week variation [41]. In older and obese men, elevated SHBG levels aberrantly raise the total serum testosterone and a more direct measurement of bioavailable testosterone is needed to diagnose hypogonadism. Measurement of free testosterone is complicated by inaccurate radioimmunoassay techniques, however [42–44]. The more involved equilibrium dialysis assay, which more consistently characterizes free testosterone levels, is only available at a few laboratories [45]. Concurrent measurement of total testosterone and SHBG would allow calculation of bioavailable testosterone, but measurement of SHBG is expensive. Until more cost-effective strategies emerge, serum total testosterone will suffice for most men with a total testosterone below 250 ng/dL or above 350 ng/dL. Those with an intermediate total testosterone of 250 to 350 ng/dL would benefit from measurement of free or bioavailable testosterone.

Further hormonal evaluation is reserved for patients with confirmed low levels of testosterone. ED secondary to hypogonadism may be a presenting complaint of pituitary disorders. These patients exhibit low serum testosterone coupled with low serum LH and follicle-stimulating hormone (FSH) concentrations or hyperprolactinemia. Most endocrinologists recommend MRI assessment of the sellae in patients with symptoms suggestive of a pituitary tumor (eg, headaches and visual loss), hyperprolactinemia, and serum testosterone levels below 150 ng/dL. Although the prevalence of hyperprolactinemia is low in screening populations of men who have ED, as many as 30% of men with low serum testosterone levels have an associated elevation in serum prolactin [32]. Of five men who had hypogonadism and hyperprolactinemia reported by Nickel and colleagues [38], imaging studies revealed large pituitary adenomas in two. Assessment with FSH, LH, and prolactin further confirms hypogonadism and screens for potential concomitant pituitary pathology.

Beyond a hormonal evaluation, a new diagnosis of hypogonadism mandates a thorough examination of any medications that may affect gonadal function. Common culprits include thiazide diuretics, long-acting oral opiates, antiepileptics, corticosteroids, and atypical antipsychotic medications such as risperidone and olanzapine [46]. Chemical castration for prostate cancer induces an immediate and near-complete hypogonadal state, and attention to the sexual and systemic effects of hypogonadism should be standard in the maintenance of patients on androgen-deprivation therapy.

Forms of testosterone replacement therapy

Current consensus recommendations suggest limiting the use of TRT to those with a serum testosterone level of less than 200 mg/dL and symptoms of hypogonadism, although evidence supporting this recommendation is lacking [47]. Treatment of hypogonadism is pharmacologic. Over the past decade, prescription rates for testosterone preparations have increased exponentially [2]. A cursory Internet search for "testosterone replacement" in February 2005 produced 842,000 hits. Although 29% of the first 100 sites listed offered nonprofit informational services, 21% of the sites endorse herbal therapies for ED or other over-the-counter supplements. The explosion in consumer interest about testosterone replacement, combined with the commercialization of herbal androgenic supplements, mandates a thorough knowledge of testosterone replacement modalities.

Currently available formulations are comprised of molecular testosterone or testosterone salts delivered in oral, intramuscular, transdermal, or implantable preparations. Although therapy may confer additional benefits beyond the effects of testosterone on sexual function, TRT also carries potential risks. An ideal formulation allows normalization of serum testosterone levels, replicates the circadian pattern of testosterone production in eugonadal men, produces normal levels of testosterone metabolites, including DHT and estradiol, and minimizes side effects.

Oral preparations available in the United States fail to achieve sufficient levels of serum testosterone because of rapid hepatic metabolism, produce inconsistent androgenic results, and are associated with excessive adverse effects, including hepatic toxicity and the potential for increased cardiovascular risk as a result of the effects on the lipid profile [48,49]. Alkylated oral testosterone preparations, such as methyltestosterone and fluoxymesterone, may induce formation of benign and malignant hepatic tumors. Furthermore, prolonged supplementation with the oral alkylated androgens may lead to cholestasis and cholestatic jaundice, and patients taking these preparations require rigorous follow-up with routine chemistry analyses including a hepatic panel [50]. Effects on the lipid profile may include elevation of the low-density lipoprotein (LDL) proportion through an increase in absolute LDL levels and a decrease in high-density lipoprotein levels, although results from several analyses demonstrate minimal impact on lipid levels when nonalkylated agents are used and testosterone is restored to physiologic levels [51].

Testosterone undecanoate, also delivered orally, is not available in the United States, but is prescribed commonly worldwide and confers improved bioavailability without the expense of major side effects. Testosterone undecanoate is absorbed preferentially through the gut lymphatics and thus is metabolized less by the liver, therefore achieving physiologic serum testosterone levels with a relatively safe side-effect profile [51]. Elevated levels of DHT can result, however, because of 5-alpha reduction in the gut; the drug is lipid-soluble, exhibits variable absorption, and must be taken with meals. Buccal testosterone, recently introduced, produces rapid rises in serum testosterone after application, but requires twice daily dosing [52]. No oral preparations of testosterone effectively reproduce the circadian pattern of physiologic testosterone secretion.

Injectable testosterone preparations require administration every 10 to 21 days with close observation for adverse effects, including mood disturbances [53]. Testosterone enanthate and testosterone cypionate are administered intramuscularly. Serum testosterone peaks at supraphysiologic levels 2 to 5 days after injection with steadily diminishing levels over the subsequent 10 to 14 days [54]. This results in a distinctly noncircadian pattern in the serum testosterone level, which may explain the side-effect profile of the injectable preparations. The supraphysiologic levels of testosterone occasionally cause breast tenderness and gynecomastia as a result of elevated levels of estradiol, and the large variability in the serum testosterone level can induce substantial mood swings. Compared with other delivery modes, intramuscular testosterone preparations are more likely to cause erythrocytosis, necessitating dose reduction in 25% of patients [55]. Furthermore, outcomes related to sexual function vary, likely because of the large variability in the serum testosterone level. The low cost of the injectable agents, however, enables continued use of these preparations.

Transdermal preparations are available as patches and gels, and effectively reproduce diurnal variation in testosterone at normal serum levels [56]. Because transdermal testosterone preparations use molecular testosterone, metabolism is not a concern and the incidence of serious adverse effects is extremely low. Patch or gel placement at night results in peak serum levels in the early morning and a nadir at bedtime before placement of a new patch or gel. Scrotal patches largely have been replaced by nonscrotal patches because of difficulty keeping the patch in place, the need to shave the scrotum weekly for patch placement, and resultant supraphysiologic levels of DHT secondary to 5-alpha reductase in the scrotal skin [57]. Nonscrotal patches produce physiologic levels of testosterone, estradiol, and DHT [58]. Similar to scrotal patches, however, nonscrotal patches require enhancers to aid in absorption of the molecular testosterone, which frequently cause contact dermatitis at the patch placement site. Testosterone gel applied to a relatively hairless part of the body avoids this complication [59]. The gel may be absorbed by a partner during physical contact, however, which can produce testosterone levels comparable to those seen in polycystic ovary syndrome, depending on the extent of exposure [60,61]. Prior reports may have overestimated the importance of gel transfer as a complication of this treatment [62]. Use is limited further by the high cost of the agent.

Implantable testosterone pellets produce stable serum testosterone levels and, barring difficulty with pellet extrusion, require replacement every 6 months. Implant extrusion occurs in 8.5% of patients, a frustrating complication given the high cost of treatment [63,64]. The inability to discontinue treatment abruptly may prolong patient exposure to the risks of testosterone replacement, especially with regard to prostate disease and polycythemia, limiting the use of these implants in aging men. Patient continuation of treatment is high despite these deterrents [63]. Dosage schedules, costs, and side-effect profiles of the available testosterone preparations are listed in Table 1.

The future may hold promise for therapies that more specifically target the androgen receptor, exerting effects on directed end organs and thus minimizing the systemic side effects of androgen therapy [65]. Although selective estrogen receptor modulators have emerged as novel hormone replacement strategies in postmenopausal women, male equivalents, or selective androgen receptor modulators (SARMs), are still in the developmental phase [66,67]. The promise of these agents is exemplified by animal studies that demonstrated improvement in bone mineral density in castrated rats on an oral SARM [68]. Effects on other androgen-dependent organs, specifically the prostate, were minimal. Confirmation of the efficacy of these agents may provide hope for a human application in the future.

Alternative androgenic supplements

Precursors to testosterone, dehydroepiandrosterone (DHEA) and androstenedione, have found use as dietary supplements in men who have ED [69]. Among the hormones examined in the Massachusetts Male Aging Study, only DHEA sulfate demonstrated a strong correlation with the prevalence of ED, with lower levels of DHEA sulfate

Table 1
Available testosterone preparations

Generic name	Trade name	Route	Dose	Cost[a]	Testosterone metabolites[b]	Circadian rhythm[c]	Side effects
Testosterone undecanoate[d]	Andriol	Oral	120–200 mg/d	N/A[d]	Elevated DHT	No	Poor absorption, gastrointestinal effects
Buccal system	Striant	Transbuccal	30 mg twice/d	$190.30	Normal	No	Gum irritation
Testosterone enanthate and cypionate	Depo-testosterone, Delatestryl, Testoviron Depot	Intramuscular	200–400 mg every 2–3 wk	$8.30	Elevated DHT	No	Mood swings, breast tenderness, polycythemia, infertility
					Elevated estradiol		
Testosterone implants	Testopel	Subcutaneous	600–1200 mg every 4–6 mo	N/A	Elevated DHT	No	Extrusion, gynecomastia, polycythemia, fluid retention
					Elevated estradiol		
Scrotal patches	Testoderm	Transdermal	10–15 mg/d	$131.54	Elevated DHT	Yes	Dermatitis, misplacement
Nonscrotal patches	Androderm, Testoderm TTS	Transdermal	4–6 mg/d	$131.54	Normal	Yes	Dermatitis
Gel	Androgel, Testogel, Androtop, Testim	Transdermal	5 g 1% gel/d	$186.00	Normal	Yes	Partner absorption

[a] Per month of treatment of the least expensive preparation in that class (generics included when possible).
[b] Effect of the testosterone preparation on testosterone metabolites estradiol and dihydrotestosterone (DHT).
[c] Efficacy of the testosterone preparation at reproducing the circadian pattern of testosterone secretion in eugonadal men.
[d] Not currently available in the United States.

conferring an increased risk for ED [70]. Despite this correlation, results of DHEA supplementation in men who have ED have been disappointing. Reiter and colleagues [71] conducted a double-blind, randomized, placebo-controlled trial of DHEA-replacement in 40 men who had ED. Although the International Index of Erectile Function (IIEF) scores improved among men taking DHEA, the statistical significance of the improvement was not documented. Furthermore, DHEA supplementation was associated with increased levels of testosterone metabolites, especially estradiol.

Androstenedione, physiologically produced in the adrenals and gonads, was believed to increase muscle mass and improve erectile function. In a randomized trial of healthy, eugonadal men, however, androstenedione supplementation had no effect on serum testosterone levels or muscle mass [72]. Serum testosterone levels may be affected with administration of higher doses of androstenedione, but effects on estradiol levels are similarly dose-dependent, with a 128% increase in serum estradiol among subjects who received a 300-mg daily dose of androstenedione [73]. The lack of a demonstrable effect on muscle growth permits continued sales of androstenedione over-the-counter, assuming the manufacturer does not espouse any unproven benefits of the supplement. Side effects can be significant, mostly secondary to supraphysiologic levels of estradiol produced by administration of androstenedione. These include breast tenderness and gynecomastia, mood disturbances, and increased cardiovascular risk. Furthermore, androstenedione does not impact libido or sexual function. With decreased effectiveness and an increased side-effect profile, precursors of testosterone seem poorly suited as agents to treat androgen deficiency. Furthermore, it seems counterintuitive to use precursors of testosterone when safe, cost-effective forms of molecular testosterone or testosterone salts are available.

Risks and benefits of testosterone replacement therapy

Risk for cardiovascular and prostate disease increases with age. The androgen dependence of benign and malignant prostate disease is well established, but it generally is accepted that TRT does not induce the development of prostate cancer [74]. A recent study examined the effect of testosterone supplementation on men who had biopsy-proven prostatic intraepithelial neoplasia, a precursor of prostate cancer [75]. Although control subjects were not included, the investigators demonstrated no increased risk for progression to prostate cancer in the men on TRT. Testosterone supplementation can exacerbate existing prostate cancers, however, and a diagnosis of prostate cancer remains a contraindication to TRT [76,77]. Case studies of TRT unmasking occult prostate cancer emphasize the need to screen for prostate disease before initiation of TRT, and to follow patients with serial digital rectal (DRE) and prostate-specific antigen (PSA) examinations. Clinicians should consider lower PSA thresholds for prostate biopsy in hypogonadal men because these men have depressed PSA levels compared with age-matched controls [4]. Furthermore, a rising PSA on TRT does not imply that an undetected prostate cancer is present. Men receiving exogenous androgens have an associated PSA increase of 0.30 ng/mL/y, with older men experiencing a larger mean increase of 0.43 ng/mL/y [4].

Testosterone, through its conversion to DHT, can exacerbate obstructive voiding symptoms secondary to benign prostatic hyperplasia. Like PSA, prostate volumes are lower in hypogonadal men [4]. Measurement of prostate volume by transrectal ultrasonography demonstrates a significant volume increase within the first 6 months of initiation of TRT. Despite the increase in prostate volume, American Urological Association (AUA) symptom scores did not increase appreciably.

With cardiovascular disease, a hormonal association is more speculative. Intuitively, elevated testosterone confers an increased risk for coronary disease; overall, men have a higher incidence of acute cardiac events than women. Studies of short-term testosterone supplementation, however, demonstrate that higher serum testosterone levels may be cardio-protective [78]. In population-based studies, serum testosterone levels were correlated inversely with cardiovascular risk: higher levels of testosterone conferred a lower risk for coronary atherosclerosis [79]. Furthermore, short-term TRT in men with stable angina produced significant improvements in treadmill stress test outcomes and general health-related quality of life compared with controls [80]. Changes in the lipid profile believed to occur in men on TRT, contributing to a presumed increased cardiovascular risk, are less relevant when testosterone is restored to physiologic as opposed to supraphysiologic levels [51,81]. No studies have evaluated the long-term effect of testosterone supplementation on cardiovascular risk.

Other adverse effects of TRT include hepatotoxicity, polycythemia, and exacerbation of sleep-disordered breathing. Hepatotoxicity derives from metabolism of oral-alkylated testosterone preparations by the liver, and is uncommon with other testosterone preparations. Polycythemia and exacerbation of obstructive sleep apnea are associated almost exclusively with parenteral testosterone therapy and may relate to the supraphysiologic androgen levels seen with injectable testosterone [82,83]. Maintenance of physiologic levels of testosterone also ameliorates mood changes common in men on injectable preparations of testosterone. Any form of testosterone therapy will inhibit spermatogenesis and hypogonadotropic infertility may result.

The documented benefits of TRT are no less equivocal. The syndrome of ADAM includes decreased lean muscle mass and increased body fat, osteoporosis, depression and cognitive deficits, decreased libido, and ED. To justify routine use of TRT, evidence is needed of improvement in the physical, mental, and sexual detriments associated with hypogonadism. Several prospective studies have shown improvement in bone density, decreased fat mass and increased lean muscle mass, improved libido, improved erectile function, and improved mood and cognitive ability following short-term trials of TRT [59,84–88]. Likewise, several prospective clinical trials have shown a lack of improvement in bone density, fat and lean muscle mass, sexual function, and cognition related to TRT [85,89–93]. Testosterone supplementation maximally benefited patients who were hypogonadal before initiation of TRT. Interpretation of most of these trials, positive and negative, is limited by the short duration of androgen therapy. This discrepancy prompted a directive from the National Institutes of Health for the IOM to evaluate the current state and future research directions of TRT. Recommendations of the IOM are as follows:

- Conduct clinical trials in older men with low testosterone levels
- Begin with short-term efficacy trials to determine benefit
- If short-term efficacy is established, perform long-term, large-scale studies to assess risks and benefits

- Ensure the safety of research participants with strict exclusion criteria and monitoring requirements
- Conduct further research into the mechanism of action of testosterone, its physiologic role, and age-related changes

Monitoring patients on testosterone replacement therapy

A baseline assessment should include a thorough history to mete out any symptoms of prostate disease or obstructive sleep apnea as well as any cardiovascular risk factors. Physical examination must include a DRE. The initial laboratory evaluation should confirm low serum testosterone levels and detect prostate cancer or other conditions that would complicate or contraindicate TRT. The authors obtain a baseline PSA and hematocrit level. In hypogonadal men the authors restrict prostate biopsy to those with a PSA density above 0.15 ng/gm, although some investigators advocate routine prostate biopsy in all patients before initiation of TRT [74]. The authors follow PSA examination with a repeat determination 6 to 12 weeks after starting androgen therapy, with semiannual monitoring thereafter. Although there is no agreement on the threshold for prostate evaluation based on an increase in PSA level after initiating testosterone therapy, the presence of a nodule on follow-up DRE or a PSA velocity greater than 0.75 ng/mL/y, regardless of the baseline PSA level, should prompt further investigation with a prostate biopsy.

Evaluation of the clinical response to TRT should include assessments of physical and sexual function and bone mineral density, especially in patients who have documented osteoporosis or osteopenia at baseline. The ADAM questionnaire has been proposed as an objective measure of clinical improvement [29]. Other instruments that may aid in the evaluation of patients on TRT include the AUA symptom index and the IIEF. Serial measurement of serum testosterone usually is not indicated unless patients demonstrate a poor clinical response or signs of any adverse effects of treatment. Other laboratory examinations obtained on a routine basis include an annual hematocrit and lipid profile.

Summary

The management of ED is evolving. As we learn more about the mechanisms that combine to promote tumescence, evaluation algorithms and therapeutic strategies require constant revision. Our understanding of the role of androgens in the mediation and potentiation of erections exemplifies that evolution. Basic science evidence suggests that testosterone contributes to the erectile response, possibly through effects on the cavernosal architecture or gene expression of members of the nitric oxide or cyclic GMP pathways. The prevalence of androgen deficiency concomitantly affects a population of men similarly predisposed to ED. Pharmacologic interventions for the management of hypogonadism, based on short-term clinical trials, are safe and efficacious, although long-term studies of the risks and benefits of testosterone therapy are lacking. The growth of consumer demand pressures the scientific obligation to confirm clinical effect before advocacy of widespread testosterone supplementation. Testosterone should be restricted to patients who have androgen deficiency clearly established with hormonal testing.

References

[1] Bhasin S, Buckwalter JG. Testosterone supplementation in older men: a rational idea whose time has not yet come. J Androl 2001;22(5):718–31.

[2] Liverman CT, Blazer DG, National Research Council (US) Committee on Assessing the Need for Clinical Trials of Testosterone Replacement Therapy. Testosterone and aging: clinical research directions. Washington (DC): National Academies Press; 2004.

[3] Centers for Disease Control and Prevention. Public health and aging: trends in aging—United States and worldwide. Available at: http://www.cdc.gov/mmwr/preview/mmwrhtml/mm5206a2.htm. Accessed August 27, 2005.

[4] Bhasin S, Singh AB, Mac RP, et al. Managing the risks of prostate disease during testosterone replacement therapy in older men: recommendations for a standardized monitoring plan. J Androl 2003; 24(3):299–311.

[5] Rajfer J, Aronson WJ, Bush PA, et al. Nitric oxide as a mediator of relaxation of the corpus cavernosum in response to nonadrenergic, noncholinergic neurotransmission. N Engl J Med 1992;326(2):90–4.

[6] Burnett AL, Lowenstein CJ, Bredt DS, et al. Nitric oxide: a physiologic mediator of penile erection. Science 1992;257(5068):401–3.

[7] Lugg JA, Rajfer J, Gonzalez-Cadavid NF. Dihydrotestosterone is the active androgen in the maintenance of nitric oxide-mediated penile erection in the rat. Endocrinology 1995;136(4):1495–501.

[8] Penson DF, Ng C, Cai L, et al. Androgen and pituitary control of penile nitric oxide synthase and erectile function in the rat. Biol Reprod 1996;55(3): 567–74.

[9] Traish AM, Park K, Dhir V, et al. Effects of castration and androgen replacement on erectile function in a rabbit model. Endocrinology 1999;140(4): 1861–8.

[10] Garban H, Marquez D, Cai L, et al. Restoration of normal adult penile erectile response in aged rats by long-term treatment with androgens. Biol Reprod 1995;53(6):1365–72.

[11] Foresta C, Caretta N, Rossato M, et al. Role of androgens in erectile function. J Urol 2004;171(6 Pt 1):2358–62.

[12] Aversa A, Isidori AM, De Martino MU, et al. Androgens and penile erection: evidence for a direct relationship between free testosterone and cavernous vasodilation in men with erectile dysfunction. Clin Endocrinol (Oxf) 2000;53(4):517–22.

[13] Gould DC, Petty R. The male menopause: does it exist?: for: some men need investigation and testosterone treatment. West J Med 2000;173(2):76–8.

[14] Lamberts SW, van den Beld AW, van der Lely AJ. The endocrinology of aging. Science 1997; 278(5337):419–24.

[15] Cooke RR, McIntosh JE, McIntosh RP. Circadian variation in serum free and non-SHBG-bound testosterone in normal men: measurements, and simulation using a mass action model. Clin Endocrinol (Oxf) 1993;39(2):163–71.

[16] Feldman HA, Longcope C, Derby CA, et al. Age trends in the level of serum testosterone and other hormones in middle-aged men: longitudinal results from the Massachusetts male aging study. J Clin Endocrinol Metab 2002;87(2):589–98.

[17] Harman SM, Metter EJ, Tobin JD, et al. Longitudinal effects of aging on serum total and free testosterone levels in healthy men. Baltimore Longitudinal Study of Aging. J Clin Endocrinol Metab 2001; 86(2):724–31.

[18] Perry HM III, Miller DK, Patrick P, et al. Testosterone and leptin in older African-American men: relationship to age, strength, function, and season. Metabolism 2000;49(8):1085–91.

[19] Neaves WB, Johnson L, Porter JC, et al. Leydig cell numbers, daily sperm production, and serum gonadotropin levels in aging men. J Clin Endocrinol Metab 1984;59(4):756–63.

[20] Gray A, Feldman HA, McKinlay JB, et al. Age, disease, and changing sex hormone levels in middle-aged men: results of the Massachusetts Male Aging Study. J Clin Endocrinol Metab 1991;73(5):1016–25.

[21] Marrama P, Carani C, Baraghini GF, et al. Circadian rhythm of testosterone and prolactin in the ageing. Maturitas 1982;4(2):131–8.

[22] Montanini V, Simoni M, Chiossi G, et al. Age-related changes in plasma dehydroepiandrosterone sulphate, cortisol, testosterone and free testosterone circadian rhythms in adult men. Horm Res 1988;29(1):1–6.

[23] Bremner WJ, Vitiello MV, Prinz PN. Loss of circadian rhythmicity in blood testosterone levels with aging in normal men. J Clin Endocrinol Metab 1983;56(6):1278–81.

[24] Vermeulen A, Kaufman JM. Ageing of the hypothalamo-pituitary-testicular axis in men. Horm Res 1995;43(1–3):25–8.

[25] Araujo AB, O'Donnell AB, Brambilla DJ, et al. Prevalence and incidence of androgen deficiency in middle-aged and older men: estimates from the Massachusetts Male Aging Study. J Clin Endocrinol Metab 2004;89(12):5920–6.

[26] Johannes CB, Araujo AB, Feldman HA, et al. Incidence of erectile dysfunction in men 40 to 69 years old: longitudinal results from the Massachusetts male aging study. J Urol 2000;163(2):460–3.

[27] Couillard C, Gagnon J, Bergeron J, et al. Contribution of body fatness and adipose tissue distribution to the age variation in plasma steroid hormone concentrations in men: the HERITAGE Family Study. J Clin Endocrinol Metab 2000;85(3):1026–31.

[28] Barrett-Connor E, Khaw KT, Yen SS. Endogenous sex hormone levels in older adult men with diabetes mellitus. Am J Epidemiol 1990;132(5):895–901.

[29] Morley JE, Charlton E, Patrick P, et al. Validation of a screening questionnaire for androgen deficiency in aging males. Metabolism 2000;49(9):1239–42.

[30] Smith KW, Feldman HA, McKinlay JB. Construction and field validation of a self-administered screener for testosterone deficiency (hypogonadism) in ageing men. Clin Endocrinol (Oxf) 2000;53(6):703–11.

[31] Ansong KS, Punwaney RB. An assessment of the clinical relevance of serum testosterone level determination in the evaluation of men with low sexual drive. J Urol 1999;162(3 Pt 1):719–21.

[32] Buvat J, Lemaire A. Endocrine screening in 1,022 men with erectile dysfunction: clinical significance and cost-effective strategy. J Urol 1997;158(5):1764–7.

[33] Replacing testosterone in men [review]. Drug Ther Bull 1999;37(1):3–6.

[34] Morley JE. Clinical diagnosis of age-related testosterone deficiency. Aging Male 2000;3(Suppl 1):55.

[35] Earle CM, Stuckey BG. Biochemical screening in the assessment of erectile dysfunction: what tests decide future therapy? Urology 2003;62(4):727–31.

[36] Bodie J, Lewis J, Schow D, et al. Laboratory evaluations of erectile dysfunction: an evidence based approach. J Urol 2003;169(6):2262–4.

[37] Johnson AR III, Jarow JP. Is routine endocrine testing of impotent men necessary? J Urol 1992;147(6):1542–3 [discussion 1543–4].

[38] Nickel JC, Morales A, Condra M, et al. Endocrine dysfunction in impotence: incidence, significance and cost-effective screening. J Urol 1984;132(1):40–3.

[39] Kalinchenko SY, Kozlov GI, Gontcharov NP, et al. Oral testosterone undecanoate reverses erectile dysfunction associated with diabetes mellitus in patients failing on sildenafil citrate therapy alone. Aging Male 2003;6(2):94–9.

[40] Aversa A, Isidori AM, Spera G, et al. Androgens improve cavernous vasodilation and response to sildenafil in patients with erectile dysfunction. Clin Endocrinol (Oxf) 2003;58(5):632–8.

[41] Morley JE, Patrick P, Perry HM III. Evaluation of assays available to measure free testosterone. Metabolism 2002;51(5):554–9.

[42] Winters SJ, Kelley DE, Goodpaster B. The analog free testosterone assay: are the results in men clinically useful? Clin Chem 1998;44(10):2178–82.

[43] Vermeulen A, Verdonck L, Kaufman JM. A critical evaluation of simple methods for the estimation of free testosterone in serum. J Clin Endocrinol Metab 1999;84(10):3666–72.

[44] Rosner W. An extraordinarily inaccurate assay for free testosterone is still with us. J Clin Endocrinol Metab 2001;86(6):2903.

[45] Matsumoto AM. Andropause: clinical implications of the decline in serum testosterone levels with aging in men. J Gerontol A Biol Sci Med Sci 2002;57(2):M76–99.

[46] Lunenfeld B. Androgen therapy in the aging male. World J Urol 2003;21(5):292–305.

[47] The Practice Committee of the American Society for Reproductive Medicine. Treatment of androgen deficiency in the aging male. Fertil Steril 2004;81(5):1437–40.

[48] Wang C. Androgen delivery systems: overview of existing methods and applications. In: Bhasin S, Gabelnick HL, Spieler JM, et al, editors. Pharmacology, biology, and clinical applications of androgens: current status and future prospects. New York: Wiley-Liss; 1996. p. 433–5.

[49] Morales A, Johnston B, Heaton JW, et al. Oral androgens in the treatment of hypogonadal impotent men. J Urol 1994;152(4):1115–8.

[50] Borhan-Manesh F, Farnum JB. Methyltestosterone-induced cholestasis. The importance of disproportionately low serum alkaline phosphatase level. Arch Intern Med 1989;149(9):2127–9.

[51] Whitsel EA, Boyko EJ, Matsumoto AM, et al. Intramuscular testosterone esters and plasma lipids in hypogonadal men: a meta-analysis. Am J Med 2001;111(4):261–9.

[52] Wang C, Swerdloff R, Kipnes M, et al. New testosterone buccal system (Striant) delivers physiological testosterone levels: pharmacokinetics study in hypogonadal men. J Clin Endocrinol Metab 2004;89(8):3821–9.

[53] Bhasin S. Clinical review 34: androgen treatment of hypogonadal men. J Clin Endocrinol Metab 1992;74(6):1221–5.

[54] Sokol RZ, Palacios A, Campfield LA, et al. Comparison of the kinetics of injectable testosterone in eugonadal and hypogonadal men. Fertil Steril 1982;37(3):425–30.

[55] Amory JK, Watts NB, Easley KA, et al. Exogenous testosterone or testosterone with finasteride increases bone mineral density in older men with low serum testosterone. J Clin Endocrinol Metab 2004;89(2):503–10.

[56] McClellan KJ, Goa KL. Transdermal testosterone. Drugs 1998;55(2):253–8.

[57] Bardin CW, Swerdloff RS, Santen RJ. Androgens: risks and benefits. J Clin Endocrinol Metab 1991; 73(1):4–7.

[58] Meikle AW, Arver S, Dobs AS, et al. Pharmacokinetics and metabolism of a permeation-enhanced testosterone transdermal system in hypogonadal men: influence of application site—a clinical research center study. J Clin Endocrinol Metab 1996; 81(5):1832–40.

[59] Wang C, Swerdloff RS, Iranmanesh A, et al. Transdermal testosterone gel improves sexual function, mood, muscle strength, and body composition parameters in hypogonadal men. Testosterone Gel Study Group. J Clin Endocrinol Metab 2000;85(8): 2839–53.

[60] Delanoe D, Fougeyrollas B, Meyer L, et al. Androgenisation of female partners of men on medroxyprogesterone acetate/percutaneous testosterone contraception. Lancet 1984;1(8371):276.

[61] Moore N, Paux G, Noblet C, et al. Spouse-related drug side effects. Lancet 1988;1(8583):468.

[62] Rolf C, Knie U, Lemmnitz G, et al. Interpersonal testosterone transfer after topical application of a newly developed testosterone gel preparation. Clin Endocrinol (Oxf) 2002;56(5):637–41.

[63] Handelsman DJ, Mackey MA, Howe C, et al. An analysis of testosterone implants for androgen replacement therapy. Clin Endocrinol (Oxf) 1997; 47(3):311–6.

[64] Kelleher S, Conway AJ, Handelsman DJ. Influence of implantation site and track geometry on the extrusion rate and pharmacology of testosterone implants. Clin Endocrinol (Oxf) 2001;55(4):531–6.

[65] Negro-Vilar A. Selective androgen receptor modulators (SARMs): a novel approach to androgen therapy for the new millennium. J Clin Endocrinol Metab 1999;84(10):3459–62.

[66] Baracat E, Haidar M, Lopez FJ, et al. Estrogen activity and novel tissue selectivity of delta8,9-dehydroestrone sulfate in postmenopausal women. J Clin Endocrinol Metab 1999;84(6):2020–7.

[67] Kanis JA, Johnell O, Black DM, et al. Effect of raloxifene on the risk of new vertebral fracture in postmenopausal women with osteopenia or osteoporosis: a reanalysis of the Multiple Outcomes of Raloxifene Evaluation trial. Bone 2003;33(3): 293–300.

[68] Rosen J, Negro-Vilar A. Novel, non-steroidal, selective androgen receptor modulators (SARMs) with anabolic activity in bone and muscle and improved safety profile. J Musculoskelet Neuronal Interact 2002;2(3):222–4.

[69] Moyad MA. Dietary supplements and other alternative medicines for erectile dysfunction. What do I tell my patients? Urol Clin North Am 2002;29(1):11–22 [vii].

[70] Reiter WJ, Pycha A, Schatzl G, et al. Serum dehydroepiandrosterone sulfate concentrations in men with erectile dysfunction. Urology 2000;55(5):755–8.

[71] Reiter WJ, Pycha A, Schatzl G, et al. Dehydroepiandrosterone in the treatment of erectile dysfunction: a prospective, double-blind, randomized, placebo-controlled study. Urology 1999;53(3):590–4.

[72] King DS, Sharp RL, Vukovich MD, et al. Effect of oral androstenedione on serum testosterone and adaptations to resistance training in young men: a randomized controlled trial. JAMA 1999;281(21): 2020–8.

[73] Leder BZ, Longcope C, Catlin DH, et al. Oral androstenedione administration and serum testosterone concentrations in young men. JAMA 2000; 283(6):779–82.

[74] Rhoden EL, Morgentaler A. Risks of testosterone-replacement therapy and recommendations for monitoring. N Engl J Med 2004;350(5):482–92.

[75] Rhoden EL, Morgentaler A. Testosterone replacement therapy in hypogonadal men at high risk for prostate cancer: results of 1 year of treatment in men with prostatic intraepithelial neoplasia. J Urol 2003;170(6 Pt 1):2348–51.

[76] Loughlin KR, Richie JP. Prostate cancer after exogenous testosterone treatment for impotence. J Urol 1997;157(5):1845.

[77] Curran MJ, Bihrle W III. Dramatic rise in prostate-specific antigen after androgen replacement in a hypogonadal man with occult adenocarcinoma of the prostate. Urology 1999;53(2):423–4.

[78] Liu PY, Death AK, Handelsman DJ. Androgens and cardiovascular disease. Endocr Rev 2003; 24(3):313–40.

[79] Hak AE, Witteman JC, de Jong FH, et al. Low levels of endogenous androgens increase the risk of atherosclerosis in elderly men: the Rotterdam study. J Clin Endocrinol Metab 2002;87(8):3632–9.

[80] English KM, Steeds RP, Jones TH, et al. Low-dose transdermal testosterone therapy improves angina threshold in men with chronic stable angina: a randomized, double-blind, placebo-controlled study. Circulation 2000;102(16):1906–11.

[81] Singh AB, Hsia S, Alaupovic P, et al. The effects of varying doses of T on insulin sensitivity, plasma lipids, apolipoproteins, and C-reactive protein in healthy young men. J Clin Endocrinol Metab 2002; 87(1):136–43.

[82] Jockenhovel F, Vogel E, Reinhardt W, et al. Effects of various modes of androgen substitution therapy on erythropoiesis. Eur J Med Res 1997;2(7):293–8.

[83] Liu PY, Yee B, Wishart SM, et al. The short-term effects of high-dose testosterone on sleep, breathing, and function in older men. J Clin Endocrinol Metab 2003;88(8):3605–13.

[84] Marin P. Testosterone and regional fat distribution. Obes Res 1995;3(Suppl 4):609S–12S.

[85] Snyder PJ, Peachey H, Hannoush P, et al. Effect of testosterone treatment on body composition and muscle strength in men over 65 years of age. J Clin Endocrinol Metab 1999;84(8): 2647–53.

[86] Tenover JS. Effects of testosterone supplementation in the aging male. J Clin Endocrinol Metab 1992; 75(4):1092–8.

[87] Morley JE, Perry HM III, Kaiser FE, et al. Effects of testosterone replacement therapy in old hypogonadal males: a preliminary study. J Am Geriatr Soc 1993;41(2):149–52.

[88] Janowsky JS, Oviatt SK, Orwoll ES. Testosterone influences spatial cognition in older men. Behav Neurosci 1994;108(2):325–32.

[89] Benkert O, Witt W, Adam W, et al. Effects of testosterone undecanoate on sexual potency and the hypothalamic-pituitary-gonadal axis of impotent males. Arch Sex Behav 1979;8(6):471–9.

[90] Sih R, Morley JE, Kaiser FE, et al. Testosterone replacement in older hypogonadal men: a 12-month randomized controlled trial. J Clin Endocrinol Metab 1997;82(6):1661–7.

[91] Janowsky JS, Chavez B, Orwoll E. Sex steroids modify working memory. J Cogn Neurosci 2000;12(3): 407–14.

[92] Kenny AM, Bellantonio S, Gruman CA, et al. Effects of transdermal testosterone on cognitive function and health perception in older men with low bioavailable testosterone levels. J Gerontol A Biol Sci Med Sci 2002;57(5):M321–5.

[93] Wolf OT, Preut R, Hellhammer DH, et al. Testosterone and cognition in elderly men: a single testosterone injection blocks the practice effect in verbal fluency, but has no effect on spatial or verbal memory. Biol Psychiatry 2000;47(7):650–4.

ELSEVIER
SAUNDERS

Urol Clin N Am 32 (2005) 469–478

UROLOGIC
CLINICS
of North America

Peyronie's Disease: Etiology, Epidemiology and Medical Treatment

Jason M. Greenfield, MD*, Laurence A. Levine, MD

Rush Univeristy Medical Center, 1725 W. Harrison Street, PB Suite 348, Chicago, IL 60612, USA

Despite increasing interest, the exact pathophysiology and epidemiology of Peyronie's disease has gone largely unstudied over the past few centuries. A review of the medical literature reveals that much is yet to be learned of this disease in addition to the pursuit of effective treatments. This article will serve to review what has been elicited so far as to the possible etiologies of the disease in addition to what is known about its epidemiology. Finally, an extensive overview of medical therapies for Peyronie's disease is presented.

Etiology

The proposed etiology of Peyronie's disease (PD) is still being elucidated today as it is one of the fastest growing areas of PD research. Historically, some of the earliest theories centered on the patient's sexual history and deviant behavior [1,2]. Other proposed theories included infection, as in the case of sexually transmitted diseases such as gonorrhea and syphilis [3,4]. In general, these etiologies have received little, if any, support in the modern literature.

A popular sentiment among researchers is that PD is a disorder of wound healing, not too dissimilar to that of a keloid scar, for example [5]. This has generated a significant amount of research into immunologic, biochemical, and cytogenetic factors that may play a role in plaque formation. Similar to a keloid scar, trauma, as an inciting factor, has been a popular theory

among urologists. Devine et al [6] formally proposed this in 1997. Despite great support for this hypothesis, other studies have pointed to its inconsistency [7]. Until more investigation can be completed, trauma, as an instigating factor, will remain a popular presumption in the urologic community.

Dupuytren's contracture has been associated with PD. Examination of the patient's hands for evidence of contracture is considered part of the routine exam of the patient presenting with PD. The association between the two diseases was first recognized in 1828 and reported by Abernathy [4]. As a genetic disorder that exhibits autosomal dominant inheritance, it was associations like this that encouraged a search for a genetic etiology of PD.

The study of gene expression profiles in PD plaques has been an area of investigation in recent years. A study comparing genetic expression between PD plaques and control tunica albuginea demonstrated upregulation of several genes that are involved in collagen synthesis, myofibroblast differentiation, tissue remodeling, inflammation, ossification, and proteolysis in PD plaques. In addition, genes responsible for inhibiting these processes were downregulated in PD plaques as was collagenase expression [8]. In 2004, Qian et al [9] compared the results of gene expression profiles in RNA samples taken from PD plaques, normal tunica albuginea, Dupuytren's nodules, and normal palmar fascia. Several gene families were found to be upregulated in both the PD and Dupuytren's tissue samples. These included matrix metalloproteinases (MMP2 and MMP9), which play a role in collagen degradation, and thymosins TMβ10 and TMβ4, which are believed to be MMP activators. This evidence seems to suggest

---

* Corresponding author.

E-mail address: jasonmgreenfield@yahoo.com (J.M. Greenfield).

common pathophysiologic pathways in PD and Dupuytren's contracture.

PD is, in essence, a disease of fibrosis. As a disorder of wound healing, collagen synthesis is abnormally increased in respect to collagen breakdown. In addition, the cells responsible for the collagen synthesis and wound contraction such as myofibroblasts seem to occur in excessive amounts. Most likely, trauma is the inciting event that activates an abnormal response to local injury in a man who has a genetic predisposition to abnormal scar formation and healing.

Wound healing may be divided into three phases. The acute phase involves enzymatic cleanup of dead, damaged, or infected tissue with concurrent release of cytokines. Fibrin has been described as being generated and deposited into tissues (including the tunica albuginea in men with PD) and has been proposed to result in the persistent stimulation of scar formation. However, fibrin does not act alone. Overexpression of other cytokines (including transforming growth factor beta [TGF-β]) may also play a role. The second or reparative phase involves strengthening of the wound through scar formation. In a normal individual, cytokines activate the migration of fibroblasts and macrophages. In PD, these fibroblasts may actually differentiate to become myofibroblasts, which respond differently to injury. In the final, or contractile, phase of wound healing, scar remodeling occurs. During this period, metalloproteinases are released (such as collagenases and gelatinases), which remodel the tissue resulting in a smaller, more organized scar. It is believed that patients with PD may have abnormal amounts or dysfunctional types of these collagenases, resulting in the abnormal scar remodeling [10].

The evaluation of pro-fibrotic factors involved in plaque formation is a recent area of interest. In 2003, Davila et al [11] investigated fibrin as a potential protein involved in the development of the Peyronie's lesion. Using a rat model in which tunica albuginea specimens were injected with fibrin, Peyronie's-like plaques did, in fact, develop. Injection of TGF-β1, which is thought to play a role in the local release of fibrin, also induced the formation of edema and fibrosis in the tunica albuginea. The authors hypothesized that fibrin may play a key role in the pathogenesis of PD. TGF-β has been described to be present in increased levels in PD plaques. Alterations in the TGF-β pathway have also been found to be altered in the plaques of PD patients, and thus may play a role in the pathogenesis of PD [12].

Other pro-fibrotic factors that have been investigated include plasminogen activator inhibitor-1, which is a known inhibitor of the breakdown of fibrin and collagen. Levels of this protein have been found to be elevated in PD plaque tissue [13]. Using the model of PD as a disorder of wound healing and remodeling, investigation into endogenous inhibitors of collagenases has led to the detection of increased levels of tissue inhibitors of metalloproteinases. This further supports the theory, as increased levels of tissue inhibitors of metalloproteinases would result in progressive scar formation without remodeling [10].

Although the etiology of PD has yet to be fully elucidated, interest in this area is increasing and expanding at a rapid rate. From the evidence that is available to us presently, it appears that PD is a result of genetic and traumatic causes in which several pro-fibrotic factors may play a role. Through further investigation, the exact etiology and factors involved may yet be identified, and may also yield a direction at which to aim future research into medical therapies. This is simply a brief review of the pathophysiology of PD, and is to provide an outline of an area of intense research that could certainly be expanded into its own article.

Epidemiology

Similar to other areas of investigation into PD research, epidemiologic data is inconsistent and limited. The first published data was reported by Polkey [14], in 1928, consisting of 550 case reports. In 1968, Ludvik [15] reported on an experience in a private clinic which demonstrated a prevalence rate of 0.3% to 0.7%. In 1997, Devine [16] reported a prevalence of symptomatic PD in two populations of male physicians of approximately 1%. This had been the widely quoted prevalence rate until recent reports indicated that it is, in fact, much higher. However, many physicians, including urologists, still hold to the false notion that 1% is the accepted rate [17].

A report by Lindsay et al [18], in 1991, provided the first cross-sectional study giving the proposed incidence and prevalence rates of PD. The reported prevalence in this study was consistent with earlier reports with a rate of 0.38%. From this study, it was estimated that there were 423,000 men with PD in the United States at that time, and that 32,000 new cases occur annually. Mean patient age at diagnosis was 53 years with a range of 19 to 83 years of age. The first prevalence rates to be reported in a European cross-sectional study were from Sommer et al [19], in 2002. In a survey of 8000 men (aged 30 to 80 years) in Cologne, Germany, 3.2% reported a palpable plaque in the penis. It is now believed that the actual prevalence rate may be closer to 7% or even higher. For example, in a study of 534 men presenting to a group of geographically diffuse urologists in the United States for prostate cancer screening, 8.9% were found to have objective evidence of PD [20]. Also of concern is the hypothesis that the true prevalence rate may be even higher and easily underestimated due to the fact that patients are likely to underreport such a condition that causes embarrassment.

Not surprisingly, controversy also exists regarding the natural history of PD. In 1990, Gelbard et al [21] reported on 97 men with PD, lasting from 3 months to 8 years, who responded to a questionnaire. According to their report, 47% of these men felt their disease had undergone little no change, 40% worsened, and only 13% felt they had gradually improved. In 2002, Kadioglu et al [22] retrospectively reviewed 63 patients who had presented with acute disease and were followed for approximately 6 months without treatment. In this group of patients, 30% felt their disease was progressively worsening while 67% had stable disease. Only two patients in this cohort were found to have any spontaneous resolution.

Most recently, Mulhall et al [23] reported on 246 men with PD who presented within 6 months of the onset of disease and were followed for at least 1 year without any treatment. At a mean follow-up of 18 months, stretched flaccid length had decreased by 0.8 cm. Of those with curvature, 12% improved, 40% remained stable, and the remaining 48% had worsened. In those who improved, curvature changed a mean of 15°, while in those who worsened, mean curvature change was 22°.

Aside from the belief that PD is a disease often of spontaneous resolution, another popular misconception is that PD is mainly a disease of older men. PD has been reported to occur over a wide range of ages, with reports in patients as young as 18 years of age [24]. In this study by Levine et al [24], patients presenting with PD under the age of 40 were more likely to present with erectile dysfunction (ED) than the standard PD patient, and all patients reported a palpable plaque. These younger patients were also less likely to recall a specific traumatic event or have pain with intercourse. In addition, they were more likely to have multiple plaques in different locations as well as multiple areas of curvature in more than one direction. In a study by Tefekli et al [25], the prevalence of PD in patients younger than 40 years of age was 8.2%. The majority had a dorsal curvature, and ED occurred in 21%. The authors of this study concluded that PD in the younger patient is generally more acute and severe, and should be treated more aggressively. Further support of these two studies was reported by Briganti et al [26], in 2003. Twenty patients less than 40 years old with PD were compared with 28 patients with PD over 40 years. Significant differences were found between International Index of Erectile Dysfunction domain scores and subjective reduction in penile length. The authors also agreed that younger patients appeared to demonstrate a more acute onset of disease and suffer less frequently from associated ED.

As research in PD has progressed, the more it appears that its prevalence has been severely underestimated. Common misconceptions about PD as a disease which is rare, seldom found in young patients, and rarely requires treatment still permeate the medical community. As more is learned about this disease, the growing impact it has on male physical and sexual health is becoming increasingly evident as the search for a cure becomes more imperative.

Medical therapy

Since the disease of acquired penile curvature was described by Francois Gigot de la Peyronie in 1743, multiple options for medical therapy have been explored. Despite this search, however, a consistent and successful medical therapy for PD continues to evade the practicing urologist. The fact that we still know so little about the pathophysiology of this disease emphasizes the need for further research to help direct future therapies.

Current nonsurgical options for the treatment of PD are based largely on anecdotal experiences, and the literature that does exist generally reports on studies characterized by a small number of patients with limited follow-up, the absence of placebo or control groups, and few, if any, objective measures of improvement. The historic reporting of spontaneous remission rates ranging from 7% to 29% also further confounds the issue [21,27,28].

Here, we review nonsurgical options that are currently available for the treatment of the pain and curvature associated with PD, including oral, topical, intralesional injection, external energy, and combination therapies.

Oral therapy

A number of oral therapies have been investigated for the treatment of PD.

Vitamin E

This vitamin was the first oral therapy to be described for this condition. First investigated by Scott and Scardino [29], in 1948, Vitamin E was suspected to be of clinical value due to its antioxidant properties. Theoretically, its use would reverse or stabilize the pathologic changes in the tunica albuginea. The study population included 23 patients, and the majority noted some benefit in curvature, plaque size, or pain.

Use of vitamin E continues today, and is the choice of many practicing urologists, largely due to its minimal side effect profile and low cost. Its possible benefit in the chemoprevention of prostate cancer has also increased its popularity. However, most studies have not taken the natural history of the disease into account nor have they involved a placebo arm. Accordingly, Gelbard et al [21] investigated vitamin E therapy in comparison to the natural history of PD. In their study of 86 patients, no significant differences between the treatment and control groups were noted for the parameters of curvature, pain, and ability to have intercourse.

Colchicine

Due to its inhibition of collagen synthesis and antifibrotic effects, colchicine has recently been used as a primary oral therapy as well as in combination with other agents for PD. Use of this agent was first proposed by Akkus et al in 1994 [30]. In their study, a gradually increasing dose was given over a 3- to 5-month period to 19 patients. Improvement in curvature was noted in 7 (36%) patients, and palpable plaque improved in 12 (63%). Of nine patients with an initial complaint of pain with erection, this symptom improved in seven (78%). Again, no placebo or control arm was used in this study. In a subsequent noncontrolled study by Kadioglu et al [31], 60 patients were treated with colchicine (1 mg) twice a day, with a mean follow-up of 11

months. Although these authors noted significant improvements in pain in 57 (95%) of the men, the percentage of patients with improvement in curvature (30%) and worsening curvature (22%) were similar. Gastrointestinal disturbances, including severe diarrhea, are the major side effects of this drug.

Potassium aminobenzoate

Another oral agent that is used as therapy for PD is potassium aminobenzoate (Potaba, Glenwood). It is also used for other conditions, including scleroderma, dermatomyositis, and pemphigus. This medication is believed to increase the activity of monoamine oxidase in tissues, thereby decreasing local levels of serotonin, which may contribute to fibrogenesis and scar formation.

Use of potassium aminobenzoate for PD was initially investigated by Zarafonatis and Horrax in 1959 [32]. Subsequently, a pooled European study published in 1978 involving 2653 patients reported a 57% success rate, with complete resolution in 9% [33]. Again, however, no control or placebo group was incorporated into the study, nor were objective measures of deformity employed.

Weidner et al [34] reported on a randomized prospective double-blind trial of potassium aminobenzoate (3 g) four times per day for 1 year versus an oral placebo. The only significant difference in improvement between the two groups was a decreased plaque size in those treated with potassium aminobenzoate. However, a reduction in plaque size has not been shown to correlate with reduction in curvature. This drug also carries a significant cost, requires taking up to 24 tablets daily, and is known for its low tolerability due to gastrointestinal side effects.

Tamoxifen citrate

The role of oral tamoxifen (Nolvadex, AstraZeneca) for the treatment of PD was first investigated in 1992 by Ralph et al [35] in patients with early-stage disease. The theory behind its potential benefit is based on its effect on the release of TGF-β from fibroblasts and blocking of TGF-β receptor sites, resulting in diminished fibrogenesis [35,36]. A dose of 20 mg was given twice a day for 3 months to 36 patients who had recently acquired PD (defined as less than 4 months). Results of this study demonstrated a reduction in pain in 29 (80%) patients, improvement in curvature in 13 (35%), and decreased plaque size in 12 (34%). However, in a controlled trial by Teloken et al [37], in 1999, a similar dosage was given, and there was no significant difference in improvement in the treatment group compared with placebo. It is unlikely that an adequate concentration of this effective antifibrotic agent can reach the plaque via oral administration.

Carnitine

Use of oral carnitine (Carnitor, Sigma-Tau) has also been investigated for the treatment of PD. Its mechanism of action is proposed to be inhibition of acetyl coenzyme-A. In a preliminary report by Biagiotti and Cavallini [38], published in 2001, 48 men were randomized to receive carnitine or tamoxifen. The first group received tamoxifen (20 mg) twice daily for 3 months, and the second group took acetyl-L-carnitine (1 g) twice daily for 3 months. Overall, men receiving carnitine saw greater benefit with respect to curvature, with significantly fewer side effects. However, the results were reported as mean deformity for the entire group without exact numbers of the men responding or degree of improvement. Further investigation of the possible role of this agent, both as monotherapy and in combination with other agents, is needed.

Topical therapy

Use of topical verapamil is based on prior reported experience using it as an intralesional therapy (discussed later in this review), as well as on experiments by Kelly [39], who demonstrated that exocytosis of extracellular matrix molecules, including collagen, fibronectin, and glycosaminoglycans (the primary components of the Peyronie's plaque), is a calcium ion-dependent process. Aggeler et al [40] noted changes in cell shape when fibroblasts were exposed to calcium antagonists in vitro. This change was associated with increased extracellular matrix collagenase secretion as well as decreased collagen and fibronectin synthesis and secretion. In 1990, Lee and Ping [41] cultured bovine fibroblasts in increasing doses of verapamil and found that the concentration necessary to inhibit extracellular matrix formation of collagen is much greater than the typical doses used in the systemic treatment of hypertension. Based on these findings, local injection of this agent is necessary to avoid systemic toxicity as well as to expose the target fibroblasts to an adequate concentration of verapamil.

To help confirm the hypothesis that topically applied verapamil gel penetrates into the tunica albuginea, a study by Martin et al [42], in 2002, investigated tissue concentrations in men who used topical verapamil gel. Men in this study were exposed to the compound before penile prosthesis implantation surgery, at which time a sample of tunica albuginea was excised and analyzed. Although some of the drug was found in the urine, no verapamil was detected in the tunica albuginea specimens. The authors concluded that transdermal application of topical verapamil has no scientific basis. When coupled with the fact that no controlled trial demonstrating benefit has been performed, topical verapamil is not currently recommended by many authorities in the filed of PD research.

Intralesional therapy

Direct injection of an agent into the Peyronie's lesion has an extensive history of investigation.

Steroids

In 1954, Teasley [43] proposed the use of intralesional injection of steroids in a study of 29 patients; however, the results were unclear. In that same year, Bodner et al [44] reported successful outcomes in 17 patients treated with intralesional hydrocortisone and cortisone injection. Although these results appeared promising, a study performed by Winter and Khanna [45], in 1975, showed no statistical difference when patients treated with intralesional dexamethasone injections were compared with the natural history of the disease in their general patient population of men with PD. In addition, no objective measurements of improvement in plaque size or curvature were reported. A prospective study by Williams and Green [46], in 1980, investigated the use of intralesional triamcinolone. All patients in the study first underwent observation for 1 year, during which time no treatment was administered, and only 3% had spontaneous resolution of symptoms. After treatment with triamcinolone, administered every 6 weeks for 36 weeks, 33% of patients reported improvement, most consistently in their pain, followed by plaque size, and then curvature.

Currently the treatment of PD with intralesional steroid injections is discouraged. The beneficial effects of this treatment are unpredictable, and may result in local tissue atrophy. Also of importance, steroid use can distort tissue planes between Buck's fascia and the tunica albuginea, making subsequent surgical correction more difficult.

Collagenase

The potential effect of collagenase on Peyronie's plaques was first studied in vitro by Gelbard et al in 1982 [47]. Subsequently, this group reported objective improvement in 20 (64%) of 31 patients within 4 weeks of treatment with collagenase injections [48]. One recurrence was noted. In 1993, Gelbard et al [49] published their findings from a double-blind trial of collagenase injections in 49 men. After stratifying patients based on severity of curvature, a statistically significant improvement was seen in curvature in the collagenase-treated group. However, maximal improvement ranged from 15° to 20°, and was only noted in patients with a bend of 30° or less and a plaque size of less than 2 cm in length. Based on these limited results and the low side-effect profile, this mode of treatment may hold promise as an alternative therapy for patients with mild to moderate disease. Further clinical trials of collagenase are in development.

Verapamil

The use of verapamil as an intralesional injection was first reported by Levine et al in 1994 [50]. In this noncontrolled study, 14 men received biweekly injections of verapamil into the Peyronie's plaques for 6 months. Subjectively, there was significant improvement in plaque-associated penile narrowing in all patients and curvature in 6 (42%). Objectively, a decreased plaque volume of >50% was noted in 4 (30%) of the subjects. Plaque softening was noted in all patients, while 12 (83%) noticed that plaque-related changes in erectile function had improved.

Rehman et al [51] published the first randomized single-blind trial of intralesional injection of verapamil versus saline. In this study of 14 patients, significant differences were noted in subjective improvement in quality of erections, as well as in objective measurements of plaque volume. A nonsignificant improvement trend was also noted in degree of curvature in the verapamil group.

More recently, Levine et al [52] published results of another nonplacebo-controlled trial involving 156 men treated with intralesional verapamil, more than three-fourths (77%) of whom had failed prior oral therapy with vitamin E,

potassium aminobenzoate, or colchicine. In this study, a local penile block using 0.5% bupivicaine (10–20 mL) was administered at the base of the penis. Next, using a short (5/8 in) needle (25-gauge to prevent needle breakage), one to five punctures were made through the skin. However, multiple passes were made through the plaque as verapamil was delivered, with the goal of leaving the drug in the tracks. The standard dose of verapamil administered was 10 mg, diluted with 6 mL of injectable saline for a total volume of 10 mL. Injections were administered every 2 weeks for a total of 12 injections [52].

Of 128 men who completed this study, 84% of those with pain had complete resolution [52]. A blinded technician assessed curvature with a protractor following creation of a full erection by papaverine injection. Measured curvature improved in 79 (62%) of the men, with a mean improvement of 31° (range, 5–75°). Only 10 (8%) of the patients had measured worsening of their initial curvature. Improvements in girth, rigidity, and sexual performance were noted in 83%, 80%, and 71%, respectively. When patients were segregated based on severity and duration of disease (greater or less than 1 year), no differences between the groups were noted in terms of improvements in curvature, rigidity, sexual function, and girth, suggesting that this therapy may be suitable for men with mild to severe deformity at various points in the course of the disease [52]. With further follow-up, no cardiovascular side effects have been noted in more than 800 patients studied.

Currently, we recommend a trial of six injections, with each injection occurring every 2 weeks. If no improvement is noted, the injection therapy may be terminated, the dose of verapamil increased to 20 mg (in men with no cardiovascular disease), or interferon (IFN) injections may be offered. It also should be noted that verapamil injection is contraindicated in patients with a ventral plaque or with extensive calcifications. For this reason, ultrasound is an important tool in the evaluation of the patient considering this therapy.

Interferons

The potential viability of IFNs as intralesional therapy for PD was first demonstrated in a study by Duncan et al in 1991 [53]. IFNs were shown to decrease the rate of proliferation of fibroblasts in Peyronie's plaques in vitro as well as to reduce the production of extracellular collagen and increase that of collagenase. Initial clinical trials published in 1995 and 1997 by Wegner et al [54,55] on the use of IFN-α-2b demonstrated low rates of improvement and high rates of side effects, most notably fever and myalgia. Also in 1997, Judge and Wisniewski [56] published results of a study in which the dose was modified. Only moderate improvements were noted with many patients still experiencing side effects, albeit less severe.

More promising results with IFN injection were demonstrated by Ahuja et al [57] in a non-randomized study of 20 men who received 1 million units biweekly for 6 months. In this trial, 100% of the men had softening of the plaque, 90% of those presenting with pain had improvement, and 55% had a subjective reduction in plaque size. In a recent study by Dang et al [58], participants received a reduced dose of IFN (2×10^6 U) biweekly for 6 weeks. Objectively measured improvements in curvature (using pharmacologic stimulation and a protractor) of >20% were noted in 67% of study participants. Of those presenting with pain, 80% claimed improvement. In addition, 71% with presenting complaints of ED also noted improvement in function. The authors conclude that these results are encouraging, and warrant further investigation given the equally efficacious and better tolerated dose regimen.

In 2003, Hellstrom et al [59] reported the preliminary results of a single-blind, multicenter, placebo-controlled study on the efficacy of IFN-α-2b injection. Patients in the treatment arm, which involved 6 biweekly injections of IFN (5×10^6 units), had encouraging results when compared with those who received placebo (saline). An improvement in curvature of more than 20% was seen in 69% of the treatment group versus only 37% of the control group. In addition, the mean reduction in curvature was 12.2° in the treatment group versus 8° in the control group. However, pain control was not significantly different between the groups, with 58% of patients treated with IFN and 50% of the control group reporting a reduction in pain.

Further investigation is clearly needed in regard to IFN therapy as well as possible effects of plaque injection in general, as it appears that saline injection itself may offer some benefit to certain patients. Although placebo-controlled trials remain the ultimate litmus test of medical treatment, due to the invasive nature of injection therapy and the sensitive nature of penile injection, it has been difficult for investigators accrue subjects to these trials.

External energy therapy

Over the past several years, various modes of external energy, both alone and in combination with other therapies, have been investigated for the treatment of PD.

Shock wave therapy

Local penile electroshock wave therapy (ESWT) has been suggested to be potentially helpful. Various hypotheses about its mechanism of action include direct damage to the plaque, resulting in an inflammatory reaction with increased macrophage activity, yielding plaque lysis; improved vascularity with plaque resorption following an inflammatory response induced by ESWT; and the creation of scarring of the penis contralateral to the plaque resulting in a "false" straightening [60].

Most studies on the efficacy of ESWT are limited to subjective reports of improvement of deformity, plaque size, or pain and objective improvement limited to autophotography [61, 62]. Hauck et al [63] controlled trial randomized 43 men to ESWT or an oral placebo for 6 months. No significant effect of treatment was noted on curvature change, plaque size, or subjective improvements in sexual function or rigidity. Although further investigation is clearly needed, enthusiasm for ESWT is waning in Europe, where much of the work in this area has been.

Iontophoresis

Several studies have recently investigated the efficacy of topically applied verapamil with or without dexamethasone with enhanced penetration using iontophoresis, or electromotive drug administration (EMDA) [64–67]. Levine et al [68] verified the efficacy of this mode of transmission of verapamil in 2002 using surgically retrieved tunica albuginea specimens after a single intraoperative exposure before partial plaque excision and grafting surgery. Di Stasi et al's [69] recent prospective study randomized 96 patients to treatment with verapamil (5 mg) plus dexamethasone (8 mg) using EMDA or 2% lidocaine also administered electromotively. A total of 73 patients completed the study, and 43% in the verapamil/dexamethasone group noted objective improvement in plaque size (as measured by ultrasound) and curvature (assessed by photography). However, there was no measured change in these parameters in the lidocaine group. All patients noted temporary erythema at the electrode site, but no other side effects were reported.

Preliminary results of iontophoresis with verapamil versus saline reported at the 2003 meeting of the American Urological Association suggested similar results in both groups [69]. This may indicate that the electric current itself may have some beneficial effect on wound healing as shown in the dermatologic literature [70]. Further investigation based on these early results continues.

Combination therapy

Various combinations of therapies have been investigated as potential treatments for PD. The goal of combination therapy is to combine different mechanisms of action to enhance improvement in deformity and function.

A recent placebo-controlled study by Prieto Castro et al [71] randomized 45 patients to receive vitamin E plus colchicine or ibuprofen (placebo). Patients in the treatment group reported a higher proportion of pain relief, although the difference was not statistically significant. Statistically significant improvements in curvature and plaque size were noted in the treatment arm as measured by photography and ultrasound, respectively. The authors concluded that although this regimen might be helpful, more extensive investigation is needed.

In a prospective trial, Mirone et al [72] examined two populations of patients with PD; one group was treated with ESWT while the other group received ESWT plus perilesional verapamil injections. A 52% improvement in plaque size for the ESWT-only group was noted compared with 19% in the combination group. A subsequent study by the same investigators involving 481 patients demonstrated a 49% improvement in plaque size deformity among those treated with both ESWT and verapamil [73]. The authors concluded that this form of combination therapy should be considered as the nonsurgical treatment of choice.

In a study of 60 men by Cavallini et al [74], patients were randomized to receive intralesional verapamil plus oral carnitine or intralesional verapamil plus oral tamoxifen. No significant difference in pain was elicited between the groups, but the group exposed to oral carnitine did demonstrate statistically significant subjective improvements in curvature, plaque size, and erectile function.

Summary

Clearly, the investigation of medical options for the treatment of PD is lacking controlled clinical trials with uniform standardized assessments and objective measures of deformity, including curvature and circumference. A key to defining the beneficial effects of various medical therapies lies in standardizing the evaluation of the Peyronie's patient across various studies so that the proposed benefits can be confirmed and applied to all populations [75]. Furthermore, basic science research into the pathophysiology of this disorder is likely to yield new insights into potential treatment options and direct future therapies.

At this time, there is no nonsurgical cure for PD in sight. However, several of the treatments reviewed appear to result in measured improvement with minor side effects in a majority of men with this condition. Due to the devastating physical and psychologic effects of this disorder, it is important to consider that improvement, or even stabilization, may be better than no treatment at all.

References

[1] Murphy LJT. Miscellanea: Peyronie's disease (fibrous cavernositis). In: The history of urology. 1st ed. Springfield (IL): Charles C. Thomas; 1972. p. 485–6.

[2] Wesson MB. Peyronie's disease (plastic induration) cause and treatment. J Urol 1943;49:350–6.

[3] Hunter J. Of the treatment of occasional symptoms of the gonorrhea. In: Nicol G, Johnson J, editors. A treatise on the venereal disease. 2nd ed. Philadelphia: J. Webster, 1818. p. 88–9.

[4] Abernethy J. The consequences of gonorrhea. Lecture on anatomy, surgery, and pathology: including observations on the nature and treatment of local diseases, delivered at St. Bartholomew's and Christ's Hospitals. 1st ed. London (England): James Balcock; 1828. p. 205.

[5] Levine LA. Treatment of Peyronie's disease with intralesional verapamil injection. J Urol 1997; 158(4):1395–9.

[6] Devine CJ Jr, Somers KD, Jordan SG, et al. Proposal: trauma as the cause of the Peyronie's lesion. J Urol 1997;157(1):285–90.

[7] Zargooshi J. Trauma as the cause of Peyronie's disease: penile fracture as a model of trauma. J Urol 2004;172(1):186–8.

[8] Magee TR, Qian A, Rajfer J, et al. Gene expression profiles in the peyronie's disease plaque. Urology 2002;59(3):451–7.

[9] Qian A, Meals RA, Rajfer J, et al. Comparison of gene expression profiles between Peyronie's disease

and Dupuytren's contracture. Urology 2004;64(2): 399–404.

[10] Cole A. Increased endogenous inhibitors of collagenases within Peyronie's plaques may represent a scar remodeling disorder [Abstr 944]. Annual Meeting of the American Urological Association; San Antonio, TX. May 21–26, 2005.

[11] Davila HH, Ferrini MG, Rajfer J, et al. Fibrin as an inducer of fibrosis in the tunica albuginea of the rat: a new animal model of Peyronie's disease. BJU Int 91(9):830–8.

[12] Haag SM, Hauck EW, Altinkilic B, et al. Alterations in the transforming-growth-factor-beta pathway as a possible risk factor in the pathogenesis of Peyronie's disease [Abstr 939]. Annual Meeting of the American Urological Association; San Antonio, TX. May 21–26, 2005.

[13] Davila HH, Magee TR, Zuniga F, et al. Plasminogen activator inhibitor-1 (PAI-1) is increased in human Peyronie's disease [Abstr 943]. Annual Meeting of the American Urological Association; San Antonio, TX. May 21–26, 2005.

[14] Polkey HJ. ID induratio penis plastica. Urol Cut Rev 1928;32:287–308.

[15] Ludvik W, Wasserburger K. Die Radiumbehandlung der induratio penis plastica. Z Urol Nephrol 1968;61:319–25.

[16] Devine CJ. Introduction to Peyronie's disease. J Urol 1997;157:272–5.

[17] La Rochelle JC, Levine LA. Survey of primary care physisicans and urologists regarding Peyronie's disease. [Abstr 941]. Annual Meeting of the American Urological Association; San Antonio, TX. May 21–26, 2005.

[18] Lindsay MB, Schain DM, Grambsch P, et al. The incidence of Peyronie's disease in Rochester, Minnesota, 1950 through 1984. J Urol 1991;146(4): 1007–9.

[19] Sommer F, Schwarzer U, Wassmer G, et al. Epidemiology of Peyronie's disease. Int J Impot Res 2002;14(5):379–83.

[20] Mulhall JP, Creech SD, Boorjian SA, et al. Subjective and objective analysis of the prevalence of Peyronie's disease in a population of men presenting for prostate cancer screening. J Urol 2004;171(6 Pt 1): 2350–3.

[21] Gelbard MK, Dorey F, James K. The natural history of Peyronie's disease. J Urol 1990;144(6):1376–9.

[22] Kadioglu A, Tefekli A, Erol H, et al. A retrospective review of 307 men with Peyronie's disease. J Urol 2002;168(3):1075–9.

[23] Mulhall JP, Guhring P, Depierro C. Intralesional verapamil prevents progression of Peyronie's disease [Abstr 936]. Annual Meeting of the American Urological Association; San Antonio, TX. May 21–26, 2005.

[24] Levine LA, Estrada CR, Storm DW, et al. Peyronie's disease in younger men: Characteristics and treatment results. J Androl 2003;24(1):27–32.

[25] Tefekli A, Kandirali E, Erol H, et al. Peyronie's disease in men under 40: characteristics and outcome. Int J Impot Res 2001;13(1):18–23.

[26] Briganti A. Clinical presentation of Peyronie's disease in young patients. Int J Impot Res 2003; 15(Suppl 6):S44–7.

[27] Williams JL, Thomas GG. The natural history of Peyronie's disease. J Urol 1970;103(1):75–6.

[28] Kadioglu A, Tefekli A, Sanly O, et al. Lessons learned from 307 men with Peyronie's disease. J Urol 2001;165(5 Suppl):202–3 [Abstract 838].

[29] Scott WW, Scardino PL. A new concept in the treatment of Peyronie's disease. South Med J 1948;41: 173–7.

[30] Akkus E, Carrier S, Rehman J, et al. Is colchicine effective in Peyronie's disease? A pilot study. Urology 1994;44(2):291–5.

[31] Kadioglu A, Tefekli A, Koksal T, et al. Treatment of Peyronie's disease with oral colchicine: long-term results and predictive parameters of successful outcome. Int J Impot Res 2000;12(3):169–75.

[32] Zarafonetis CJ, Horrax TM. Treatment of Peyronie's disease with potassium para-aminobenzoate (potaba). J Urol 1959;81(6):770–2.

[33] Hasche-Klunder R. Treatment of peyronie's disease with para-aminobenzoacidic potassium (POTOBA) (author's transl). Urologe A 1978;17(4):224–7.

[34] Weidner W, Schroeder-Printzen I, Rudnick J, et al. Randomized prospective placebo-controlled therapy of Peyronie's disease (IPP) with Potaba* (aminobenzoate potassium). J Urol 1999;6(4 Suppl):205 [Abstr 785].

[35] Ralph DJ, Brooks MD, Bottazzo GF, et al. The treatment of Peyronie's disease with tamoxifen. Br J Urol 1992;70(6):648–51.

[36] Colletta AA, Wakefield LM, Howell FV, et al. Antioestrogens induce the secretion of active transforming growth factor beta from human fetal fibroblasts. Br J Cancer 1990;62(3):405–9.

[37] Teloken C, Rhoden EL, Grazziotin TM, et al. Tamoxifen versus placebo in the treatment of Peyronie's disease. J Urol 1999;162(6):2003–5.

[38] Biagiotti G, Cavallini G. Acetyl-L-carnitine vs tamoxifen in the oral therapy of Peyronie's disease: a preliminary report. BJU Int 2001;88(1):63–7.

[39] Kelly RB. Pathways of protein secretion in eukaryotes. Science 1985;230(4721):25–32.

[40] Aggeler J, Frisch SM, Werb Z. Changes in cell shape correlate with collagenase gene expression in rabbit synovial fibroblasts. J Cell Biol 1984;98(5):1662–71.

[41] Lee RC, Ping JA. Calcium antagonists retard extracellular matrix production in connective tissue equivalent. J Surg Res 1990;49(5):463–6.

[42] Martin DJ, Badwan K, Parker M, et al. Transdermal application of verapamil gel to the penile shaft fails to infiltrate the tunica albuginea. J Urol 2002; 168(6):2483–5.

[43] Teasley GH. Peyronie's disease a new approach. J Urol 1954;71(5):611–4.

[44] Bodner H, Howard AH, Kaplan JH. Peyronie's disease: cortisone-hyaluronidase-hydrocortisone therapy. J Urol 1954;72:400–31.

[45] Winter CC, Khanna R. Peyronie's disease: results with dermo-jet injection of dexamethasone. J Urol 1975;14:898–900.

[46] Williams G, Green NA. The non-surgical treatment of Peyronie's disease. Br J Urol 1980;52:392–5.

[47] Gelbard MK, Walsh R, Kaufman JJ. Collagenase for Peyronie's disease: experimental studies. Urol Res 1982;10:135–40.

[48] Gelbard MK, Lindner A, Kaufman JJ. The use of collagenase in the treatment of Peyronie's disease. J Urol 1985;134:280–3.

[49] Gelbard MK, James K, Riach P, et al. Collagenase versus placebo in the treatment of Peyronie's disease: a double-blind study. J Urol 1993;149(1):56–8.

[50] Levine LA, Merrick PF, Lee RC. Intralesional verapamil injection for the treatment of Peyronie's disease. J Urol 1994;151(6):1522–4.

[51] Rehman J, Benet A, Melman A. Use of intralesional verapamil to dissolve Peyronie's disease plaque: a long-term single-blind study. Urology 1998;51(4):620–6.

[52] Levine LA, Goldman KE, Greenfield JM. Experience with intraplaque injection of verapamil for Peyronie's disease. J Urol 2002;168(2):621–5.

[53] Duncan MR, Berman B, Nseyo UO. Regulation of the proliferation and biosynthetic activities of cultured human Peyronie's disease fibroblasts by interferons-alpha, -beta and -gamma. Scand J Urol Nephrol 1991;25(2):89–94.

[54] Wegner HE, Andresen R, Knispel HH, et al. Treatment of Peyronie's disease with local interferon-alpha 2b. Eur Urol 1995;28(3):236–40.

[55] Wegner HE, Andresen R, Knispel HH, et al. Local interferon-alpha 2b is not an effective treatment in early-stage Peyronie's disease. Eur Urol 1997;32(2):190–3.

[56] Judge IS, Wisniewski ZS. Intralesional interferon in the treatment of Peyronie's disease: a pilot study. Br J Urol 1997;79(1):40–2.

[57] Ahuja S, Bivalacqua TJ, Case J, et al. A pilot study demonstrating clinical benefit from intralesional interferon alpha 2B in the treatment of Peyronie's disease. J Androl 1999;20(4):444–8.

[58] Dang G, Matern R, Bivalacqua TJ, et al. Intralesional interferon-alpha-2B injections for the treatment of Peyronie's disease. South Med J 2004;97(1):42–6.

[59] Hellstrom W, Eichelberg C, Pryor JL, et al. A single-blind, multi-center, placebo-controlled study to assess the safety and efficacy of intralesional interferon alpha-2b in the non-surgical treatment of Peyronie's disease. J Urol 2003;169(4 Suppl):274 [Abstr 1065].

[60] Levine LA. Review of current nonsurgical management of Peyronie's disease. Int J Impot Res 2003;15(Suppl 5):S113–20.

[61] Manikandan R, Islam W, Srinivasan V, et al. Evaluation of extracorporeal shock wave therapy in Peyronie's disease. Urology 2002;60(5):795–9.

[62] Lebret T, Loison G, Herve JM, et al. Extracorporeal shock wave therapy in the treatment of Peyronie's disease: experience with standard lithotriptor (siemens-multiline). Urology 2002;59(5):657–61.

[63] Hauck EW, Altinkilic BM, Ludwig M, et al. Extracorporeal shock wave therapy in the treatment of Peyronie's disease. First results of a case-controlled approach. Eur Urol 2000;38(6):663–9.

[64] Riedl CR, Plas E, Engelhardt P, et al. Iontophoresis for treatment of Peyronie's disease. J Urol 2000;163(1):95–9.

[65] Montorsi F, Salonia A, Guazzoni G, et al. Transdermal electromotive multi-drug administration for Peyronie's disease: preliminary results. J Androl 2000;21(1):85–90.

[66] Di Stasi SM, Giannantoni A, Capelli G, et al. Transdermal electromotive administration of verapamil and dexamethasone for Peyronie's disease. BJU Int 2003;91(9):825–9.

[67] Di Stasi SM, Giannantoni A, Stephen RL, et al. A prospective, randomized study using transdermal electromotive administration of verapamil and dexamethasone for Peyronie's disease. J Urol 2004;171(4):1605–8.

[68] Levine LA, Estrada CR, Shou W, et al. Tunica albuginea tissue analysis after electromotive drug administration. J Urol 2003;169(5):1775–8.

[69] Levine LA, Sevier VL. A double-blind, placebo-controlled trial of electromotive drug administration (EMDA) using verapamil vs. saline for Peyronie's disease: preliminary results. J Urol 2003;169(4 Suppl):274–5 [Abstr 1066].

[70] Ojingwa JC, Isseroff RR. Electrical stimulation of wound healing. J Invest Dermatol 2003;121(1):1–12.

[71] Prieto Castro RM, Leva Vallejo ME, Regueiro Lopez JC, et al. Combined treatment with vitamin E and colchicine in the early stages of Peyronie's disease. BJU Int 2003;91(6):522–4.

[72] Mirone V, Palmieri A, Granata AM, et al. Ultrasound-guided ESWT in Peyronie's disease plaques. Arch Ital Urol Androl 2000;72(4):384–7.

[73] Mirone V, Imbimbo C, Palmieri A, et al. Our experience on the association of a new physical and medical therapy in patients suffering from induratio penis plastica. Eur Urol 1999;36(4):327–30.

[74] Cavallini G, Biagiotti G, Koverech A, et al. Oral propionyl-l-carnitine and intraplaque verapamil in the therapy of advanced and resistant Peyronie's disease. BJU Int 2002;89(9):895–900.

[75] Levine LA, Greenfield JM. Establishing a standardized evaluation of the man with Peyronie's disease. Int J Impot Res 2003;15(Suppl 5):S103–12.

ELSEVIER
SAUNDERS

Urol Clin N Am 32 (2005) 479–485

UROLOGIC
CLINICS
of North America

Surgical Treatment of Peyronie's Disease

Chris Tornehl, MD*, Culley C. Carson, MD

*Division of Urology, University of North Carolina–Chapel Hill, 2140 Bio informatics Building,
Chapel Hill, NC 27599-7235, USA*

Peyronie's Disease (PD) afflicts middle-aged men resulting in an acquired plaque-induced penile deformity. Plaque formation on the tunica albuginea can cause penile curvature, indentation, or hour-glass shape. The prevalence of PD is 3.2% among men, mainly occurring in Caucasians with a mean age of 57.4 years [1]. Symptoms include pain with erections, erectile dysfunction, inability to have intercourse secondary to penile deformity, and a palpable plaque. The etiology of PD is suspected to be from trauma to the penis leading to subtunical bleeding, inflammation, and fibrosis along the tunica albuginea and subsequent scar or plaque formation [2].

Various treatments are available for PD: oral medications, topical agents, intralesional injections, extracorporeal shock wave lithotripsy, and surgery have all been employed [3]. Understandably, most patients opt for conservative medical treatments before surgery, although medications frequently prove ineffective. Regardless of patient and physician choices in therapies, the ultimate treatment goal is a satisfactory erection for the patient and his partner for comfortable, successful coitus.

Surgery

PD regresses spontaneously in 13% of men, while progressing in 40% of untreated men and showing no change over time in 47% of men [4]. Penile deformity precluding intercourse or severe erectile dysfunction refractory to medical treatments is an indication for surgery in appropriate candidates. Timing of surgery is critical in achieving satisfactory results. PD involves both an active and quiescent phase. The active phase occurs with the onset of the PD, characterized by painful erections and evolving plaque, curvature, or deformity. The later quiescent phase is characterized by stable deformity, lack of pain, and possibly new onset erectile dysfunction. Surgery should be avoided during active PD, as the penile deformity evolves. Montorsi et al [5] recommend waiting at least 1 year from the onset of stable disease before surgery, finding that a large number of patients with stable disease for 6 months or less suffer recurrence postoperatively.

Three surgical categories exist for PD: tunica lengthening procedures, tunica shortening procedures, and implantation of penile prosthesis. Surgical choices for patients require individualization. Penile prosthesis implantation is reserved for men with refractory erectile dysfunction. Men with satisfactory erectile function with or without medications are candidates for tunica lengthening or shortening procedures. Tunica shortening procedures include Nesbit or modified Nesbit, and plication techniques and tunica lengthening procedures include plaque incision/excision and grafting.

Assessing a patient's erectile status is a key step in selecting the appropriate surgery. Potency may be determined by history, a phosphodiesterase-5 (PDE-5) inhibitor take-home test, or intracavernosal injection/Doppler ultrasound (ICI/DUS) examination. Reports of a rigid erection are sufficient to proceed with a tunica lengthening or shortening procedure. However, many men with PD have avoided sexual contact due to penile deformity, and are uncertain of their potency. In these individuals, a trial of PDE-5 inhibitors and subsequent follow-up reports on the adequacy of erections can be valuable in surgical decision making. When erectile status is unclear or erectile dysfunction (ED) is likely, ICI/DUS is helpful in

---

* Corresponding author.
 E-mail address: ctornehl@yahoo.com (C. Tornehl).

0094-0143/05/$ - see front matter © 2005 Elsevier Inc. All rights reserved.
doi:10.1016/j.ucl.2005.08.009

revealing abnormalities in penile hemodynamics, plaque location and size, and degree of curvature. Large calcified plaques are poor prognostic indicators for spontaneous resolution of PD or response to medications. Additionally, Montorsi et al [5] noted that DUS shows subclinical penile abnormalities and communicating vessels that could contribute to ED if transected during surgery. Severe hemodynamic anomalies should promote prosthesis implantation. Digital photography at the time of ICI/DUS or at home by patients can be valuable in determining the severity of PD, planning surgery, and counseling patients and partners.

Tunica lengthening procedures are appropriate in men with adequate erectile function, shorter penis, cuvature >45°, or hour-glass deformity. Meanwhile, tunica shortening procedures are indicated in men with good erectile function, adequate penile length, or curve <45°. Figure 1 reveals the University of North Carolina (UNC) algorithm for selecting treatment for PD [6].

Preoperative discussions should include patients' and partners' expectations, risks, and complications of surgery. Patient satisfaction will be greater if they have a realistic understanding of their postoperative symptoms and possible complications. The most frequent complications of

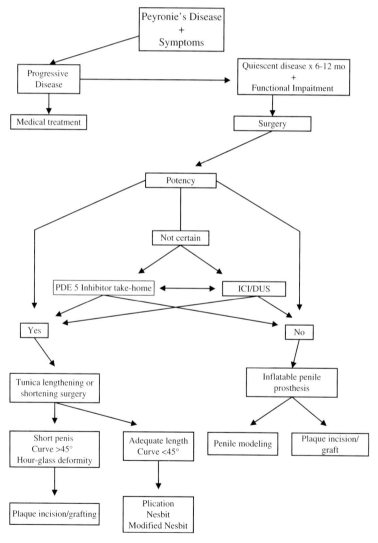

Fig. 1. The UNC algorithm for treatment of Peyronie's disease. *From* Tornehl CK, Carson CC. Surgical alternatives for treating Peyronie's disease. BJU Int 2004;94(6):774–83; with permission.

procedures are: penile shortening, glans hypoesthesia, ED, curve recurrence, and hematoma.
Further complications will be identified below.

Tunica shortening

*The Nesbit, modified Nesbit, and other plication
procedures*

The Nesbit procedure was first described in
1965 for treating congenital penile curvature
caused by corporal disproportion [7], and later applied to PD by Pryor and Fitzpatrick [8]. With this
procedure, the tunica opposite the Peyronie's
plauque and penile curvature is excised or plicated
to straighten the penis. An initial circumcision incision is made followed by degloving the penis. A
ventral incision may be used for ventral lexposure
in very proximal dorsal curvature. Longitudinal
penile shaft incisions should be avoided. Buck's
fascia is dissected from the tunica albuginea with
the corpus spongiosum in patients with dorsal
curvature or it is dissected off the neurovascular
bundles for ventral curvatures. An artificial erection is induced and the point of maximum curvature is marked on the convex side of the penis. A
5 to 10-mm transverse ellipse on the tunica albuginea may be excised in the classic Nesbit procedure
(~1 mm for every 10° of curvature). Rehman et al
[9] modified this technique by using a partial
thickness shaving of the tunica to avoid possible
bleeding and cavernosal injury. Next, the tunica
is closed watertight and horizontally using inter-
rupted, nonabsorbable, braided suture with buried knots. Absorbable suture may fail, allowing
the curvature to return. A circumcision is recommended in men with redundant foreskin due to
the increased risk for edema and phimosis postoperatively. An artificial erection is again induced
and if the penis is straight, Buck's fascia and the
skin are closed. If not adequately straight, subsequent plications or tunica incision/excision and
closure are necessary. Patients may be discharged
home the same day with this surgery, and should
avoid sexual activity for 6 weeks.

Yachia [10] modified the Nesbit procedure
making single or multiple 1 to 1.5-cm longitudinal
incisions along the convex side of the tunica,
which are subsequently closed horizontally, apply-
ing the Heineke-Mikulicz principle. Yachia felt his
modification would reduce injury to the neurovascular bundle and glans hypoesthesia, although
this complication is still possible. The authors prefer a longitudinal incision with horizontal closure

in the Heineke-Mikulicz technique as tunical de-
formities and palpable suture lines appear to be
fewer. Licht and Lewis [11] compared the Nesbit,
modified Nesbit, and tunical incision with grafting
and found the highest satisfaction rates (83%) and
lowest ED rates (0%) with the modified Nesbit.

Recent studies show patient satisfaction rates
for the Nesbit procedure between 75% to 88%
and rates of complete straightening between
61.9% to 82.1% [9,11–14]. Similar rates of satisfaction (78–83%) and straightening (93%) have
been found with Yachia's modification to the Nesbit procedure [10,15,16].

Despite these high satisfaction and straightening rates, penile shortening remains problematic
with the Nesbit, modified Nesbit, and plication
procedures. In a study involving 359 men, Pryor
reported shortening <1 cm in 86.6% of the men,
between 1 to 2 cm in 8.6% of the men, and >2 cm
in 4.7% of the men [12]. Similarly, in another
large study including 157 men, Savoca reported
shortening <1.5 cm in 86% of the men and between 1.5 to 3 cm in 14% of the men [13]. Pryor
argues that the degree of shortening rarely pre-
cludes sexual activity, only occurring in 1.7% of
men in his study [12]. Analyzing other studies,
the range for reported sexual dysfunction secondary to shortening is 1.3% to 11.9% for the Nesbit
and modified Nesbit procedures [11–14,16]. Complications with the procedures include: curve recurrence (7.7–10.6%), ED (0–22.9%), penile
induration or narrowing (0–16.7%), suture granu-
loma (0–1.9%), and glans hypoesthesia (0–21.4%)
[9–16]. Glans hypoesthesia is common postoperatively, although frequently resolves after several
months.

Plication

Plication of the tunica albuginea is the least
invasive technique for correction of PD, often
completed under local anesthetic. Gholami and
Lue [17] describe a plication method with a high
patient satisfaction rate. Following induction of
an artificial erection, a dorsal longitudinal or cir-
cumcising incision is made for ventral curvatures.
Longitudinal incisions are reserved for uncircum-
cised men desiring to keep their foreskin. Buck's
fascia is incised medial to the neurovascualar bundle and an intervascular space developed bluntly
between the dorsal vein and arteries. Nerve fibers
travel lateral to the dorsal arteries, so plication sutures may be placed in the developed space. For

men with a dorsal curvature, a ventral longitudinal incision is made down to dartos fascia overlying the corpus cavernosum. Sutures are placed 2 mm lateral to the corpus spongiosum. After marking the center of the curve and entry and exit sites for the plicating sutures, two to three pairs of 2-0 braided polyester sutures are placed through the tunica albuginea (four entry and exit points per suture). Van der Horst et al [18] found that polytetrafluoroethylene sutures result in significantly less patient complaints of discomfort than polypropylene sutures (13% versus 52%) using a similar plication technique. The sutures are gradually tied with one surgical knot placed and subsequent clamping. Once all plications are partly tied and clamped, the erect penis is examined. If the penis is straight, the knots are completed and buried, ideally under minimal tension. The Buck's or dartos fascia is then reapproximated and the skin closed. Patients are discharge on the same day of surgery.

Gholami and Lue report 85% of patients maintained a straight erection, while 15% suffered curve recurrence in a study of 124 patients at a mean follow-up of 2.6 years. Forty-one percent of patients in their series reported shortening from 0.5 to 1.5 cm, causing sexual dysfunction in 7% of patients. Twelve percent reported bothersome knots, 11% erectile pain, 9% penile indentation, 6% glans hypoesthesia, and 6% worsened ED [17]. Results vary for plication procedures, with straightening rates ranging from 57% to 85% and satisfaction rates ranging from 58% to 82% [17,19–23]. Cahall et al [19] reported significantly worse outcomes than Gholami and Lue, with 57% of patients reporting a deterioration in their quality of life, 55% with severe penile shortening, 48% with glans hypoesthesia, and 34% with bothersome nodules.

Tunica lengthening procedures

Plaque incision/excision with placement of grafts has been used for patients with severe penile curvature, complex or hour-glass deformity, or in men with a shortened penis from PD. In 1950, Lowsley and Boyce [24] first reported a series in patients with PD who underwent plaque excision with a fat graft but no report of follow-up. Various materials have since been applied including dermis [25], temporalis fasica [26], vein [5,27–30], cadaveric or bovine pericardium [31–33], duramater [34], synthetic material [11], and porcine

small intestine submucosa (SIS) [35]. The ideal graft should be: pliable, easy to handle, packaged in various sized, good tensile strength, low inflammatory response, low patient morbidity, low risk of disease transmission, and low cost. At UNC, we employ the use of porcine SIS (Cook Urological, Inc., Spencer, Indiana) as described by Knoll. SIS is processed into a reliably packaged, acellular matrix, consistent in thickness and compliance. One drawback for the use of SIS is that Jewish and Muslim patients may not accept a porcine graft materials for religious reasons. Synthetic materials, such as Dacron and GoreTex, may cause increased postoperative inflammation leading to fibrosis. Licht and Lewis [11] reported poor patient satisfaction with synthetic grafts. Sampaio et al [34] report 95% of the men achieved a straight penis with duramater; however, this material has not been widely accepted because of concerns for prion transmission. Although rare, the media have increased the concern regarding human tissues and prion transmission. Use of vein grafts is well documented, with good results ranging from 60% to 95% straightening and 88% to 92% satisfaction [5,27–30], although these risk harvest-site infection, lymphatic leak, and require longer operative time. Begun with the deep dorsal penis vein, more recent vein grafts have used the saphenous vein. Use of a vein requires creation of a patchwork graft to fill larger tunical defects. Although we prefer SIS, no material has emerged as the superior graft.

The procedure begins with an artificial erection to assess penile curvature. For dorsal plaques, a circumcision incision and degloving of the penis is performed. Ventral plaques are accessed via a direct incision longitudinally over the plaque. These incisions are only appropriate if performed ventrally. The neurovascular bundles, located lateral to the dorsal arteries of the penis, should be carefully avoided. The plaque can be approached through the bed of the deep dorsal vein with venous ligation 1 cm proximal and distal to the plaque and excised between. Bucks fascia can also be incised at the 3 and 9 o'clock positions and dissected to retract the neurovascular area from the plaque. Buck's fascia and the contained dorsal penile nerves are then elevated. A relaxing H-shaped incision is then made in the plaque with subsequent grafting, a technique described by Lue and El-Sakka [36]. Egydio [37] describes a "tripod-shaped forks of 120°" incision to produce a geometrically optimal relaxing tunical defect for easy graft suturing. The incision resembles end-on-end Mercedes-Benz emblems. Larger or calcified plaques may require complete excision. The SIS graft is cut 20% larger than the measured defect and sutured to the tunica with a running locking 4-0 PDS suture. An artificial erection is induced to check straightening and when necessary; plications are placed on the contralateral side of the penis to correct any residual curvature. Large residual curves may require a second incision and grafting. After straightening is achieved, Buck's fascia and the skin are closed. A penile block is injected, a fine suction drain is kept beneath the skin overnight, and the patient is discharged the following morning. Ice is maintained on the operative site for 48 to 72 hours.

Patients are discharged home on nightly diazepam to prevent nocturnal erections, and amyl nitrate may be used as needed to prevent erections for 2 weeks following surgery. Patients are advised to avoid sexual activity for 6 weeks following surgery for adequate healing. If patients experience mild curvature recurrence in the postoperative period, a vacuum device is employed twice daily for 10 minutes without the constriction device once the patient has recovered from surgery.

Reported satisfaction and straightening rates vary widely. Complications include worsening erectile dysfunction with most studies reporting 0% to 15% [5,11,27–35], although this often takes up to 6 months to improve and may require assistance with a vacuum device or PDE-5 inhibitors. Because this "penile shock" is expected in most patients, the authors use a PDE-5 inhibitor for 6 to 9 months following surgery. Other complications include penile shortening (0–40%), glans and penile hypoesthesia (0–16.7%), curve recurrence (0–16.7%), and hematoma [5,11,27–35]. Although the risk for penile shortening is less with these procedures, patients still need to be warned of this outcome. Yurkanin [29] reported average penile lengthening of 2.1 cm. Interestingly, over half the patients in this study reported subjective shortening.

Penile prosthetic implantation

Severe erectile dysfunction and PD is best treated with implantation of an inflatable penile prosthesis. The previously discussed tunica lengthening and shortening procedures may provide a straight penis, although a completely impotent patient will not benefit if ED is severe and PDE-5 inhibitors do not resolve ED.

Montorsi et al [38] found that implantation of a semirigid prosthesis in men with PD had very poor 5-year patient (48%) and partner (40%) satisfaction rates despite a high satisfaction rate (90%) at 3 months. Complaints included poor erection quality and girth with erections, unnatural sensation, and partner pain. Meanwhile, these and other authors report good results with inflatable penile prosthesis, with patient satisfaction rates ranging from 75% to 93% [33,39,40].

Following penile prosthesis implantation, patients with continued curvature should be treated with modeling, plaque incision and grafting, or a modified Nesbit. Wilson and Delk [41] first described modeling in a large 138-patient retrospective study. Before pump placement in the scrotum, the cylinders are distended maximally and the connector tubings to the pump are clamped to prevent excessive back-pressure. Additionally, pressure is placed over the corporotomies to protect the sutures. The penis is bent manually for 90 seconds directly opposite the curve. This results in plaque splitting and often an audible crack. Wilson and Delk [41] reported this technique as being successful in 118 of 138 patients, avoiding plaque incision and grafting. They also reported that modeling was associated with greater postoperative pain, swelling, and possibly related to urethral perforation in four patients. Carson described the technique in 28 of 30 patients, none of whom suffered complications from modeling at a mean follow-up of 31.4 months [42]. The remaining two patients in this study required plaque incision and grafting. Chaudhary et al [39] reported the use of modeling in 28 of 46 patients undergoing prosthesis implantation for PD. The remaining 18 patients achieved adequate straightening merely with the prosthetic implantation. Furthermore, a recent study showed slightly higher patient (88% versus 81%) and partner (80% versus 72%) satisfaction rates for modeling versus corporoplasty with insertion of inflatable penile prosthesis [33]. AMS 700CX and Mentor alpha-1 prostheses are optimal for patients with PD because these higher pressure cylinders provide adequate rigidity to straighten the penis across the Peyronie's plaque.

Complications of inflatable penile prosthesis implantation such as infection and device breakdown are not more common in men with PD. As mentioned above, 4 of 138 patients in Wilson and Delk's study suffered urethral perforation possibly linked to modeling, although none of the patients in Carson's or Chaudhary's reports experienced this complication [39,41,42]. Regardless, all men undergoing prosthetic implantation should be warned of risks for infection and device malfunction before surgery.

Summary

PD is a sexually debilitating disease resulting in significant psychologic stress for many men. Urologists have an opportunity to help men suffering from PD to improve their lives. Appropriate treatment should be individualized and tailored to the patient's expectations, disease history, physical examination findings, and erectile function. This review is intended to share the experiences of other urologists in the surgical approach to PD.

References

[1] Schwarzer U, Sommer F, Klotz T, et al. The prevalence of Peyronie's disease: result of a large survey. BJU Int 2001;88:727–30.

[2] Devine CJ Jr, Somers KD, Jordan SG, et al. Proposal; trauma as cause of Peyronie's lesion. J Urol 1997;157:285–90.

[3] Gholami SS, Gonzalez-Cadavid NF, Lin CS, et al. Peyronie's disease: a review. J Urol 2003;169: 1234–41.

[4] Gelbard MK, Dorey F, James K. The natural history of Peyronie's disease. J Urol 1990;144:1376–9.

[5] Montorsi F, Salonia A, Maga T, et al. Evidence based assessment of long-term results of plaque incision and vein grafting for Peyronie's disease. J Urol 2000;163:1704–8.

[6] Tornehl CK, Carson CC. Surgical alternatives for treating Peyronie's disease. BJU Int 2004;94:774–83.

[7] Nesbit RM. Congenital curvature of the phallus: report of thre cases with description of corrective operation. J Urol 1965;93:230–2.

[8] Pryor JP, Fitzpatrick JM. A new approach to correction of the penile deformity in Peyronie's disease. J Urol 1979;122:622–3.

[9] Rehman J, Benet A, Minsky LS, et al. Results of surgical treatment for abnormal penile curvature: Peyronie's disease and congenital deviation by modified Nesbit plication. J Urol 1997;157:1288–91.

[10] Yachia D. Modified corporoplasy for the treatment of penile curvature. J Urol 1990;143:80–2.

[11] Licht MR, Lewis RW. Modified Nesbit procedure for the treatment of Peyronie's disease: a comparative outcome analysis. J Urol 1997;158:460–3.

[12] Pryor JP. Correction of penile curvature in Peyronie's disease: why I prefer the Nesbit technique. Int J Impot Res 1998;10:129–31.

[13] Savoca G, Thrombetta C, Ciampalini S, et al. Long-term results with Nesbit's procedure as treatment of Peyronie's disease. Int J Impot Res 2000;12:289–93.

[14] Syed AH, Abbasi Z, Hargreave TB. Nesbit procedure for disabling Peyronie's curvature: a median follow up of 84 months. Urology 2003;61: 999–1003.

[15] Daitch JA, Angermeier KW, Montague DK. Modified corporoplasty for penile curvature: long term results and patient satisfaction. J Urol 1999;162: 2006–9.

[16] Sulaiman MN, Gingell JC. Nesbit's procedure for penile curvature. J Androl 1994;15(suppl):54S–6S.

[17] Gholami SS, Lue TF. Correction of penile curvature using the 16-dot plication technique: a review of 132 patients. J Urol 2002;167:2066–9.

[18] van der Horst C, Martinez-Portillo FJ, Melchior D, et al. Polytetrafluoroethylene versus polyproplylene sutures for Essed-Schroeder tunical plication. J Urol 2003;170:472–5.

[19] van der Drift DG, Vroege JA, Groendijk PM, et al. The plication procedure for penile cuvature: surgical outcome and postoperative sexual functioning. Urol Int 2002;69:120–4.

[20] Chahal R, Gogoi NK, Sundaram SK, et al. Corporal plication for penile curvature caused by Peyronie's disease: the patient's perspective. BJU Int 2001;87: 352–6.

[21] Thiounn N, Missirliu A, Zerbib M, et al. Corporal plication for surgical correction of penile curvature of penile curvature: experience with 60 patients. Eur Urol 1998;33:401–4.

[22] Geertsen UA, Brok KE, Andersen B, et al. Penile curvature treated by plication of the penile fascia. BJU 1996;77:733–5.

[23] Nooter RI, Bosch JL, Schroeder FH. Peyronie's disease and congenital penile curvature: long-term results of operative treatment with the plication procedure. BJU 1994;74:497–500.

[24] Lowsley O, Boyce W. Further experience to cure Peyronie's disease. J Urol 1950;63:888.

[25] Devine CJ, Horton CE. The surgical treatment of Peyronie's disease with a dermal graft. J Urol 1974; 111:44–9.

[26] Gelbard MK. Relaxing incisions in the correction of penile deformity due to Peyronie's disease. J Urol 1995;154:1457–60.

[27] El-Sakka AL, Rashawn HM, Lue TF. Venous patch graft for Peyronie's disease. Part II: outcome analysis. J Urol 1998;160:2050–3.

[28] Backhaus BO, Muller SC, Albers P. Corporoplasty for advanced Peyronie's disease using venous and/ or dermis patch grafting: new surgical technique and longterm patient satisfaction. J Urol 2003;169: 981–4.

[29] Yurkanin JP, Dean R, Wessells H. Effect of incision and saphenous vein grafting for Peyronie's disease on penile length and sexual satisfaction. J Urol 2001;166:1769–73.

[30] Adenyi AA, Goorney SR, Pryor JP, et al. The Lue procedure: an analysis of the outcome in Peyronie's disease. BJU Int 2002;89:404–8.

[31] Egydio PH, Lucon AM, Arap S. Treatment of Peyronie's disease by incomplete circumferential incision of the tunica albuginea and plaque with bovine pericardium. Urology 2002;59:570–4.

[32] Chun JL, McGregor A, Krishan R, et al. A comparison of dermal and cadaveric pericardial grafts in the modified Horton-Devine procedure for Peyronie's disease. J Urol 2001;166:185–8.

[33] Usta MF, Bivalacqua TJ, Sanabria J, et al. Patient and partner satisfaction and longterm results after surgical treatment for Peyronie's disease. Urology 2003;62:105–9.

[34] Sampaio JS, Fonesca J, Passarinho A, et al. Peyronie's disease: surgical correction of 40 patients with relaxing incision and duramater graft. Eur Urol 2002;41:551–5.

[35] Knoll LD. Use of porcine small intestinal submucosa graft in the surgical management of Peyronie's disease. Urology 2001;57:753–7.

[36] Lue TF, El Sakka AL. Venous patch graft for Peyronie's disease. Part I. technique. J Urol 1998;160:2047–9.

[37] Egydio PH, Lucon AM, Sami A. A single relaxing incision to correct different types of penile curvature: surgical technique based on geometrical principles. BJU Int 2004;94:1147–57.

[38] Montorsi F, Guazzoni G, Bergamashci F, et al. Patient–partner satisfaction with semi-rigid penile prosthesis for Peyronie's disease: a 5-year follow-up study. J Urol 1993;150:1819–21.

[39] Chaudhary M, Sheikh N, Asterling S, et al. Peyronie's disease with erectile dysfunction: penile modeling over inflatable penile prosthesis. Urology 2005;65:760–4.

[40] Montorsi F, Guazzoni G, Barbieri L, et al. AMS 700 CX inflatable penile implants for Peyronie's disease: functional results, morbidity and patient–partner satisfaction. Int J Impot Res 1996;8:81–6.

[41] Wilson SK, Delk JR. A new treatment for Peyronie's disease: modeling the penis over an inflatable penile prosthesis. J Urol 1994;152:1121–3.

[42] Carson CC. Penile prosthesis implantation in the treatment of Peyronie's disease. Int J Impot Res 1998;10:125–8.

ELSEVIER
SAUNDERS

Urol Clin N Am 32 (2005) 487–501

UROLOGIC
CLINICS
of North America

Central Nervous System Agents in the Treatment of Erectile Dysfunction

Muammer Kendirci, MD, Melissa M. Walls, MD,
Wayne J.G. Hellstrom, MD, FACS*

*Department of Urology, Tulane University, Health Sciences Center, 1430 Tulane Avenue,
SL-42, New Orleans, LA 70112, USA*

A fully rigid erection is the end result of cavernosal smooth muscle relaxation in the penis. This process is mediated by a spinal reflex process and involves the central nervous system (CNS), integrating numerous tactile, olfactory, auditory, and mental stimuli; various central neurotransmitters participate in its modulation. Autonomic and somatic efferent nerve fibers also receive contributions from the peripheral nervous system. A balance between contractile and relaxing influences controls the degree of tone in the penile vasculature and cavernosal smooth muscle, and determines the functional state of the penis, ranging between complete detumescence to a full erection [1].

The evolution of basic concepts of erectile physiology and a better understanding of the pathophysiologies underlying erectile dysfunction (ED) in recent decades have produced several pharmacologic approaches for the treatment of ED. The recognized efficacy of certain oral erectogenic agents with peripheral (phosphodiesterase type-5 [PDE5] inhibitors) and CNS (apomorphine) sites of action has motivated researchers to investigate the mechanisms of penile erection further. One can anticipate that as our appreciation of the CNS pathways involved in the genesis of ED expands, CNS-based therapies will become more common.

Using animal models, a significant database has been established regarding neurotransmission, impulse propagation, and intracellular transduction of neural signals to induce cavernosal smooth muscle relaxation. These studies have identified several putative CNS agents for the potential therapy of ED. Overall, current PDE5-inhibitor therapy has been efficacious in 40% to 90% of patients, depending on the etiology and duration of ED. Comparatively, patients with a history of pelvic surgery (eg, radical prostatectomy) and diabetes mellitus show a reduced responsivity to this class of drugs (40%–65%); hence the need to develop, support, and evaluate further novel alternatives for the treatment of ED, specifically CNS agents [2–5].

This article reviews the current understanding of central mechanisms involved in penile erection and focuses on various CNS-based agents for the treatment of ED (Fig. 1).

Dopamine

Central dopaminergic neurons comprise the incertohypothalamic system that connects the medial preoptic area (MPOA) and the paraventricular nucleus (PVN) to the lumbosacral spinal cord [6]. Dopaminergic receptors, D_1-like (D_1 and D_5) and D_2-like (D_2, D_3 and D_4), are postulated to regulate the central relay components of the autonomic and somatic penile reflex arc [1]. The D_2 receptor is responsible for many behavioral effects of dopamine, including stretching, yawning, and penile erection. The injection of apomorphine, a dopamine D_1/D_2 agonist, into the MPOA and

* Corresponding author.
  E-mail address: whellst@tulane.edu
(W.J.G. Hellstrom).

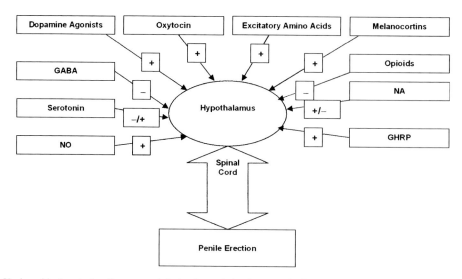

Fig. 1. Various biochemical pathways modulating hypothalamic control of penile erection and sexual behavior. Serotonin facilitates penile responses through 5-HT$_{1C}$ receptors and inhibts sexual behavior through 5-HT$_{1A}$ receptors. Excitatory amino acids, N-methyl-D-aspartate, L-aspartate; GABA, gamma aminobutyric acid; GHRP, growth hormone–releasing peptide; NA, noradrenalin (α_1-AR produces stimulation; α_1-AR inhibits sexual behavior); NO, nitric oxide.

PVN facilitates sexual function and causes the stretching/yawning/penile erection response [7,8]. In the MPOA, dopaminergic transmission mediates erectile responses mainly through D$_1$ receptors, whereas in the PVN, D$_2$ receptors are the primary facilitators of penile erection [8–10].

Penile erections induced by paraventricular D$_2$-receptor stimulation can be blocked by oxytocin antagonists and by electrical lesions of the PVN that deplete central oxytocin content. Hence, D$_2$-receptor stimulation is recognized to function through the oxytocinergic pathway [11,12]. Furthermore, nitric oxide (NO) also is involved in dopaminergic transmission because subcutaneous administration of apomorphine increases nitric oxide synthase (NOS) and NO production in the PVN. As expected, NO concentration and erectile response to apomorphine can be attenuated by NOS inhibition [13]. Intrathecal administration of apomorphine promotes erections in normal male rats and in spinalized animals, suggesting that the dopaminergic system can induce penile erections at supraspinal and spinal levels [14,15].

Apomorphine

Apomorphine, a D$_1$/D$_2$ postsynaptic dopamine receptor agonist, can induce penile erections in male rats, healthy men, and men who have ED through receptor activation in the hypothalamus

[7]. In 1984, Lal and colleagues [16] showed in a placebo-controlled, double-blind study in healthy volunteers that subcutaneous apomorphine (0.25–0.75 mg) could cause penile erection. Later, Danjou and colleagues [17] demonstrated that apomorphine could induce penile erections and potentiate erections induced by visual sexual stimulation. NO seems to be a necessary cofactor in this process [18]. These studies and observations led to the development of apomorphine as a therapeutic option for the treatment of ED.

Apomorphine is formed by the dehydration of morphine, but has no recognized opiate analgesic or addictive properties. In vivo rat studies reveal a supraspinal pathway for apomorphine action. In the rat, intracerebroventricular and subcutaneous injections of apomorphine at nanomolar doses induced penile erections, whereas intrathecal injections at 30× this dose had less efficacy. Haldol and clozapine, centrally acting dopamine antagonists, readily can inhibit the apopmorphine response, whereas domperidone, a periphally acting dopamine antagonist, cannot block this pathway.

Sublingual apomorphine has been marketed in the 2- and 3-mg doses in the European market. When administered through this route, it avoids first-pass metabolism with mean dissolution of the pill occurring in 7 minutes. Clearance is predominately through glucuronidation in the liver and its peak plasma concentration is reached at

15 to 20 minutes [19]. Studies show no tolerance to repeat administrations of apomorphine and no interaction with food, alcohol, or nitrates [20]. The effectiveness of apomorphine in causing erections was dose-dependent, and repeated injections have documented increasing responsiveness [21].

A double-blind, placebo-controlled, crossover study lasting 10 to 12 weeks in 252 volunteers who had ED assessed apomorphine at a dose of 2 mg; 10% more of the apomorphine-treated men achieved erections firm enough for intercourse compared with placebo ($P < .001$) [22]. The rate for completion of successful intercourse was also higher in the apomorphine group compared with placebo. In another double-blind, randomized, crossover study, Dula and colleagues [23] investigated the efficacy of apomorphine, 3 mg, with placebo in patients who had ED of various causes and degrees of severity. Apomorphine, 3 mg, was significantly more effective than placebo ($P < .001$) for the endpoints of erections firm enough for intercourse (49.9% versus 32.3%) and the completion-of-intercourse rate (48% versus 34%).

A dose-response effect was evident in another double-blind dose-escalation study in 507 randomized patients prescribed escalating doses of apomorphine versus placebo over 8 weeks. Forty-one percent of participants who received the 3-mg dose achieved successful intercourse in more than 50% of attempts, compared with 33% who received apomorphine, 2 mg [24]. Increasing the dose to 4 mg did not provide further efficacy. Buvat and colleagues [25] compared the 3- and 4-mg doses of apomorphine in a double-blind, crossover study but observed no statistically significant difference in either the proportion of erections firm enough for penetration (49.4% versus 50.2%; $P > .4$) or completion of intercourse rate (48.4% versus 49.6%; $P > .4$). Another multicenter, uncontrolled, open-label, phase-III dose-optimization study of apomorphine in 849 men who had ED documented at least a 20% increase in the number of successful sexual encounters compared with baseline [26].

It is important to comment on the rapid onset of action in patients taking apomorphine. Dula and colleagues [27] showed that 34% of responders to apomorphine exhibit penile erection within the first 10 minutes of administration and 37% in the second 10 minutes. Thus, in patients who are apomorphine-responsive, 71% responded in the first 20 minutes.

With the advent of PDE5 inhibitors, several studies have compared the efficacies of apomorphine and sildenafil. Perimenis and colleagues [28] evaluated 40 men who had ED in a prospective, unblinded, two-arm, crossover study. The overall success for sexual encounters with apomorphine was 62.7%, whereas it was 73.1% with sildenafil. Another similar study documented the overall success, regardless of dose, as 63.7% and 32.1% for sildenafil and apomorphine, respectively [29]. These investigators noted that the response in arteriogenic ED was 76% for sildenafil and only 14% for apomorphine. In this study, 80% of the study participants titrated their doses of apomorphine from 2 mg to 3 mg, whereas 58% of men remained at the initial 50-mg dose of sildenafil [29]. In an open-label, randomized, flexible-dose comparison of apomorphine to sildenafil over an 18-week period with a 2-week washout, there was a 75% success rate for sildenafil and 35% for apomorphine [30]. Of the 117 men in this study, 90% preferred sildenafil over apomorphine.

The predominant side effects documented with apomorphine are nausea, headache, yawning, and dizziness. In a multicenter, randomized, double-blind, parallel group study evaluating the safety and efficacy of sublingual apomorphine, 3 and 4 mg, the most common side effect was nausea in 9.8% [31]. Eighty-seven percent of participants completed the study, with only 1.2% discontinuing because of nausea. Other common side effects were dizziness (7.1%) and headache (6.7%). There was a marked increase in the incidence of treatment-related emergent nausea at the higher doses, escalating from 3.3% to 14.1%, demonstrating the overall benefit–to–adverse effect ratio favoring the lower 3-mg dose. Dose optimization at 3 mg causes nausea, headache, and dizziness rates below the 5% threshold [25].

Data from patients enrolled in long-term extension studies revealed that among those who received apomorphine 2 mg or 3 mg, 92% of attempts at intercourse resulted in sufficiently firm erections at 1 month and 90% after 6 months of treatment. The best efficacy results were reported in patients who had mild-to-moderate ED. To minimize the risk for adverse events, patients are instructed to initiate therapy at the 2-mg dose and repeat twice before titrating up to the 3-mg dose. Heaton and colleagues [24] maintain that maximal efficacy is achieved only if the final dose is attempted at least eight times.

There are no specific contraindications or interactions of apomorphine with alcohol, nitrates, or antihypertensive agents [25]. In individuals with severe renal insufficiency, the 2-mg dose is not to be exceeded, and because plasma concentrations of apomorphine are elevated significantly in patients with severe hepatic dysfunction, it must be prescribed with caution under these circumstances.

Apomorphine exhibits maximum efficacy in patients maintaining some residual erectile function at the time of diagnosis—especially in younger men and those with mild-to-moderate ED. For different pharmacodynamic (side effects) and pharmacokinetic reasons, however, apomorphine has exhibited limited therapeutic acceptance [32]. To circumvent some of apomorphine's limitations, researchers have developed an intranasal route of application to prolong its half-life and decrease its side-effect profile [33]. A combination of apomorphine and sildenafil also has been proposed, based on data from the rat model that document a synergistic increase in intracavernous pressure when using both agents together [34].

Serotonin

Serotonin (5-hydroxytriptamine, 5-HT) participates in the modulation of sexual behavior in animals and humans. Neurons containing serotonin involved in sexual function are localized to the supraspinal levels [35]. The bulbar spinal cord in the rat and cat is innervated heavily by bulbospinal neurons containing 5-HT [7]. Some 5-HT–containing fibers have synaptic connections with sacral preganglionic neurons and motoneurons [36]. Although 5-HT pathways exert a general inhibitory effect on male sexual behavior, some pathways can be either inhibitory or facilitatory, depending on the subtype of 5-HT receptor [37–39]. 5-HT_{1A}, 5-HT_{1B}, 5-HT_{2A}, and 5-HT_{2C} receptor subtypes are localized to different levels in the spinal cord [40,41]. 5-HT_{1A}–receptor stimulation inhibits erections, whereas 5-HT_{1C} and 5-HT_{2C} receptors facilitate this response [42–44]. Selective 5-HT_{2C} agonist–induced penile erection in studies with male rats suggests the integral role of the 5-HT_{2C} receptor in modulation of erection [45]. Elegant studies on these receptors implicate oxytocin and NO involvement in the 5-HT_{1C} receptor–mediated erectile responses [42,46].

Preliminary investigations with selective inhibitors of 5-HT uptake, such as trazodone, have reported improved erectile function [47]. The major metabolite of trazodone, m-chlorophenypiperazine (mCCP), displays agonist activity at the 5-HT_{2C} receptor and can induce erections and display spontaneous discharge from the cavernous nerves [48,49]. Trazodone and its metabolite, mCCP, also have been reported to exhibit α-antagonist activity on isolated human cavernosal tissue. When injected intracavernosally in men who have ED, it can induce penile erection [47]. Oral administration of trazodone has been associated with priapism, and increases nocturnal erections in healthy volunteers [50]. Despite these positive reports, evidenced-based studies have not shown a general benefit in most men having ED of various causes [51,52]. Recent reports with RSD 992, a 5-HT_{2C} receptor agonist, has documented proerectile activity and facilitated copulatory behavior [53]. The role of 5-HT_{2C} agonists on erectile function needs further investigation, because this receptor may become truly beneficial for the treatment of ED.

Noradrenaline

Noradrenergic neurons involved in penile erection arise from the A5 region and the locus coeruleus and project to nuclei in the spinal cord [15]. Noradrenergic neurotransmission exhibits activity on α_1- and α_2-adrenergic receptors (AR). Animal studies have suggested that increased central noradrenergic activity stimulates copulatory behavior through α_1-AR, whereas it suppresses sexual activity through α_2-AR [38]. Direct injection of clonidine, an α_2-AR agonist, into the MPOA suppresses sexual behavior in male rats, and this action can be inhibited by a selective α_2-AR antagonist [54]. Yohimbine, an α_2-AR antagonist, facilitates sexual behavior in male rats by increasing sexual motivation and reducing ejaculatory latency [35].

In a small group study using RigiScan monitoring [55], the clinical efficacy of yohimbine was evaluated in 18 nonsmoking men who had organic ED. Nine of these men (50%) were successful in completing intercourse in more than 75% of attempts. The yohimbine responders, however, had less severe ED, higher sexual function scores, and slightly higher levels of serum testosterone. In another study, the efficacy and safety of yohimbine therapy was evaluated in a double-blind, placebo-controlled, three-way crossover, randomized clinical trial to treat organic ED in 45 men, consisting of the combination of 6 g of L-arginine glutamate and 6 mg of yohimbine hydrochloride, 6 mg of yohimbine hydrochloride alone, and placebo [56]. Drugs were administered orally on-demand 1 to 2 hours before intended sexual intercourse, and the endpoint was assessed using the erectile function domain of the International Index of Erectile Function. The success rates evaluated by the investigators were reported as 35.6% in the L-arginine glutamate and yohimbine group, 26.7% in the yohimbine-alone group, and 13.3% in the placebo group. When stratified according to baseline scores, patients with erectile function domain scores of 14 or below showed no statistical difference among all three groups. In another prospective, randomized, controlled, double-blind, crossover study by Kuneilis and colleagues [57], a high dose of yohimbine did not establish clinical success over placebo for the treatment of ED.

Growth hormone–releasing peptide

Growth hormone–releasing peptides (GHRP) can affect erectile function. Two analogs of GHRP hexarelin, EP 60,761 and EP 50,885, when administered into the PVN of male rats, can induce penile erections similar to those caused by the dopamine receptor agonists, oxytocin and N-methyl-D-aspartate (NMDA) [58–60]. This beneficial effect on erectile function was observed irrespective of growth hormone release. The mechanisms of action of EP 60,761 and EP 50,885 on inducing erections are hypothesized to involve central oxytocinergic neurotransmission. Again, NOS producing NO in the cell bodies of oxytocinergic neurons in the PVN seems to be responsible for the activity of GHRP in producing erections.

Amino acids

Excitatory amino acids influence sexual behavior and penile erection. Studies have demonstrated that NMDA increases the number of penile erections and intracavernosal pressure when injected into the PVN [61–64]. As validation, the effects of NMDA can be blocked by intracerebroventricular administration of an oxytocin antagonist [62]. Increased concentration of NO metabolites in the PVN following administration of NMDA suggests that the NOS signal transduction pathway mediates the effect of NMDA on sexual behavior [65]. Further support

for this theory is that injection of NOS inhibitors into the PVN and intracerebroventricular area prevents the effect of NMDA [62,66]. L-glutamate also exhibits an effect on penile erection. Microinjection of L-glutamate into the MPOA causes increased intracavernosal pressure and penile erection [67].

In contrast, γ-aminobutyric acid (GABA) acts as an inhibitory amino acid on mediating penile erection in the autonomic and somatic reflex pathways [1]. GABAergic nerve fibers and receptors are localized to the sacral parasymphathetic nucleus and bulbocavernous motor nucleus [68,69]. High concentrations of GABA have been documented in the MPOA [70]. $GABA_A$ and $GABA_B$ receptors are responsible for the effects of GABA on erectile function. Studies in male rats have shown that $GABA_A$ agonists injected into the MPOA reduce copulatory behavior, whereas $GABA_A$ antagonists increase this activity [71,72]. Similarly, systemic or intrathecal administration of baclofen, a $GABA_B$ receptor agonist, decreased the number of penile erections in male rats [38].

The PVN also plays a role in mediating GABAergic neurotransmission. Stimulation of $GABA_A$ receptors in the PVN reduces penile erection and causes yawning, a response that is similar to those of apomorphine, NMDA, and oxytocin in male rats [73]. Excitatory and inhibitory amino acids play a role in erectile function and have potential as future treatments for ED.

Oxytocin

Oxytocin induces penile erection when injected into the PVN, lateral cerebral ventricle, or hypothalamus in animals [74–76]. Following sexual stimulation in humans, plasma levels of oxytocin are increased [77]. The effect of oxytocin on erectile activity can be blocked by oxytocin antagonists, electrical lesions of the PVN, and castration [12,76,78,79]. This inhibition on erectile function by low serum androgen levels can be restored readily by testosterone replacement.

Dopamine activates and opioid peptides inhibit the central neurotransmission of the oxytocinergic pathway [7]. Calcium functions as the second messenger in modulating oxytocin-mediated penile erections originating from the PVN [80]. Because inhibition of the NOS pathway prevents oxytocin-induced penile erections, the oxytocinergic signal transduction system is influenced strongly by NOS [81]. Although various centrally acting agents stimulate penile erection through oxytocinergic mechanisms, systemic administration of oxytocin fails to produce an erection in healthy young men [7]. Potential exploitation of the oxytocinergic system in the treatment of ED needs further exploration.

Opioid peptides

Because sexual behavior often is depressed in men with chronic opioid use, endogenous opioid peptides have been implicated in modulating sexual function [82]. This same observation has been documented in laboratory animals following chronic administration of opioids [83]. Morphine blocks noncontact penile erections and reduces copulatory behavior in male rats when injected into the PVN [84]. In addition, systemic injection or intracerebroventricular administration of morphine inhibits penile erections induced by the intracerebroventricular injection of oxytocin or subcutaneous dopamine [84]. The inhibitory effect of systemic morphine administration on erectile function can be blocked by the opioid antagonist naloxane [85]. Furthermore, reduced NO concentration in the PVN, inhibition of noncontact penile erections, and decreased copulatory behavior following morphine administration suggests that morphine somehow inhibits NO-mediated erections at the level of hypothalamus [85–87].

Nitric oxide

Aside from its crucial role in modulating penile erections in the periphery, NO is an important CNS neurotransmitter, specifically in the MPOA and PVN [46,88–90]. NOS inhibitors, when injected into the PVN or intracerebroventricularly, prevent penile erections induced by dopamine agonists, adrenocorticotropic hormone (ACTH), NMDA, and $5-HT_{2C}$ agonists [46,63,81,91–93]. Concomitant administration of L-arginine with NOS inhibitors, however, abolishes the effect of the NOS inhibitor. Another observation suggesting a central involvement of NO in penile erections is the increased production of NO in the PVN during noncontact penile erection and during increased sexual behavior in rats [94]. Furthermore, nitroglycerin, an NO donor, induces penile erections and yawning in the male rat following injection into the PVN. This mechanism involves central oxytocinergic neurotransmission in the PVN through a cyclic GMP–independent mechanism [92]. NO release in the MPOA, associated with copulatory behavior, supports a role of the MPOA in the regulation of centrally NO-mediated erectile function. In contrast to the intercellular modulatory effect of NO in the periphery, NO acts as an intracellular neurotransmitter to mediate erectile function in the PVN [46]. Distribution studies on NOS-containing neurons in the spinal cord suggest that NO plays a major role in spinal cord pathways, particularly preganglionic sympathetic and parasympathetic, somatosensory, visceral sensory, and possibly motor pathways [95–97]. These results confirm the physiologic role of NO in mediating penile erection at the level of the CNS. Potential modulation of central NO pathways in the regulation of penile erection for the treatment of ED has not been established clearly, however.

The melanocortin system

The melanocortin system consists of the melanocortin peptides (α-, β-, and γ-melanocyte-stimulating hormone [MSH]), ACTH, G protein–coupled melanocortin receptors (MCRs), melanocortin antagonists, and two ancillary proteins [98]. The melanocortins are involved in various physiologic functions, including pigmentation, steroidogenesis, energy homeostasis, exocrine secretions, analgesia, inflammation, immunomodulation, temperature control, cardiovascular regulation, neuromuscular regeneration, and sexual function. Given the important regulatory role in these functions, the development of melanocortin-based drugs is under consideration for the treatment of various disease states, including ED.

The melanocortins are tissue-specific post-translational products of the proopiomelanocortin (POMC) prohormone. The POMC gene is expressed primarily in the pituitary gland, arcuate nucleus of the hypothalamus, and nucleus of the solitary tract in the brain stem [98]. Furthermore, POMC mRNA and immunoreactivity have been documented in several peripheral human tissues, including the gastrointestinal tract, adrenal gland, spleen, lung, thyroid, immune system, and genitourinary tract [99]. POMC cleaving by prohormone convertases is tissue-specific, creating a mechanism for tissue selectivity for the action of a common prohormone.

In animals, neuropeptides have been implicated in the induction of penile erection and the regulation of sexual behavior [100]. The involvement of the melanocortin system in controlling sexual function was first reported in the 1960s by Ferrari and colleagues [101], when direct intraventricular injection of ACTH or α-MSH induced penile erections in dogs, rabbits, monkeys, and cats. After observing the unexpected erections in men receiving melanotan-II (MT-II) for tanning in a dermatologic study, a formal study for this MCR agonist was investigated in men who had ED [102]. Recently, microinjection of ACTH and α-MSH into distinct periventricular nuclei surrounding the third ventricle has produced penile erections in rats [103]. Among the five MCRs, penile erection seems to be mediated by MC4R and possibly MC3R [104]. MC4R expression has been demonstrated throughout the brain, particularly in the hypothalamus [105]. The role of MC4R in the hypothalamus and PVN is consistent with known erectile pathways defined by classic tracing techniques [103].

Receptor subtypes

Five G protein–coupled MCRs are defined, which are linked to cyclic AMP generation through the stimulatory G protein, G_s, and adenylate cyclase [99]. MCR signaling is associated with increased intracellular Ca^{2+} levels secondary to activation of inositol triphosphate [106], influx of extracellular Ca^{2+} [107], and protein kinase C pathways [108]. These receptors have different affinities for the melanocortins (Table 1). Only MC3R and MC4R are expressed in regions participating in the regulation of erectile function [98]. SHU9119, a synthetic peptide antagonist to MC3R and MC4R, abolishes MT-II–induced increases in intracavernous pressure [109]. In a mouse model, the role of tetrahydroisoquinolone

(THIQ), a highly selective MC4R agonist (> 500-fold selective for MC4R in binding assays and > 1000-fold selective in functional assays), in mediating the action of MC4R on erectile function and copulatory behavior was elucidated using electrical stimulation of the cavernous nerve (Table 2) [110]. THIQ augmented neurogenic-mediated intracavernosal pressure increases in wild-type mice but not in MC4R-null mice. In a behavioral model of sexual function, the absence of MC4R led to diminished copulatory behavior (mounting and intromission latency), whereas activation of MC4R agonists improved sexual function in wild-type mice for motivation and performance parameters.

MC4R mRNA has been demonstrated in the spinal cord and pelvic ganglion of male rats, and in the penis of male rats and humans, providing an anatomic basis for the effect of melanocortin on sexual function. Further characterizing the involvement of MC4R in erectile function, Martin and colleagues [111] demonstrated in the ex copula male rat model that THIQ exhibited marked increases in erectile activity. This was determined by increases in intracavernous pressure and the number of penile erections, following retraction of the preputial sheath. These proerectile effects were elicited by central and systemic administration of THIQ. THIQ increased the magnitude and number of erectile episodes in which intracavernous pressure remained above a predetermined threshold for more than 15 seconds, a requirement for penile erection. The duration of each interval recorded following THIQ treatment was significantly longer than that observed after vehicle treatment. Because central injection of the endogenous nonsubtype-specific MCR antagonist agouti-related protein (AgRP) and intravenous injection of MBP10, a MC4R antagonist, blocked the penile erections induced by intravenous THIQ administration, MC4R may mediate the effect of THIQ. In addition, these investigators showed

Table 1
Melanocortin receptors, ligand potencies, and physiologic functions

Receptor type	Potency of ligands	Function
MCR1	α-MSH=ACTH>β-MSH>γ-MSH	Inflammation, pigmentation
MCR2	ACTH	Steroidogenesis
MCR3	α-MSH=β-MSH=γ-MSH=ACTH	Energy homeostasis, erectile function (?)
MCR4	α-MSH=ACTH>β-MSH>γ-MSH	Energy homeostasis, erectile function
MCR5	α-MSH>ACTH>β-MSH>γ-MSH	Sebaceous gland secretion

Data from Gantz I, Fong TM. The melanocortin system. Am J Physiol Endocrinol Metab 2003;284(3):E468–74.

Table 2
Melanocortins and their receptor binding profiles

Melanocortin	Type	MCR binding profile	Potency (KI) for human MC4R	Selectivity ratio (MC3R:MC4R)[a]
α-MSH [134]	Endogenous peptide agonist	MC1R, MC3R, MC4R, MC5R	900 nM	0.04
ACTH [135]	Endogenous peptide agonist	MC1R, MC2R, MC3R, MC4R, MC5R	755 nM	0.04
MT-II [136]	Synthetic peptide agonist	MC1R, MC3R, MC4R, MC5R	6.6 nM	5.2
PT-141 [112]	Synthetic peptide agonist	MC1R, MC3R, MC4R	10.0 nM	?
THIQ [137]	Synthetic small molecule agonist	MC4R	1.2 nM	634
SHU9119 [134]	Synthetic peptide antagonist	MC3R, MC4R	0.4 nM	3.3
HS014 [114]	Synthetic peptide antagonist	MC1R, MC3R, MC4R, MC5R	3.2 nM	17.2
AgRP [124]	Endogenous peptide antagonist	MC3R, MC4R	2.6 nM	1.3
MB10 [125]	Synthetic peptide antagonist	MC4R	6.2 nM	125

[a] No Ki reported for PT-141 against MC3R [74].

Data from Martin WJ, MacIntyre DE. Melanocortin receptors and erectile function. Eur Urol 2004;45(6):706–13.

that MC4R-mediated erections required activation of central oxytocinergic pathways that modulate erectile activity.

Current data on experiments in mice and rats indicate that the affinities of the clinically effective MT-II and PT-141 are highest for MC4R, suggesting the importance of MC4R in penile erection (Table 2) [112,113]. Several studies, however, showed that the administration of a melanocortin MC4R antagonist, HS014, failed to block penile erections produced by α-MSH and ACTH or influence sexual behavior in rats [103,114–116]. Given the data on the MC4R-null mutant mouse that suggest MC4R activation is required for the pro-erectile effects of melanocortins, however, an incomplete blockade of MC4R by HS014 may account for the failure to block penile erections in the rat [117]. It is postulated that concomitant activation of MC3R, MC4R, and MC5R could be responsible for increasing erectile activity more than activation of the MC4R subtype alone.

Sites of action

The generation and modulation of penile erection requires the integration of information from supraspinal, spinal, and peripheral origins. Intravenous administration of ^{125}I-MT-II, similar in pharmacologic profile to MT-II, exhibits

limited brain penetration and predominantly labels circumventricular organs [118]. Inhibition of the specific binding of ^{125}I-MT-II by an MC4R agonist indicates that MC4R is the predominant MCR subtype expressed in the penis. Transcripts encoding MC4R were not identified in penile corpus cavernosal cells, however, suggesting that cavernosal smooth muscle cells were not the source of MC4R expression in the rat penis. Available data suggest that MCR activity in the penis does not act on cavernous smooth muscle, although the MC4R mRNA is localized to nerve fibers, nerve endings, and mechanoreceptors. Hence, MC4R agonists, such as MT-II and THIQ, do not have a relaxatory effect on cavernous smooth muscle strips and do not change intracavernous pressure when administered through direct injection [109,110]. Molecular studies using an NOS hybridization probe failed to demonstrate colocalization of NOS and MC4R [110]. These data indicate that MCR modulation of erectile function in the periphery is not mediated through a direct action on cavernosal smooth muscle cells, but rather through activation of peripheral proerectile pathways.

Vergoni and colleagues [115] demonstrated that intracerebroventricular injections of α-MSH and ACTH produced stretching, yawning, and penile erection. Binding studies have shown a potential for multiple sites of action for melano-cortins in the brain [119]. Receptor subtype–specific studies demonstrated that only MC3R and MC4R are expressed in the CNS regions related to the modulation of erectile function [120,121]. MCR expression, particularly MC4R, was especially dense in the hypothalamus [105].

Parallel to this localization of MCRs, micro-injection of α-MSH and ACTH into specific hypothalamic regions, including the PVN, reproduces stretching, yawning, and penile erections [103]. Intracerebroventricular administration of MT-II and PT-141 exhibits erections in male rats at 100- to 1000-fold lower doses than those required to produce erectile activity when administered systematically [112,122]. Given the inhibitory effect of L-NAME on α-MSH–induced penile erections in anesthetized rats, the supra-spinally mediated erectogenic effects of the melanocortin agonist may require NO [123]. Because intracerebroventricular administration of SHU9119, MC3R, and MC4R antagonists inhibits penile erection, activation of MC3R or MC4R may induce erectile activity [122]. This finding was characterized further by the intracere-broventricular administration of the endogenous nonsubtype-specific melanocortin receptor antagonist (AgRP) and the melanocortin MC4R-preferring antagonist (MBP10) that inhibits penile erections induced by intravenous administration of the MC4R-selective agonist, THIQ [124,125]. Collectively these data indicate that MCRs in the brain, particularly the MC4R subtype, modulate penile erection.

Mechanisms of action

The recognized modulatory effect of MCR agonists at the supraspinal, spinal, and peripheral levels raises the potential interactions of MCRs with the biochemical and pharmacologic pathways that control erectile function. Most studies have focused primarily on the role of oxytocin. Oxytocin plays an integral role in the modulation of erectile function and is a viable target for therapy of ED [126]. The presence of MCRs in the hypothalamus raises the possibility that oxytocin release is important in melanocortin-induced penile activity [127]. The effects of intracerebroven-tricular administration of α-MSH– and ACTH-induced penile erections and increased intracavernous pressure in anesthetized male rats, however, failed to be blocked by oxytocin antagonists [78,123]. On the contrary, Martin and colleagues

demonstrated that central and systemic adminis-tration of an oxytocin receptor antagonist, L-368899, significantly reduced the number of penile erections induced by MC4R agonists [111]. Data show that MT-II increases the number of penile erections and induces Fos expression in the hypothalamic nuclei, from which oxytocin is released. These findings suggest that oxyto-cinergic mechanisms may participate in MCR-mediated erectile function at the supraspinal level [118,122,128]. Furthermore, oxytocin and melano-cortins modulate erectile activity at the level of the spinal cord [122,129]. In contrast to oxytocin, cur-rent data on the role of the dopaminergic system in melanocortin-mediated erectile function are not available.

Preclinical studies

The main endogenous MCR agonists, ACTH and α-MSH, contain the amino acid sequence His-Phe-Arg-Trp, which is essential for the phar-macobiologic activity of melanocortins. The US Patent and Trademark Office reports on 21 di-rectly relevant issued patents regarding melano-cortins and sexual function. At least six pharmaceutical companies have direct involve-ment in melanocortin-based drug patents that have been issued in the last 4 years. The current synthetic analogs of the MC4R agonists, which are being investigated for their role in sexual function and dysfunction in animal and preclini-cal human studies, are MT-II, a cyclic peptide analog; PT-141, a cyclic heptapeptide analog; and THIQ, a highly selective small molecule MC4R agonist.

MT-II, the nonselective cyclic peptide analog of α-MSH, exhibits agonist activity at four of the five known MCRs (MC1R, MC3R, MC4R, and MC5R). In a double-blind, placebo-controlled, crossover study of 10 men having psychogenic ED using RigiScan monitoring, MT-II and saline vehicle were administered twice to each subject through a subcutaneous abdominal wall injection for a total of four injections (crossover). In 8 of the 10 subjects treated with MT-II, clinical erec-tions developed [130]. The mean duration of tip rigidity greater than 80% was 38 minutes with MT-II and 3 minutes with placebo ($P = .0045$). The mean time of onset to the first erection was approximately 2 hours (range 15–270 min). Tran-sient side effects of nausea, stretching, yawning, and decreased appetite were reported more frequently after injections of MT-II than placebo, none requiring treatment.

In another double-blind, placebo-controlled, crossover study in patients with organic risk factors for ED, including obesity, hypercholesterolemia, and hypertension, the effect of MT-II on erectile response was evaluated [131]. MT-II (0.025 mg/kg) and the vehicle were each administered twice, again by subcutaneous injection; real-time RigiScan monitoring and a visual analog scale were used to quantify the erections during the ensuing 6-hour period. The level of sexual desire and side-effect profile were recorded through a validated questionnaire. MT-II–initiated erections were witnessed in 12 of 19 injections (63.1%) versus only 1 of 21 doses with placebo (4.7%). The mean rigidity score of the responders was 6.9 on a scale of 0 to 10 and the mean duration of tip rigidity greater than 80% was 45.3 minutes with MT-II versus 1.9 minutes for placebo ($P = .047$). The level of sexual desire after injection of the agent was significantly higher in the MT-II group compared with placebo. Nausea, decreased appetite, and stretching/yawning occurred more frequently with MT-II. Of the 19 injections, four were associated with severe nausea (21%). This study demonstrates that the erectogenic properties of MT-II are not limited to cases of psychogenic ED; men with a variety of organic risk factors attained normal penile erections with this medication.

PT-141, a cyclic heptapeptide analog with high affinity for MC4R, is clinically effective in producing positive erectile effects [113]. Recently, subcutaneous injection of PT-141 (0.3–10 mg) was evaluated using RigiScan in healthy male subjects without sexual stimulation [132]. A statistically significant erectile response was documented at doses greater than 1 mg despite a lack of visual sexual stimulation. In the same study, sildenafil-responsive patients who had ED were subjected to visual sexual stimulation and monitored by RigiScan. The erectile response induced by PT-141 at 4- or 6-mg doses was statistically significant.

Further development of PT-141 for intranasal administration has been evaluated in similar phase-1 testing in healthy male subjects and phase-2a testing in patients who have ED who were sildenafil-responders [133]. The erectile response in these patients was assessed by RigiScan in healthy subjects with and without visual sexual stimulation. In healthy subjects, mean C_{max} and the area under the curve increased in a dose-dependent manner. The median C_{max} values measured were 14.9 (4 mg), 50.5 (7 mg), 90.1 (10 mg), and 140.5 (20 mg) ng/mL. The median T_{max} was 30 minutes and the mean $t_{1/2}$ ranged from 1.85 to 2.09 hours.

In both studies, the erectile response (rigidity and duration) induced by PT-141 was statistically significant compared with placebo at doses greater than 7 mg in a dose-dependent manner. The onset of the first erection occurred at approximately 30 minutes. PT-141 was safe and well tolerated in both studies. Flushing (up to 50%) and nausea (up to 33%) were the most common adverse events reported in doses greater than 7 mg. There were no clinically significant changes noted in vital signs, laboratory tests, electrocardiograms, and physical examinations. Given its central initiating activity for erections in the absence of sexual stimulation and tolerability profile, PT-141 is a candidate for further investigation as a potential therapy of ED.

When comparing the mechanisms of action of apomorphine and MCR agonists, there are some notable differences: (1) the PVN is required for apomorphine-induced erections, but not for ACTH [12]; (2) apomorphine is more effective when injected systemically or intraventricularly, whereas MT-II is more effective through spinal administration; and (3) apomorphine reduces latency times between erections, whereas melanocortins do not. The involvement of the oxytocinergic pathway is a necessary component of the signaling cascade for apomorphine-induced erections. There may be possible parallels to the actions of the melanocortins.

It is believed that melanocortin modulation of sexual function is caused by central and peripheral actions. Because melanocortin-mediated sexual function can be observed after peripheral administration of a selective MC4R agonist, these results document a role for the melanocortinergic pathways in mediating penile erections. These observations may lead to more efficacious melanotropin-based therapies for ED in the near future.

Summary

In the last two decades, a better understanding of the mechanisms governing erectile function and the pathophysiologies underlying ED have led researchers to investigate novel concepts for its treatment. Development of and commercial success with PDE5 inhibitors in the therapy of ED have spurred interest in new therapies for ED. All authorities recognize, however, the fundamental role of the CNS in mediating sexual behavior. Experiments with various animal models have advanced our understanding of the neuroanatomic and neuropharmacologic basis of centrally induced penile erections. Clinical research with apomorphine has demonstrated efficacy in men who have wide ranges of ED. Recent interest has focused on other centrally acting agents for ED treatment, including the melanocortin receptor agonists (MT-II and PT-141), which have shown promise in several preclinical studies. Further investigation of the CNS will continue to provide novel CNS-based agents for the potential treatment of sexual dysfunction.

References

[1] Andersson KE. Pharmacology of penile erection. Pharmacol Rev 2001;53(3):417–50.

[2] Padma-Nathan H, Steers WD, Wicker PA. Efficacy and safety of oral sildenafil in the treatment of erectile dysfunction: a double-blind, placebo-controlled study of 329 patients. Sildenafil Study Group. Int J Clin Pract 1998;52(6):375–9.

[3] Rendell MS, Rajfer J, Wicker PA, et al. Sildenafil for treatment of erectile dysfunction in men with diabetes: a randomized controlled trial. Sildenafil Diabetes Study Group. JAMA 1999;281(5):421–6.

[4] McCullough A, Woo K, Telegrafi S, et al. Is sildenafil failure in men after radical retropubic prostatectomy (RRP) due to arterial disease? Penile duplex Doppler findings in 174 men after RRP. Int J Impot Res 2002;14(6):462–5.

[5] Hatzichristou DG. Sildenafil citrate: lessons learned from 3 years of clinical experience. Int J Impot Res 2002;14(Suppl 1):S43–52.

[6] Bjorklund A, Lindvall O, Nobin A. Evidence of an incerto-hypothalamic dopamine neurone system in the rat. Brain Res 1975;89(1):29–42.

[7] Andersson KE, Wagner G. Physiology of penile erection. Physiol Rev 1995;75(1):191–236.

[8] Chen KK, Chan JY, Chang LS. Dopaminergic neurotransmission at the paraventricular nucleus of hypothalamus in central regulation of penile erection in the rat. J Urol 1999;162(1):237–42.

[9] Hull EM, Eaton RC, Markowski VP, et al. Opposite influence of medial preoptic D1 and D2 receptors on genital reflexes: implications for copulation. Life Sci 1992;51(22):1705–13.

[10] Markowski VP, Eaton RC, Lumley LA, et al. D1 agonist in the MPOA facilitates copulation in male rats. Pharmacol Biochem Behav 1994;47(3):483–6.

[11] Carter CS. Oxytocin and sexual behavior. Neurosci Biobehav Rev 1992;16(2):131–44.

[12] Argiolas A, Melis MR, Mauri A, et al. Paraventricular nucleus lesion prevents yawning and penile erection induced by apomorphine and oxytocin but not by ACTH in rats. Brain Res 1987;421(1–2):349–52.

[13] Melis MR, Succu S, Argiolas A. Dopamine agonists increase nitric oxide production in the paraventricular nucleus of the hypothalamus: correlation with penile erection and yawning. Eur J Neurosci 1996;8(10):2056–63.

[14] Giuliano F, Rampin O. Central neural regulation of penile erection. Neurosci Biobehav Rev 2000;24(5):517–33.

[15] Giuliano F, Rampin O. Central noradrenergic control of penile erection. Int J Impot Res 2000;12(S1):S13–9.

[16] Lal S, Ackman D, Thavundayil JX, et al. Effect of apomorphine, a dopamine receptor agonist, on penile tumescence in normal subjects. Prog Neuropsychopharmacol Biol Psychiatry 1984;8(4–6):695–9.

[17] Danjou P, Alexandre L, Warot D, et al. Assessment of erectogenic properties of apomorphine and yohimbine in man. Br J Clin Pharmacol 1988;26(6):733–9.

[18] Rampin O. Mode of action of a new oral treatment for erectile dysfunction: apomorphine SL. BJU Int 2001;88(Suppl 3):22–4.

[19] Mulhall JP. Sublingual apomorphine for the treatment of erectile dysfunction. Expert Opin Investig Drugs 2002;11(2):295–302.

[20] Hsieh GC, Hollingsworth PR, Martino B, et al. Central mechanisms regulating penile erection in conscious rats: the dopaminergic systems related to the proerectile effect of apomorphine. J Pharmacol Exp Ther 2004;308(1):330–8.

[21] Rampin O, Jerome N, Suaudeau C. Proerectile effects of apomorphine in mice. Life Sci 2003;72(21):2329–36.

[22] Mirone VG, Stief CG. Efficacy of apomorphine SL in erectile dysfunction. BJU Int 2001;88(Suppl 3):25–9.

[23] Dula E, Bukofzer S, Perdok R, et al. Double-blind, crossover comparison of 3 mg apomorphine SL with placebo and with 4 mg apomorphine SL in male erectile dysfunction. Eur Urol 2001;39(5):558–63 [discussion 564].

[24] Heaton JP, Dean J, Sleep DJ. Sequential administration enhances the effect of apomorphine SL in men with erectile dysfunction. Int J Impot Res 2002;14(1):61–4.

[25] Buvat J, Montorsi F. Safety and tolerability of apomorphine SL in patients with erectile dysfunction. BJU Int 2001;88(Suppl 3):30–5.

[26] Mulhall JP, Bukofzer S, Edmonds AL, et al. An open-label, uncontrolled dose-optimization study

of sublingual apomorphine in erectile dysfunction. Clin Ther 2001;23(8):1260–71.

[27] Dula E, Keating W, Siami PF, et al. Efficacy and safety of fixed-dose and dose-optimization regimens of sublingual apomorphine versus placebo in men with erectile dysfunction. The Apomorphine Study Group. Urology 2000;56(1):130–5.

[28] Perimenis P, Markou S, Gyftopoulos K, et al. Efficacy of apomorphine and sildenafil in men with nonarteriogenic erectile dysfunction. A comparative crossover study. Andrologia 2004;36(3): 106–10.

[29] Perimenis P, Gyftopoulos K, Giannitsas K, et al. A comparative, crossover study of the efficacy and safety of sildenafil and apomorphine in men with evidence of arteriogenic erectile dysfunction. Int J Impot Res 2004;16(1):2–7.

[30] Eardley I, Wright P, MacDonagh R, et al. An open-label, randomized, flexible-dose, crossover study to assess the comparative efficacy and safety of sildenafil citrate and apomorphine hydrochloride in men with erectile dysfunction. BJU Int 2004; 93(9):1271–5.

[31] Von Keitz AT, Stroberg P, Bukofzer S, et al. A European multicentre study to evaluate the tolerability of apomorphine sublingual administered in a forced dose-escalation regimen in patients with erectile dysfunction. BJU Int 2002;89(4):409–15.

[32] Andersson KE, Hedlund P. New directions for erectile dysfunction therapies. Int J Impot Res 2002;14(Suppl 1):S82–92.

[33] Kendirci M, Hellstrom WJ. Intranasal apomorphine. Nastech Pharmaceutical. IDrugs 2004;7(5): 483–8.

[34] Andersson KE, Gemalmaz H, Waldeck K, et al. The effect of sildenafil on apomorphine-evoked increases in intracavernous pressure in the awake rat. J Urol 1999;161(5):1707–12.

[35] Andersson KE. Pharmacology of erectile function and dysfunction. Urol Clin North Am 2001;28(2): 233–47.

[36] Tang Y, Rampin O, Calas A, et al. Oxytocinergic and serotonergic innervation of identified lumbosacral nuclei controlling penile erection in the male rat. Neuroscience 1998;82(1):241–54.

[37] Rehman J, Kaynan A, Christ G, et al. Modification of sexual behavior of Long-Evans male rats by drugs acting on the 5–HT1A receptor. Brain Res 1999;821(2):414–25.

[38] Bitran D, Hull EM. Pharmacological analysis of male rat sexual behavior. Neurosci Biobehav Rev 1987;11(4):365–89.

[39] de Groat WC, Booth AM. Neural control of penile erection. Vol. 6. London: Harwood Academic Publishers; 1993.

[40] Marlier L, Teilhac JR, Cerruti C, et al. Autoradiographic mapping of 5–HT1, 5–HT1A, 5–HT1B and 5–HT2 receptors in the rat spinal cord. Brain Res 1991;550(1):15–23.

[41] Thor KB, Nickolaus S, Helke CJ. Autoradiographic localization of 5-hydroxytryptamine1A, 5-hydroxytryptamine1B and 5-hydroxytryptamine1C/2 binding sites in the rat spinal cord. Neuroscience 1993;55(1):235–52.

[42] Bagdy G, Kalogeras KT, Szemeredi K. Effect of 5–HT1C and 5–HT2 receptor stimulation on excessive grooming, penile erection and plasma oxytocin concentrations. Eur J Pharmacol 1992;229(1):9–14.

[43] Bancila M, Verge D, Rampin O, et al. 5-Hydroxytryptamine2C receptors on spinal neurons controlling penile erection in the rat. Neuroscience 1999; 92(4):1523–37.

[44] Millan MJ, Peglion JL, Lavielle G, et al. 5–HT2C receptors mediate penile erections in rats: actions of novel and selective agonists and antagonists. Eur J Pharmacol 1997;325(1):9–12.

[45] Bos M, Jenck F, Martin JR, et al. Novel agonists of 5HT2C receptors. Synthesis and biological evaluation of substituted 2-(indol-1-yl)-1-methylethylamines and 2-(indeno[1,2-b]pyrrol-1-yl)-1-methylethylamines. Improved therapeutics for obsessive compulsive disorder. J Med Chem 1997; 40(17):2762–9.

[46] Melis MR, Argiolas A. Role of central nitric oxide in the control of penile erection and yawning. Prog Neuropsychopharmacol Biol Psychiatry 1997; 21(6):899–922.

[47] Azadzoi KM, Payton T, Krane RJ, et al. Effects of intracavernosal trazodone hydrochloride: animal and human studies. J Urol 1990;144(5):1277–82.

[48] Monsma FJ Jr, Shen Y, Ward RP, et al. Cloning and expression of a novel serotonin receptor with high affinity for tricyclic psychotropic drugs. Mol Pharmacol 1993;43(3):320–7.

[49] Steers WD, de Groat WC. Effects of m-chlorophenylpiperazine on penile and bladder function in rats. Am J Physiol 1989;257(6 Pt 2):R1441–9.

[50] Saenz de Tejada I, Ware JC, Blanco R, et al. Pathophysiology of prolonged penile erection associated with trazodone use. J Urol 1991; 145(1):60–4.

[51] Meinhardt W, Schmitz PI, Kropman RF, et al. Trazodone, a double blind trial for treatment of erectile dysfunction. Int J Impot Res 1997;9(3): 163–5.

[52] Costabile RA, Spevak M. Oral trazodone is not effective therapy for erectile dysfunction: a double-blind, placebo controlled trial. J Urol 1999;161(6): 1819–22.

[53] Hayes ES, et al. Pro-erectile effect of novel seratonin agonists. Int J Impot Res 2000;12(Suppl 3):S62.

[54] Clark JT, Smith ER, Davidson JM. Evidence for the modulation of sexual behavior by alpha-adrenoceptors in male rats. Neuroendocrinology 1985; 41(1):36–43.

[55] Guay AT, Spark RF, Jacobson J, et al. Yohimbine treatment of organic erectile dysfunction in a dose-escalation trial. Int J Impot Res 2002;14(1):25–31.

[56] Lebret T, Herve JM, Gorny P, et al. Efficacy and safety of a novel combination of L-arginine glutamate and yohimbine hydrochloride: a new oral therapy for erectile dysfunction. Eur Urol 2002; 41(6):608–13 [discussion 613].

[57] Kunelius P, Hakkinen J, Lukkarinen O. Is high-dose yohimbine hydrochloride effective in the treatment of mixed-type impotence? A prospective, randomized, controlled double-blind crossover study. Urology 1997;49(3):441–4.

[58] Melis MR, Spano MS, Succu S, et al. EP 60761-and EP 50885-induced penile erection: structure-activity studies and comparison with apomorphine, oxytocin and N-methyl-D-aspartic acid. Int J Impot Res 2000;12(5):255–62.

[59] Melis MR, Succu S, Spano MS, et al. Penile erection induced by EP 80661 and other hexarelin peptide analogues: involvement of paraventricular nitric oxide. Eur J Pharmacol 2001;411(3):305–10.

[60] Melis MR, Succu S, Spano MS, et al. EP 60761 and EP 50885, two hexarelin analogues, induce penile erection in rats. Eur J Pharmacol 2000;404(1–2): 137–43.

[61] Melis MR, Stancampiano R, Argiolas A. Prevention by NG-nitro-L-arginine methyl ester of apomorphine- and oxytocin-induced penile erection and yawning: site of action in the brain. Pharmacol Biochem Behav 1994;48(3):799–804.

[62] Melis MR, Stancampiano R, Argiolas A. Penile erection and yawning induced by paraventricular NMDA injection in male rats are mediated by oxytocin. Pharmacol Biochem Behav 1994;48(1): 203–7.

[63] Melis MR, Stancampiano R, Argiolas A. Nitric oxide synthase inhibitors prevent N-methyl-D-aspartic acid-induced penile erection and yawning in male rats. Neurosci Lett 1994;179(1–2):9–12.

[64] Zahran AR, Vachon P, Courtois F, et al. Increases in intracavernous penile pressure following injections of excitatory amino acid receptor agonists in the hypothalamic paraventricular nucleus of anesthetized rats. J Urol 2000;164(5):1793–7.

[65] Melis MR, Succu S, Iannucci U, et al. N-methyl-D-aspartic acid-induced penile erection and yawning: role of hypothalamic paraventricular nitric oxide. Eur J Pharmacol 1997;328(2–3):115–23.

[66] Argiolas A. Nitric oxide is a central mediator of penile erection. Neuropharmacology 1994;33(11): 1339–44.

[67] Giuliano F, Rampin O, Brown K, et al. Stimulation of the medial preoptic area of the hypothalamus in the rat elicits increases in intracavernous pressure. Neurosci Lett 1996;209(1):1–4.

[68] Bowery NG, Hudson AL, Price GW. GABAA and GABAB receptor site distribution in the rat central nervous system. Neuroscience 1987;20(2): 365–83.

[69] Magoul R, Onteniente B, Geffard M, et al. Anatomical distribution and ultrastructural organization of the GABAergic system in the rat spinal cord. An immunocytochemical study using anti-GABA antibodies. Neuroscience 1987;20(3): 1001–9.

[70] Elekes I, Patthy A, Lang T, et al. Concentrations of GABA and glycine in discrete brain nuclei. Stress-induced changes in the levels of inhibitory amino acids. Neuropharmacology 1986;25(7):703–9.

[71] Fernandez-Guasti A, Larsson K, Beyer C. GABAergic control of masculine sexual behavior. Pharmacol Biochem Behav 1986;24(4):1065–70.

[72] Fernandez-Guasti A, Larsson K, Beyer C. Comparison of the effects of different isomers of bicuculline infused in the preoptic area on male rat sexual behavior. Experientia 1985;41(11):1414–6.

[73] Melis MR, Succu S, Spano MS, et al. Effect of excitatory amino acid, dopamine, and oxytocin receptor antagonists on noncontact penile erections and paraventricular nitric oxide production in male rats. Behav Neurosci 2000;114(4):849–57.

[74] Argiolas A, Melis MR, Gessa GL. Oxytocin: an extremely potent inducer of penile erection and yawning in male rats. Eur J Pharmacol 1986;130(3): 265–72.

[75] Argiolas A. Oxytocin stimulation of penile erection. Pharmacology, site, and mechanism of action. Ann N Y Acad Sci 1992;652:194–203.

[76] Chen K, Chang LS. Oxytocinergic neurotransmission at the hippocampus in the central neural regulation of penile erection in the rat. Urology 2001; 58(1):107–12.

[77] Murphy MR, Seckl JR, Burton S, et al. Changes in oxytocin and vasopressin secretion during sexual activity in men. J Clin Endocrinol Metab 1987; 65(4):738–41.

[78] Argiolas A, Melis MR, Vargiu L, et al. (CH2)5Tyr(Me)-[Orn8]vasotocin, a potent oxytocin antagonist, antagonizes penile erection and yawning induced by oxytocin and apomorphine, but not by ACTH-(1–24). Eur J Pharmacol 1987; 134(2):221–4.

[79] Melis MR, Mauri A, Argiolas A. Apomorphine-and oxytocin-induced penile erection and yawning in intact and castrated male rats: effect of sexual steroids. Neuroendocrinology 1994; 59(4):349–54.

[80] Argiolas A, Melis MR, Stancampiano R, et al. Oxytocin-induced penile erection and yawning: role of calcium and prostaglandins. Pharmacol Biochem Behav 1990;35(3):601–5.

[81] Melis MR, Succu S, Iannucci U, et al. Oxytocin increases nitric oxide production in the paraventricular nucleus of the hypothalamus of male rats: correlation with penile erection and yawning. Regul Pept 1997;69(2):105–11.

[82] Cushman P Jr. Sexual behavior in heroin addiction and methadone maintenance. Correlation with plasma luteinizing hormone. N Y State J Med 1972;72(11):1261–5.

[83] McIntosh TK, Vallano ML, Barfield RJ. Effects of morphine, beta-endorphin and naloxone on catecholamine levels and sexual behavior in the male rat. Pharmacol Biochem Behav 1980;13(3): 435–41.

[84] Melis MR, Stancampiano R, Gessa GL, et al. Prevention by morphine of apomorphine- and oxytocin-induced penile erection and yawning: site of action in the brain. Neuropsychopharmacology 1992;6(1):17–21.

[85] Melis MR, Succu S, Iannucci U, et al. Prevention by morphine of apomorphine- and oxytocin-induced penile erection and yawning: involvement of nitric oxide. Naunyn Schmiedebergs Arch Pharmacol 1997;355(5):595–600.

[86] Melis MR, Succu S, Argiolas A. Prevention by morphine of N-methyl-D-aspartic acid-induced penile erection and yawning: involvement of nitric oxide. Brain Res Bull 1997;44(6):689–94.

[87] Melis MR, Succu S, Spano MS, et al. Morphine injected into the paraventricular nucleus of the hypothalamus prevents noncontact penile erections and impairs copulation: involvement of nitric oxide. Eur J Neurosci 1999;11(6):1857–64.

[88] Sato Y, Christ GJ, Horita H, et al. The effects of alterations in nitric oxide levels in the paraventricular nucleus on copulatory behavior and reflexive erections in male rats. J Urol 1999;162(6): 2182–5.

[89] Sato Y, Horita H, Kurohata T, et al. Effect of the nitric oxide level in the medial preoptic area on male copulatory behavior in rats. Am J Physiol 1998;274(1 Pt 2):R243–7.

[90] Chen KK, Chan SH, Chang LS, et al. Participation of paraventricular nucleus of hypothalamus in central regulation of penile erection in the rat. J Urol 1997;158(1):238–44.

[91] Melis MR, Argiolas A. Nitric oxide synthase inhibitors prevent apomorphine- and oxytocin-induced penile erection and yawning in male rats. Brain Res Bull 1993;32(1):71–4.

[92] Melis MR, Argiolas A. Nitric oxide donors induce penile erection and yawning when injected in the central nervous system of male rats. Eur J Pharmacol 1995;294(1):1–9.

[93] Poggioli R, Benelli A, Arletti R, et al. Nitric oxide is involved in the ACTH-induced behavioral syndrome. Peptides 1995;16(7):1263–8.

[94] Melis MR, Succu S, Mauri A, et al. Nitric oxide production is increased in the paraventricular nucleus of the hypothalamus of male rats during non-contact penile erections and copulation. Eur J Neurosci 1998;10(6):1968–74.

[95] Burnett AL, Saito S, Maguire MP, et al. Localization of nitric oxide synthase in spinal nuclei innervating pelvic ganglia. J Urol 1995;153(1):212–7.

[96] Saito S, Kidd GJ, Trapp BD, et al. Rat spinal cord neurons contain nitric oxide synthase. Neuroscience 1994;59(2):447–56.

[97] Dun NJ, Dun SL, Wu SY, et al. Nitric oxide synthase immunoreactivity in the rat, mouse, cat and squirrel monkey spinal cord. Neuroscience 1993; 54(4):845–57.

[98] Gantz I, Fong TM. The melanocortin system. Am J Physiol Endocrinol Metab 2003;284(3): E468–74.

[99] Wikberg JE. Melanocortin receptors: perspectives for novel drugs. Eur J Pharmacol 1999;375(1–3): 295–310.

[100] Wessells H, Hruby VJ, Hackett J, et al. MT-II induces penile erection via brain and spinal mechanisms. Ann N Y Acad Sci 2003;994:90–5.

[101] Bertolini A, Gessa GL. Behavioral effects of ACTH and MSH peptides. J Endocrinol Invest 1981;4(2): 241–51.

[102] Gura T. Having it all. Science 2003;299(5608):850.

[103] Argiolas A, Melis MR, Murgia S, et al. ACTH- and alpha-MSH-induced grooming, stretching, yawning and penile erection in male rats: site of action in the brain and role of melanocortin receptors. Brain Res Bull 2000;51(5):425–31.

[104] Argiolas A. Neuropeptides and sexual behaviour. Neurosci Biobehav Rev 1999;23(8):1127–42.

[105] Mountjoy KG, Mortrud MT, Low MJ, et al. Localization of the melanocortin-4 receptor (MC4-R) in neuroendocrine and autonomic control circuits in the brain. Mol Endocrinol 1994;8(10): 1298–308.

[106] Konda Y, Gantz I, DelValle J, et al. Interaction of dual intracellular signaling pathways activated by the melanocortin-3 receptor. J Biol Chem 1994; 269(18):13162–6.

[107] Kojima I, Kojima K, Rasmussen H. Role of calcium and cAMP in the action of adrenocorticotropin on aldosterone secretion. J Biol Chem 1985;260(7): 4248–56.

[108] Kapas S, Purbrick A, Hinson JP. Role of tyrosine kinase and protein kinase C in the steroidogenic actions of angiotensin II, alpha-melanocyte-stimulating hormone and corticotropin in the rat adrenal cortex. Biochem J 1995; 305(Pt 2):433–8.

[109] Vemulapalli R, Kurowski S, Salisbury B, et al. Activation of central melanocortin receptors by MT-II increases cavernosal pressure in rabbits by the neuronal release of NO. Br J Pharmacol 2001; 134(8):1705–10.

[110] Van der Ploeg LH, Martin WJ, Howard AD, et al. A role for the melanocortin 4 receptor in sexual function. Proc Natl Acad Sci USA 2002;99(17): 11381–6.

[111] Martin WJ, McGowan E, Cashen DE, et al. Activation of melanocortin MC(4) receptors increases erectile activity in rats ex copula. Eur J Pharmacol 2002;454(1):71–9.

[112] Molinoff PB, Shadiack AM, Earle D, et al. PT-141: a melanocortin agonist for the treatment of sexual dysfunction. Ann N Y Acad Sci 2003;994:96–102.

[113] Wikberg JE, Muceniece R, Mandrika I, et al. New aspects on the melanocortins and their receptors. Pharmacol Res 2000;42(5):393–420.

[114] Schioth HB, Mutulis F, Muceniece R, et al. Discovery of novel melanocortin4 receptor selective MSH analogues. Br J Pharmacol 1998;124(1):75–82.

[115] Vergoni AV, Bertolini A, Mutulis F, et al. Differential influence of a selective melanocortin MC4 receptor antagonist (HS014) on melanocortin-induced behavioral effects in rats. Eur J Pharmacol 1998;362(2–3):95–101.

[116] Vergoni AV, Bertolini A, Guidetti G, et al. Chronic melanocortin 4 receptor blockage causes obesity without influencing sexual behavior in male rats. J Endocrinol 2000;166(2):419–26.

[117] Martin WJ, MacIntyre DE. Melanocortin receptors and erectile function. Eur Urol 2004;45(6):706–13.

[118] Trivedi P, Jiang M, Tamvakopoulos CC, et al. Exploring the site of anorectic action of peripherally administered synthetic melanocortin peptide MT-II in rats. Brain Res 2003;977(2):221–30.

[119] Tatro JB, Entwistle ML. Heterogeneity of brain melanocortin receptors suggested by differential ligand binding in situ. Brain Res 1994;635(1–2):148–58.

[120] Lindblom J, Schioth HB, Larsson A, et al. Autoradiographic discrimination of melanocortin receptors indicates that the MC3 subtype dominates in the medial rat brain. Brain Res 1998;810(12):161–71.

[121] Gantz I, Miwa H, Konda Y, et al. Molecular cloning, expression, and gene localization of a fourth melanocortin receptor. J Biol Chem 1993;268(20):15174–9.

[122] Wessells H, Hruby VJ, Hackett J, et al. Ac-Nle-c[Asp-His-DPhe-Arg-Trp-Lys]-NH2 induces penile erection via brain and spinal melanocortin receptors. Neuroscience 2003;118(3):755–62.

[123] Mizusawa H, Hedlund P, Andersson KE. alpha-Melanocyte stimulating hormone and oxytocin induced penile erections, and intracavernous pressure increases in the rat. J Urol 2002;167(2 Pt 1):757–60.

[124] Yang YK, Thompson DA, Dickinson CJ, et al. Characterization of Agouti-related protein binding to melanocortin receptors. Mol Endocrinol 1999;13(1):148–55.

[125] Bednarek MA, MacNeil T, Kalyani RN, et al. Selective, high affinity peptide antagonists of alpha-melanotropin action at human melanocortin receptor 4: their synthesis and biological evaluation in vitro. J Med Chem 2001;44(22):3665–72.

[126] Melis MR, Argiolas A. Central oxytocinergic neurotransmission: a drug target for the therapy of psychogenic erectile dysfunction. Curr Drug Targets 2003;4(1):55–66.

[127] Adan RA, Gispen WH. Brain melanocortin receptors: from cloning to function. Peptides 1997;18(8):1279–87.

[128] Sabatier N, Caquineau C, Dayanithi G, et al. Alpha-melanocyte-stimulating hormone stimulates oxytocin release from the dendrites of hypothalamic neurons while inhibiting oxytocin release from their terminals in the neurohypophysis. J Neurosci 2003;23(32):10351–8.

[129] Giuliano F, Bernabe J, McKenna K, et al. Spinal proerectile effect of oxytocin in anesthetized rats. Am J Physiol Regul Integr Comp Physiol 2001;280(6):R1870–7.

[130] Wessells H, Fuciarelli K, Hansen J, et al. Synthetic melanotropic peptide initiates erections in men with psychogenic erectile dysfunction: double-blind, placebo controlled crossover study. J Urol 1998;160(2):389–93.

[131] Wessells H, Gralnek D, Dorr R, et al. Effect of an alpha-melanocyte stimulating hormone analog on penile erection and sexual desire in men with organic erectile dysfunction. Urology 2000;56(4):641–6.

[132] Rosen RC, Diamond LE, Earle DC, et al. Evaluation of the safety, pharmacokinetics and pharmacodynamic effects of subcutaneously administered PT-141, a melanocortin receptor agonist, in healthy male subjects and in patients with an inadequate response to Viagra. Int J Impot Res 2004;16(2):135–42.

[133] Diamond LE, Earle DC, Rosen RC, et al. Double-blind, placebo-controlled evaluation of the safety, pharmacokinetic properties and pharmacodynamic effects of intranasal PT-141, a melanocortin receptor agonist, in healthy males and patients with mild-to-moderate erectile dysfunction. Int J Impot Res 2004;16(1):51–9.

[134] Schioth HB, Bouifrouri AA, Rudzish R, et al. Pharmacological comparison of rat and human melanocortin 3 and 4 receptors in vitro. Regul Pept 2002;106(1–3):7–12.

[135] Schioth HB, Muceniece R, Wikberg JE. Selectivity of [Phe-I7], [Ala6], and [D-Ala4,Gln5,Tyr6] substituted ACTH(4–10) analogues for the melanocortin receptors. Peptides 1997;18(5):761–3.

[136] Hruby VJ, Lu D, Sharma SD, et al. Cyclic lactam alpha-melanotropin analogues of Ac-Nle4-cyclo[Asp5, D-Phe7,Lys10] alpha-melanocyte-stimulating hormone-(4–10)-NH2 with bulky aromatic amino acids at position 7 show high antagonist potency and selectivity at specific melanocortin receptors. J Med Chem 1995;38(18):3454–61.

[137] Sebhat IK, Martin WJ, Ye Z, et al. Design and pharmacology of N-[(3R)-1,2,3,4-tetrahydroisoquinolinium- 3-ylcarbonyl]-(1R)-1-(4-chlorobenzyl)-2-[4-cyclohexyl-4-(1H–1,2,4-triazol- 1-ylmethyl) piperidin-1-yl]-2-oxoethylamine (1), a potent, selective, melanocortin subtype-4 receptor agonist. J Med Chem 2002;45(21):4589–93.

ELSEVIER
SAUNDERS

Urol Clin N Am 32 (2005) 503–509

UROLOGIC
CLINICS
of North America

Penile Prosthesis Implantation: Surgical Implants in the Era of Oral Medication

Culley C. Carson, MD

*Division of Urology, Department of Surgery, University of North Carolina–Chapel Hill,
2140 Bioinformatics Building, CB 7235, Chapel Hill, NC 27599-7235, USA*

The introduction of phosphodiesterase-5 inhibitors to treat erectile dysfunction (ED) with oral agents has revolutionized the treatment of ED throughout the world. Before the introduction of these oral agents, however, surgical implantation of a penile prosthesis was the most reliable method for treatment of patients who had ED. Penile prostheses were introduced as a result of synthetic material developed by the space program and the National Aeronautics and Space Administration in the 1960s. These new materials provided the baseline for the development of many human prosthetic devices including those for the treatment of ED. The idea of penile prosthetic surgery has long been envisioned, with early prosthetic devices constructed from rib cartilage and plastic devices. Because these implants were poorly tolerated and provided only limited erectile function, the widespread use of penile prostheses did not begin until the early 1970s. Investigators in the early 1970s developed two of the current classes of penile prosthetic devices. It was the development of synthetic materials, along with the concept of implantation of prosthetic devices into the corpus cavernosum, that allowed the current penile prosthesis designs to be implanted. Small and colleagues [1] described a pair of semirigid silicone cylinders that filled the corpora cavernosa from the glans penis to the crura. This landmark publication in 1973 reported the successful implantation of a semirigid rod penile prosthesis and use for coitus in 72% to 91% of patients. The development of the Small-Carrion penile prosthesis laid the groundwork for the development of subsequent semirigid rod and mechanical implants that are currently in use.

The second group of penile prosthesis implants was the inflatable variety developed by Scott and colleagues [2], also in 1973. Because the inflatable design was more physiologic, with a more natural appearing flaccid penis and an erection during inflation that produced more girth and flexibility, this design of prosthesis has become the most popular implant available worldwide. Early designs of this inflatable prosthesis had significant mechanical malfunction complications, and many physicians and patients chose the semirigid rod device because of its better reliability. Changes to the inflatable prosthesis in design, materials, and construction have reduced the mechanical malfunction risk to that of semirigid rod prostheses [3]. Today, inflatable prosthesis implantation is performed more commonly than any other penile prosthesis implantation [4]. Inflatable penile prostheses are currently available in two- or three-piece designs constructed of Silastic or Bioflex cylinders, a fluid-filled scrotal pump, and in the three-piece design, a fluid-filled reservoir placed beneath the rectus muscle.

Patient selection

In this era of oral agents for the treatment of ED and minimally invasive surgery, patients who choose the surgical implantation of a penile prosthesis do so when less invasive options are unavailable, unsuccessful, or provide inadequate erectile function. Penile prostheses continue to be

E-mail address: culley_carson@med.unc.edu

doi:10.1016/j.ucl.2005.09.002

used widely for complex penile reconstruction and for men who do not respond or are dissatisfied with pharmacologic treatment. Penile prostheses have been used for Peyronie's disease since their introduction. Many patients who have penile curvature, Peyronie's disease, and inadequate erection who cannot be treated with a straightening procedure such as the Horton-Devine or Nesbit procedure and who have inadequate penile rigidity are best served by treatment with implantation of a penile prosthesis. Because penile prosthesis implantation is a single surgical procedure that provides excellent penile rigidity and penile straightening, patients can resume sexual function within weeks of surgery [5].

In most ED clinics, patients are initially treated with first-line therapy of oral phosphodiesterase-5 inhibitors, followed by second- and third-line therapies including intraurethral pharmacotherapy, pharmaco-active agents injected into the corpus cavernosum, and if tolerated, vacuum erection device. After these therapies have been tried but discarded because of patient preference or functional failure, penile prostheses can be chosen. Uses of these devices require a motivated patient and are best tolerated in patients who have supportive partners. Similarly, patients who have severe ED appear to respond best to the implantation of penile prostheses. Before implantation, however, it is critically important to counsel patients regarding outcomes and expectations for penile prostheses. Because the penile prosthesis implantation serves only to provide penile shaft rigidity, patients must not expect improvements in libido, sensation, ejaculatory function, or penile length. The irreversibility of this procedure should be carefully discussed in addition to cost, infection risk, and mechanical malfunction possibilities. After having prosthetic devices demonstrated and model devices discussed, most patients select an inflatable penile prosthesis. In patients who have significantly reduced penile sensation, an inflatable penile prosthesis decreases the possibility of erosion over semirigid rods because between uses, pressure and penile tissues are reduced. Patients who have peripheral neuropathy or paraplegia should be encouraged to choose among the inflatable penile prosthesis devices.

Penile implant design

Penile prostheses are currently available in two general designs: inflatable and semirigid rod.

Widely available prostheses include the semirigid rod implants AMS 600-650 (American Medical Systems, Minnetonka, Minnesota) and Mentor Acu-Form (Mentor, Santa Barbara, California). Both designs consist of malleable rods constructed of silicone elastomer, with central metal cables facilitating positionability of the device. These devices, usually implanted by a distal corporal incision, are sized to the patient at the time of surgery. Because these devices have no mechanical parts, mechanical malfunction is rare. In patients who have these devices in place for more than 5 years, however, microfractures of the internal metal cables can lead to decreased penile rigidity [6]. Although surgery performed using local anesthesia has been reported, spinal or general anesthesia provides better patient comfort and tolerability during surgery. A similar but slightly more complex mechanical device—the Dura-II (American Medical Systems)—is also available. This device functions like a gooseneck lamp and is constructed of polyethylene disks connected by a central metal cable. It provides an erection similar to that of a semirigid rod prosthesis, with improved positionability. Satisfaction rates with these noninflatable devices, although not frequently reported in large series, appear to be satisfactory [7].

Inflatable penile prostheses are available in two- and three-piece designs. The only two-piece inflatable penile prosthesis design currently available for clinical use is the Ambicor (American Medical Systems). A newer two-piece design (Mentor) is currently undergoing clinical trials and testing. The Ambicor prosthesis consists of two inflatable cylinders implanted in the corpus cavernosum and a pump placed in the scrotum. The cylinder design includes an inflatable portion and a proximal reservoir portion. Patients obtain erection by compressing the scrotal pump several times, which transfers saline from reservoir areas of the pump and proximal cylinders into the inflatable portion of the cylinder and produces cylinder rigidity. Because of the small amount of fluid contained in these devices, distention of the cylinders and corpus cavernosum is less than that of the three-piece prosthesis designs.

The three-piece inflatable penile prostheses currently available are the AMS 700 series (American Medical Systems) and the Mentor three-piece inflatable prosthesis (Titan). Each of these designs consists of a reservoir of 65 to 100 mL, a scrotal pump with inflation and deflation portions, and two cylinders with conical rear-tip extenders to size them to the individual within 0.5 to 1 cm. The cylinders are inflatable; by activating the scrotal pump, the cylinders are inflated to pressure adequate for coitus without change in penile sensation or ejaculatory ability. Implantation of these devices is performed through an infrapubic incision or penoscrotal incision. The penoscrotal incision, the most commonly performed approach, provides enhanced patient comfort and excellent exposure of scrotum, corpora cavernosa, and access to the infrapubic area for reservoir positioning. Through this latter incision, a simultaneous artifical urinary sphincter implantation can be performed as described by Wilson and colleagues [8]. Ultrex cylinders, available through American Medical Systems, are similar to the AMS 700CX cylinders that have controlled expansion but have a three-layer design consisting of a middle woven layer. Because of their unidirectional weaving, girth expansion is the only possible expansion in the AMS 700CX cylinders. The Ultrex cylinders, however, have bidirectionally woven middle layers that permit girth and length expansion. In many patients who do not have corporal scarring, as much as a 15% increase in length can be experienced [9]. These cylinders are excellent choices, except for patients who have significant curvature from Peyronie's disease requiring modeling because the compliance of these cylinders does not permit modeling as effectively as the controlled expansion of AMS 700CX cylinders. In patients who have severe corpus cavernosum scarring from previous infection or priapism, reduced-size penile prosthesis cylinders are available as AMS CXR cylinders. These are similar in design to the AMS 700CX but require only a 10 French dilation. Availability of these cylinders is critical in patients being implanted for severe corpus cavernosum scarring. Construction of the cylinders is the main difference between the Mentor and American Medical Systems designs. The American Medical Systems cylinders are made from three-layer silicone elastomer and woven fabric, whereas Mentor cylinders are made from Bioflex material that is an inert aromatic polyether urea urethane elastomer that is constructed in a single layer. Compared with silicone, Bioflex resists abrasion and demonstrates high tensile strength but is less distensible.

Newer models of American Medical Systems and Mentor three-piece inflatable penile prostheses include designs coated with special materials to decrease prosthesis infection. The AMS 700CX InhibiZone model provides a coating of rifampin and minocycline to inhibit bacterial cell growth. This antibiotic combination targeted at gram-positive organisms such as *Staphylococcus epidermidis* and *S aureus* elutes from the surface of the prosthesis within 72 hours of implantation. These prosthetic devices are placed without soaking in the operating room to maintain the viability of the antibiotic combination. Results from large clinical studies have demonstrated a decrease in infection risk of more than 60% [10]. Adverse events associated with this coating have been few and limited. The Mentor Titan model contains a lockout valve on the prosthesis reservoir to decrease the chances of penile cylinder autoinflation. These implants are likewise coated with a hydrophilic material called Resist applied to the entire prosthesis. This hydrophilic coating permits soaking in an antibiotic solution of the surgeon's choice, with adherence of this antibiotic solution for 24 to 72 hours. Solutions such as gentamycin and bacitracin, when applied to these prostheses, have demonstrated a reduced risk of infection in clinical studies [11].

Surgical implantation of penile prostheses

Surgical implantation of penile prostheses can be performed with a variety of surgical approaches and incisions. Semirigid rod prostheses are best implanted by distal penile circum coronal incisions. Multipiece inflatable prostheses can be implanted by infrapubic or penoscrotal approaches. Although individual surgeons prefer their most familiar approach, there does not appear to be a significant difference in outcomes or patient satisfaction based on incision choice [3]. Often, however, patient anatomy may be best served by a specific approach. Infrapubic approaches may have advantages in patients in whom reservoir placement may be difficult following significant abdominal surgical procedures. Patients who are massively obese may be more efficiently implanted through a penoscrotal incision. When the prosthesis needs to be removed due to infection, using the alternate incision for reimplantation may provide a less scarred portion of the corpus cavernosa (ie, if an infrapubic-implanted penile prosthesis becomes infected and is removed, reimplantation through a penoscrotal incision may facilitate implantation).

Perioperative preparation is critical for prosthesis success. Only patients who do not have remote infection and are in reasonable health should be considered. Perioperative antibiotics targeted at the most common prosthesis infectious agents such as *S epidermidis* or *S aureus* should be administered within 2 hours of prosthesis implantation. Careful skin preparation, such as shaving in the operating room, also facilitates surgery and decreases infection risk. Although general surgical principles dictate that patients be in optimal condition before undergoing elective surgery, increased infection for patients who have elevated hemoglobin A1c is no longer a reported risk [12]. Postoperatively, early Foley catheter removal is best for patient comfort, and discharge from the hospital the morning following surgery is usually the norm. Oral antibiotics can be continued by physician choice. Patients are asked to ensure that the pump remains in their scrotum during the healing process, and activation of the prosthesis can be performed 3 to 6 weeks following surgery. Most patients are able to resume sexual activity within 6 weeks of surgery.

Penile prosthesis results have been satisfactory. Carson and colleagues [3] reported a satisfaction rate of more than 90% with the AMS 700CX prosthesis, and Levine and coworkers [13] reported similar patient/partner satisfaction results for the two-piece Ambicor inflatable penile prosthesis. Recently, Mulhall and colleagues used validated instruments including the International Index of Erectile Function (IIEF) and the Erectile Dysfunction Index for Treatment Satisfaction (EDITS) at 3-month intervals following implantation of inflatable penile prostheses. This study of two- and three-piece prostheses followed patients for 1 year to assess outcomes. These investigators demonstrated that there was a continued improvement in scores for the IIEF and EDITS stabilized 9 to 12 months following surgery. All variables, including erection, ejaculation, orgasm, and overall sexual satisfaction, improved above baseline values at 1 year post surgery. At 3 months following surgery, however, results were less satisfactory, suggesting that postoperative counseling and encouragement of patients is important to obtain ultimate satisfaction and positive outcomes at 9 to 12 months. In the long-term multicenter study of the AMS 700CX three-piece inflatable prosthesis, with a median follow-up of 48 months, 79% of patients were using their device at least twice monthly and 88% would recommend the prosthesis to a friend or relative [3]. A further study of AMS 700 series prostheses that followed a group of patients who had CX, CXM, and

Ultrex prostheses for a mean 59 months was published by Montorsi and colleagues [14]. At almost 5 years post surgery, 92.5% of patients were using their prosthesis an average of 1.7 times weekly and excellent or satisfactory results were reported by patients and their partners. Brinkman and coworkers [15] studied the satisfaction rate of 330 patients undergoing implantation of inflatable penile prostheses from American Medical Systems or Mentor. The overall satisfaction rate in their series was 69%. Although there was a trend for increased sexual satisfaction and natural feeling with the Mentor inflatable penile prosthesis, no highly statistically significant differences could be identified in this series. Jensen and colleagues [16] reviewed 46 patients implanted with the Mentor Alpha-1 inflatable penile prosthesis. Partner acceptance was reported as good, and overall satisfaction by patient and partner was high, with 95% of patients recommending the procedure to other patients or family members. The two-piece Ambicor has also been reported to produce greater than 90% patient/partner satisfaction [13].

Semirigid rod penile prostheses likewise have significant satisfaction rates, although complaints of unnaturalness and pain are more common. Ferguson and Cespedes [17] reviewed the results of the Dura-II semirigid penile prosthesis. Of implanted patients, 76% reported satisfactory rigidity, whereas 87% reported satisfactory concealment.

It is important with the implantation of any penile prosthesis to maintain rigorous sterility, surgical technique, and pre- and postimplantation antibiotics. Similarly, it is critical to counsel patients regarding device function, expectations, outcomes, and possible complications. In some patients, sexual counseling following prosthesis implantation may improve outcomes. Similarly, in patients who have decreased distal penile sensation or "cold glans" syndrome, combination therapy with intraurethral alprostadil or sildenafil citrate may increase sexual satisfaction [18,19].

Rajpurkar and Dhabuwala [20] compared total satisfaction rates in erectile function in patients treated with sildenafil, injection therapy, or penile prosthesis implantation. In this study, patients were administered standardized questionnaires (including the EDITS) with appropriate counseling. Although these treatment modalities differ substantially in their invasiveness and requirements for patient motivation, these authors demonstrated that the highest satisfaction rate and erectile function occurred among patients undergoing penile prosthesis implantation.

Complications following penile prosthesis implantation and their management

The most significant and severe complication following implantation of any prosthetic device is device infection. Penile prosthesis infections result in the most morbidity of any postoperative outcome, often resulting in device loss and complete loss of erectile function. Infections are most commonly sustained within the first 6 months following surgery and are most often caused by *S epidermadis* and other gram-positive organisms. Because the prosthetic devices are connected with a tubing system, colonization and infection in one portion of the device is expected to affect all portions of the implant. Bacteria such as staphylococci produce a glycocalix or biofilm that surrounds the prosthetic device. Bacteria can live in this biofilm, insulated from the effects of common antibiotics administered systemically. Because of this glycocalix or biofilm formation, prosthetic infections can be treated only by removal of the device, with later reimplantation or a salvage procedure as popularized by Mulcahy [21]. With the salvage procedure, success rates of 85% or greater can be expected. After a penile prosthesis infection has been identified by periprosthetic pain and discomfort, induration, erythema, or erosion, the prosthesis is removed. Thorough irrigation is performed with half-strength Betadine, half-strength hydrogen peroxide, and an antibiotic solution with pressure irrigation. Gowns, gloves, and instruments are changed, the patient is scrubbed again with antiseptic solution, and a new, preferably antibiotic-coated penile prosthesis is implanted.

The infection risk appears to be higher when performing penile prosthesis revision for noninfectious mechanical malfunction than the infection risk at initial implantation [22]. In a multicenter study, Henry and colleagues [23] cultured all portions of removed clinically uninfected penile prostheses taken from 77 patients. At least one organism (most commonly, 1 of 10 different species of *Staphylococcus*) grew in 70% of the cultures. All of these staphylococci, however, were sensitive to rifampin and tetracycline. In this same multicenter series (modified salvage procedures with intraoperative washout following removal of mechanically malfunctioning penile prostheses), infection risks could be reduced by a modified salvage technique including thorough irrigation with multiple antiseptic solutions. This series demonstrated a significantly decreased infection rate in patients who were irrigated. In those in whom infections occurred, less common organisms such as *Candida* were responsible for infection [24].

Mechanical problems occur in penile prosthesis devices less commonly than reported with only inflatable devices. Redesigned cylinders, pumps, reservoirs, and new materials have reduced mechanical malfunctions that usually consisted of fluid leaks [25]. Because most mechanical failures occur more than 4 years after initial implantation, removal and replacement of the entire device produces the least likelihood of early repeat failure. Because the surgical time and intervention associated with complete removal and reimplantation is not significantly more than it is for troubleshooting and replacing a single part, the authors prefer to remove and replace all portions of a penile implant in patients who have mechanical malfunction and perform modified salvage procedures as recommended by Henry and colleagues [23].

Difficult implantations can also result in excellent function and satisfaction. Implantation of penile prostheses for Peyronie's disease is a common indication for surgical management. Wilson and Delk [26] revolutionized this surgical procedure by introducing penile modeling in patients in whom penile prostheses were implanted for Peyronie's disease and who had persistent penile curvature. By inflating the implanted prosthesis, clamping the input tubes to the cylinders, and deflecting the penis away from the curvature for 90 seconds (repeating if necessary), more than 90% of patients experienced penile straightening without subsequent incision or further procedures. Other investigators have likewise demonstrated excellent results. Of the authors' own series of 30 men who had Peyronie's disease of 12 to 72 months duration undergoing penile prosthesis implantation, 93% implanted with an AMS 700CX prosthesis were successfully straightened, with modeling requiring only 2 men (7%) to undergo plaque incision following prosthesis implantation. Infection risks and mechanical malfunctions were not observed in this series [27]. Penile prostheses can be safely implanted into patients who have Peyronie's disease with excellent expected satisfaction and mechanical outcomes. In reviewing outcomes of patients who had Peyronie's disease in a multicenter study, however, patient satisfaction was less than it was for patients who did not have Peyronie's disease, with the dominant complaint being penile-length shortening [28]. Montorsi and colleagues [29,30] also reported the best functional and patient/partner satisfaction results with inflatable penile prostheses.

Implantation of penile prostheses in patients who have severe corpus cavernosum fibrosis is the most difficult and challenging experience for an implanting surgeon. Before treatment of these difficult cases, some improvement in penile length, in girth, and occasionally in tissue induration can be obtained with the regular use of the vacuum erection device. Moul and McLeod [31] demonstrated an improvement in penile length and fibrosis in these patients. Patients who suffer significant corpus cavernosum fibrosis from previous prosthesis infection, priapism, Peyronie's disease, or a history of pharmacologic injection therapy require careful, patient, and expert implantation. Although reservoir and pump placement is usually straightforward and can be in nonoperated areas, placement of the cylinders can be more difficult. Use of the AMS 700CXR or Mentor narrow-base implants for these patients may be helpful because dilation may be difficult. Careful corpus cavernosum dilation using multiple corporotomy incisions; excision of fibrotic corpus cavernosum; and tunneling with scissors, Otis urethrotome, and the Rosillo cavernotomes may facilitate this implantation. Similarly, reconstruction of areas of severe scarring using grafts of Gore-Tex or other materials may be necessary to adequately position a penile prosthesis for sexual function. Further discussions of surgical technique and options have been reported elsewhere [32–36].

Summary

In the twenty-first century, most patients who have ED will be satisfactorily treated with oral agents such as phosphodiesterase-5 inhibitors. In patients who are not satisfied with the results of these oral agents or in whom oral agents or other medical treatment fails to produce an adequate response, penile prosthesis implantation continues to be an excellent treatment modality for restoring erectile function. Patient/partner acceptance, use, and satisfaction rates of penile prostheses are better than for many other alternatives including pharmacologic injections. Inflatable penile prostheses are most frequently used and their satisfaction rates are highest, with most patients using their devices more than three times monthly even after 5 years of use [3]. Complications of these multipiece prostheses continue to decline, and patient satisfaction rates, tolerability, and longevity continue to increase.

References

[1] Small MP, Carrion HM, Gordon JA. Small-Carrion penile prosthesis. New implant for management of impotence. Urology 1975;5:479–86.

[2] Scott FB, Bradley WE, Timm GW. Management of erectile impotence. Use of implantable inflatable prosthesis. Urology 1973;2:80–2.

[3] Carson CC, Mulcahy JJ, Govier FE. Efficacy, safety and patient satisfaction outcomes of the AMS 700CX inflatable penile prosthesis: results of a long-term multicenter study. AMS 700CX Study Group. J Urol 2000;164:376–80.

[4] Jhaveri FM, Rutledge R, Carson CC. Penile prosthesis implantation surgery: a statewide population based analysis of 2354 patients. Int J Impot Res 1998;10:251–4.

[5] Tornehl CK, Carson CC. Surgical alternatives for treating Peyronie's disease. BJU Int 2004;94:774–83.

[6] Cohan RH, Dunnick NR, Carson CC. Radiology of penile prostheses. AJR Am J Roentgenol 1989;152:925–31.

[7] Steege JF, Stout AL, Carson CC. Patient satisfaction in Scott and Small-Carrion penile implant recipients: a study of 52 patients. Arch Sex Behav 1986;15:393–9.

[8] Wilson SK, Delk JR II, Henry GD, et al. New surgical technique for sphincter urinary control system using upper transverse scrotal incision. J Urol 2003;169:261–4.

[9] Milbank AJ, Montague DK, Angermeier KW, et al. Mechanical failure of the American Medical Systems Ultrex inflatable penile prosthesis: before and after 1993 structural modification. J Urol 2002;167:2502–6.

[10] Carson CC III. Efficacy of antibiotic impregnation of inflatable penile prostheses in decreasing infection in original implants. J Urol 2004;171:1611–4.

[11] Hellstrom WJ, Hyun JS, Human L, et al. Antimicrobial activity of antibiotic-soaked, Resist-coated Bioflex. Int J Impot Res 2003;15:18–21.

[12] Wilson SK, Carson CC, Cleves MA, et al. Quantifying risk of penile prosthesis infection with elevated glycosylated hemoglobin. J Urol 1998;159:1537–9 [discussion: 1539–40].

[13] Levine LA, Estrada CR, Morgentaler A. Mechanical reliability and safety of, and patient satisfaction with the Ambicor inflatable penile prosthesis: results of a 2 center study. J Urol 2001;166:932–7.

[14] Montorsi F, Rigatti P, Carmignani G, et al. AMS three-piece inflatable implants for erectile dysfunction: a long-term multi-institutional study in 200 consecutive patients. Eur Urol 2000;37:50–5.

[15] Brinkman MJ, Henry GD, Wilson SK, et al. A survey of patients with inflatable penile prostheses for satisfaction. J Urol 2005;174:253–7.

[16] Jensen JB, Madsen SS, Larsen EH, et al. Patient and partner satisfaction with the Mentor Alpha-1 inflatable penile prosthesis. Scand J Urol Nephrol 2005;39:66–8.

[17] Ferguson KH, Cespedes RD. Prospective long-term results and quality-of-life assessment after Dura-II penile prosthesis placement. Urology 2003;61: 437–41.

[18] Benevides MD, Carson CC. Intraurethral application of alprostadil in patients with failed inflatable penile prosthesis. J Urol 2000;163:785–7.

[19] Mulhall JP, Jahoda A, Aviv N, et al. The impact of sildenafil citrate on sexual satisfaction profiles in men with a penile prosthesis in situ. BJU Int 2004; 93:97–9.

[20] Rajpurkar A, Dhabuwala CB. Comparison of satisfaction rates and erectile function in patients treated with sildenafil, intracavernous prostaglandin E1 and penile implant surgery for erectile dysfunction in urology practice. J Urol 2003;170:159–63.

[21] Mulcahy JJ. Treatment alternatives for the infected penile implant. Int J Impot Res 2003;15(Suppl 5): S147–9.

[22] Carson CC. Penile prosthesis implantation and infection for Sexual Medicine Society of North America. Int J Impot Res 2001;13(Suppl 5):S35–8.

[23] Henry GD, Wilson SK, Delk JR II, et al. Penile prosthesis cultures during revision surgery: a multicenter study. J Urol 2004;172:153–6.

[24] Henry GD, Wilson SK, Delk JR II, et al. Revision washout decreases penile prosthesis infection in revision surgery: a multicenter study. J Urol 2005;173: 89–92.

[25] Woodworth BE, Carson CC, Webster GD. Inflatable penile prosthesis: effect of device modification on functional longevity. Urology 1991;38: 533–6.

[26] Wilson SK, Delk JR II. A new treatment for Peyronie's disease: modeling the penis over an inflatable penile prosthesis. J Urol 1994;152:1121–3.

[27] Carson CC. Penile prosthesis implantation in the treatment of Peyronie's disease. Int J Impot Res 1998;10:125–8.

[28] Carson CC. Reconstructive surgery using urological prostheses. Curr Opin Urol 1999;9:233–9.

[29] Montorsi F, Guazzoni G, Barbieri L, et al. AMS 700 CX inflatable penile implants for Peyronie's disease: functional results, morbidity and patient-partner satisfaction. Int J Impot Res 1996;8:81–5 [discussion: 85–6].

[30] Montorsi F, Guazzoni G, Bergamaschi F, et al. Patient-partner satisfaction with semirigid penile prostheses for Peyronie's disease: a 5-year followup study. J Urol 1993;150:1819–21.

[31] Moul JW, McLeod DG. Negative pressure devices in the explanted penile prosthesis population. J Urol 1989;142:729–31.

[32] Carson CC. Complications of penile prosthesis and complex implantations. In: Carson CC, Kirby RS, Goldstein I, editors. Textbook of erectile dysfunction. Oxford: Isis Medical Media; 1999. p. 435–500.

[33] George VK, Shah GS, Mills R, et al. The management of extensive penile fibrosis: a new technique of 'minimal scar-tissue excision'. Br J Urol 1996; 77:282–4.

[34] Knoll LD. Use of porcine small intestinal submucosal graft in the surgical management of tunical deficiencies with penile prosthetic surgery. Urology 2002;59:758–61.

[35] Knoll LD, Fisher J, Benson RC Jr, et al. Treatment of penile fibrosis with prosthetic implantation and flap advancement with tissue debulking. J Urol 1996;156:394–7.

[36] Carson CC, Noh CH. Distal penile prosthesis extrusion: treatment with distal corporoplasty or Gortex windsock reinforcement. Int J Impot Res 2002;14:81–4.

ELSEVIER
SAUNDERS

Urol Clin N Am 32 (2005) 511–525

UROLOGIC
CLINICS
of North America

PDE-5 Inhibitors: Current Status and Future Trends

Puneet Masson, MD, Sarah M. Lambert, MD,
Melissa Brown, MPH, Ridwan Shabsigh, MD*

*Department of Urology, College of Physicians and Surgeons, Columbia University,
161 Fort Washington Avenue, New York, NY 10032, USA*

In 2000, the World Health Organization (WHO) has recognized erectile dysfunction (ED) as a worldwide public health concern. Based on an international consensus meeting, the WHO recognized fundamental individual rights to sexual health that include: (1) a capacity to enjoy and control sexual and reproductive behavior in accordance with a personal social ethic; (2) freedom from fear, shame, guilt, false beliefs, and other factors that inhibit sexual response and impair sexual relationships; and (3) freedom from organic disorders, diseases, and deficiencies that interfere with sexual and reproductive functioning [1]. This announcement not only legitimized ED as a legitimate medical problem, but validated the development of treatment options for men who suffer from this condition. Moreover, this announcement was also instrumental for the development of a clinical paradigm regarding the treatment of ED, with a stepwise approach using available medical and surgical options. This new class of drugs—phosphodiesterase-5 (PDE-5) inhibitors—which were the first ever oral agents to receive Food & Drug Administration approval (FDA) for the treatment of ED—became first-line agents. Second-line agents included intracavernous injection and intraurethral therapies, while the third-line and final treatment option remained surgical prosthesis.

Furthermore, this event succeeded as a major milestone in medicine, which also allowed for a breakthrough in the field of ED. This event was the March 1998 FDA approval of the first ever oral agent in the management of ED, sildenafil (Viagra; Pfizer US Pharmaceutical Group). Before this time, many EDs were treated with more invasive therapies.

Since the implementation of sildenafil, two new agents have been introduced for the treatment of ED, including the PDE-5 inhibitors vardenafil (Levitra; Bayer Health Care Pharmaceuticals) and tadalafil (Cialis; Lilly ICOS LLC). This article reviews current information and advances in PDE-5 inhibitors for the treatment of ED in men.

Phosphodiesterase-5 inhibitors

Phosphodiesterase (PDE) inhibitors are drugs that block one or more of the subtypes of the enzyme PDE [2]. There are 21 mammalian PDE genes cloned to date, organized into 11 different gene families of PDEs that are structurally related yet functionally distinct. As these can be derived from multiple genes that are capable of generating a number of isoforms, currently there are over 50 known PDE enzymes. Differences in tissue expression patterns and spatial compartmentalization within cells, resulting in unique functional roles and mechanisms, are believed to explain the requirement for a large number of enzymes performing a similar process [3]. PDEs function by slicing the intracellular second messenger's cyclic AMP (cAMP) or cyclic GMP (cGMP). Attributing to their key roles in physiologic processes, PDEs are targets for many drugs that are used for different diseases, such as cardiovascular diseases, asthma, ED, and many others [2]. Most cells contain representatives of multiple gene families but in different amounts, proportions, and subcellular locations, thus forming a complex network among different PDE regulatory pathways.

---

* Corresponding author.
E-mail address: rs66@columbia.edu (R. Shabsigh).

Selectivity of phosphodiesterase inhibitors

The most obvious distinguishing feature between the 11 PDE families is their substrate specificity. Some PDEs specifically hydrolyze cAMP; others are highly specific for cGMP, whereas some are able to hydrolyze both cAMP and cGMP. Each PDE has multiple isoforms and varying degrees of selectivity for cAMP and cGMP.

Relatively nonselective phosphodiesterase inhibitors include the minor stimulant caffeine and the bronchodilator theophylline. These two drugs, as well as thousands of synthetic PDE inhibitors, have been used to investigate the physiologic effects of cyclic nucleotides and PDE activity. Many have also been tested for therapeutic effects. As a group, many of these inhibitors lack potency and specificity because they block PDE catalytic activity in several PDEs, including PDE-5 [4].

Based on their central role in regulating the intracellular concentration of cyclic nucleotides, PDEs have been targets for pharmacologic interventions. The first clinically available selective PDE inhibitor was the PDE-3 inhibitor milrinon, which was used to treat hypertension and certain types of cardiac failure. It is no longer in use, however, owing to its presumed ability to induce life-threatening arrhythmias.

Among the PDEs, PDE-4 is the major cAMP-metabolizing enzyme found in inflammatory and immune cells. PDE-4 inhibitors have proven potential as anti-inflammatory signals and also as inhibitors of the production of reactive oxygen species. PDE-4 inhibitors have a high therapeutic and commercial potential as nonsteroidal disease controllers in inflammatory airway diseases such as chronic obstructive pulmonary disease. Development of PDE-4 inhibitors for the treatment of asthma, such as Rolipram, or the PDE-4A selective inhibitors, Roflumilast and Cliomilast, are in the pipeline. Enoximone, which inhibits PDE-4, and milrinone, which inhibits PDE3c, are useful for short-term treatment of cardiac failure. Clinically, these drugs mimic sympathetic stimulation and increase cardiac output. PDE6 located in the rods and the cons of the retina is attributable to visual phototransduction. PDE11 found in the anterior pituitary, testes, prostate, and the penis has no known functions.

Although five PDE isoenzymes have been reported in penile tissues (PDE2, 3, 4, 5, and 11) the predominant isoform is PDE-5. The most prominent PDE in the human corpus cavernosum is the cGMP-specific phosphodiesterase-5 (PDE-5). It is this specificity that makes PDE-5 the germane goal for the management of ED. The PDE-5 enzyme is present in small concentrations in the systemic vasculature. Sildenafil, a potent inhibitor of PDE-5, was originally studied for the treatment of angina before its effectiveness in treating ED was serendipitously discovered. Sildenafil has several transient side effects, such as headache, nasal congestion, dyspepsia, flushing, and visual disturbances. These side effects may be attributed to the presence of small amounts of PDE-5 in organs other than the penis and in the case of visual disturbances to its weak inhibition of PDE6 [5].

Due to the increasing understanding of the important role of the nitric oxide cGMP-signaling pathway during sexual stimulation, the development of sildenafil citrate (Viagra) in the early 1990s, and its introduction into the market in the 1998 as an oral treatment of ED, the therapeutic potential of PDE5 inhibitors was reaffirmed. Five years later, two more potent PDE5 inhibitors, vardenafil (Levitra) and tadalafil (Cialis), came to the market.

Thus, the need exists for PDE5 inhibitors possessing improved PDE isoenzyme selectivity. In addition, the potential use of PDE5 inhibitors in other indications such as pulmonary hypertension, stroke, and cardiovascular protection is also fuelling interest in this field.

Sildenafil

Sildenafil (Viagra; Pfizer US Pharmaceutical Group, New York, New York) was the first oral phosphodiesterase-5 (PDE-5) inhibitor approved by the FDA in 1998. In the subsequent 7 years, 23 million men worldwide have used sildenafil for treatment of ED. Sildenafil has been evaluated for safety and efficacy in over 130 clinical trials involving over 13,000 patients [5]. Sildenafil acts as an orally active, potent, and selective inhibitor of cGMP-specific PDE-5, which represents the predominant isoform in human erectile tissue [6]. For example, it is 4000-fold more selective for PDE-5 than PDE-3, the isoenzyme involved in regulation of cardiac contractility [6]. PDE-5 is not expressed in cardiac tissue, but is expressed in the systemic vasculature. Clinical trials reveal that Sildenafil can result in small clinically insignificant reduction in blood pressure in healthy volunteers [6,7]. PDE-5 activity has also been established in the genitourinary tract, gastrointestinal tract, vascular, cerebral, and pulmonary tissues, and there is potential for PDE-5 inhibitors effects on these systems. By inhibiting PDE-5, sildenafil potentates the relaxant effects necessary for erection initiated by nitric oxide release from the nonadrenergic-noncholinergic (NANC) autonomic nerves of the parasympathetic system and the vascular endothelium during sexual stimulation. Specifically, sildenafil inhibits PDE-5, the enzyme responsible for degradation of cGMP, thereby potentiating relaxant of the corporeal arterial and sinusoidal smooth muscle [8].

Pharmacokinetics and pharmacodynamics

Sildenafil is administered orally with a bioavailability of 40%. Peak plasma concentration (t_{max}) is 30 to 120 minutes, with a median time of 60 minutes [5]. Onset of action for sildenafil typically occurs 1 hour after oral ingestion, but effects can be seen as early as 30 minutes. High-fat meals decrease the rate of absorption, delay peak plasma concentrations, and may reduce peak plasma concentrations by 29%. Therefore, it is recommended that sildenafil be ingested 1 hour before sexual activity and not in association with heavy meals or the depressant effects of alcohol consumption. The plasma half-life of sildenafil is 3 to 5 hours [9]. Recommended dosage of sildenafil ranges from 25 to 100 mg with a starting dose of 50 mg. In the American flexible-dose study, 75% of patients chose the 100 mg dose, 23% the 50 mg dose, and 2% the 25 mg dose [10].

Sildenafil is degraded in the liver by cytochrome P-450 3A4 and 2C9 [11]. Therefore, patients with hepatic dysfunction, >65 years of age, or taking cytochrome P-450 3A4 or 2C9 inhibitors have increased plasma levels of sildenafil. Potent cytochrome P-450 3A4 or 2C9 inhibitors include grapefruit, cimetidine, ketoconazole, and erythromycin. Patients taking ritonavir, a protease inhibitor with two metabolic pathways shared with sildenafil, should not be prescribed sildenafil doses >25 mg every 48 hours. Severe renal insufficiency is also associated with elevated serum levels of sildenafil [5]. Patients with the above conditions should be prescribed a starting dose of 25 mg secondary to their decreased metabolism of sildenafil. Dose escalation can be performed under medical supervision. Of note, side effect profiles for sildenafil do not increase with higher serum concentrations seen in these patients [5].

Efficacy

The efficacy of sildenafil in alleviating ED has been demonstrated in >3000 patients in 21 American and European randomized, double-blind, placebo-controlled phase III trials [11]. The initial efficacy data for sildenafil are based upon the New Drug Application to the FDA. This data includes 4526 patients with 576 patients from phase I trials, 3003 patients from phases II to III, 769 patients from extension studies, and 178 patients from Japanese studies. Mean patient age was 55 years, ranging from 18 to 87 years; 51.8% of patients were diagnosed with organic ED, 25.7% mixed ED, and 18% psychogenic ED. Efficacy was determined using the International Index of Erectile Dysfunction (IIEF), a global efficacy question, an erectile activity log, a four-point penile rigidity scale (American fixed-dose study), and an optional partner assessment survey [12,13]. In all 21 studies, sildenafil improved the ability to achieve and maintain an erection, reflecting the National Institute of Health definition of ED. The ability to achieve and maintain an erection increased by 100% and 130%, respectively [10]. Fifty-nine percent of patients receiving sildenafil reported the ability to achieve and maintain erections on most to all occasions compared with 15% of patients receiving placebo [13]. The long-term efficacy and safety of sildenafil was evaluated in 1008 patients with ED in a flexible-dose, open-label, study revealing that after 36 and 52 weeks 92% and 89% of patients, respectively, felt that their erections had improved [14]. Subgroup analyses revealed that these results were demonstrated in all patients irrespective of age, race, severity of ED, or etiology of ED. In addition, sildenafil improved erections in patients with significant comorbidities such as coronary artery disease, peripheral vascular disease, coronary artery bypass grafts, hypertension, spinal cord injury, radical prostatectomy, and transurethral resection of the prostate. The results of the IIEF were supported by the data obtained from the global efficacy question and activity log. When asked, "Did the treatment improve your erections," 74% of patients receiving sildenafil compared with 16% of patients receiving placebo responded "yes." In addition, the number of men with improved erections increased as the dose of sildenafil increased: 63%, 74%, and 82% of men receiving 25 mg, 50 mg, 100 mg, respectively, of sildenafil reported improved erections. This dose response was also demonstrated in patients' activity logs [5]. Therefore, sildenafil improves the ability to achieve and maintain erections that are satisfactory to patients in all subgroups and this result can be sustained for > 4 years. Patients initially labeled as nonresponders can often be converted into responders with further instructions. Many patients may only have tried sildenafil once, only used lower doses, or lacked sexual stimulation during the therapeutic window [15].

Safety, contraindications, and precautions

The primary adverse effects of sildenafil in clinical trials include headache 15.8%, flushing 10.5%, dyspepsia 6.5%, nasal congestion 4.5%, altered vision 2.7%, and diarrhea [16]. The fixed-dose, randomized, placebo-controlled trial determined that these adverse effects are dose related, and can therefore be minimized by using the lowest effective dose [17]. There have not been any reported cases of priapism during clinical trials. Post-FDA approval, 25 cases of priapism have been reported mostly related to the use of sildenafil in conjunction with other therapies for ED. A review of 18 clinical trials involving 3700 patients revealed a total of 574 adverse events in the 734 patients treated with sildenafil with 62% described as mild and transient. In addition, the overall discontinuation rate for sildenafil was 2.5% with a discontinuation rate for placebo of 2.3% [18]. In long-term studies incorporating 2199 patients headache accounts for the primary reason for discontinuation [19].

Sildenafil's vasodilatory action can potentiate the hypotensive effects of nitrates, and is therefore contraindicated in patients using organic nitrates or other nitric oxide donors including recreational nitric oxide use [20]. Additionally, sildenafil should be taken with caution in patients with coronary ischemia, congestive heart failure, borderline low blood pressure, low cardiac output states, or an intensive multidrug regimen for systemic hypertension [21]. Postrelease product labeling from the FDA also cautions use of sildenafil in patient subgroups not included in clinical trials such as men with myocardial infarction, stroke, life-threatening arrhythmia within 6 months, resting blood pressure less than 90/50 or > 170/110 mmHg, cardiac failure, unstable angina, or retinitis pigmentosa. Although the original clinical trials of sildenafil did not include patients with cardiac disease, subsequent studies have evaluated the cardiovascular effects of sildenafil in men with coronary artery disease. An examination of

cardiovascular effects of sildenafil during exercise in men with known coronary artery disease revealed that men with stable coronary artery disease had no adverse effects from sildenafil. There was no effect on symptoms, exercise duration, or exercise-induced ischemia as determined by exercise stress echocardiography [22]. These results are supported by a review of 18 placebo-controlled studies in which the incidence of adverse cardiac events was 3.0% in the sildenafil group and 3.5% in the placebo group [16]. Recently, 43 reported cases of nonarteritic anterior ischemia optic neuropathy (NAION) have been suggested in association with use of PDE-5 inhibitors: 38 of these cases occurring with sildenafil, 4 with vardenafil, 1 with tadalafil. There have been no reported cases of NAION during clinical trials, and 23 million patients have been treated with sildenafil in the past 7 years since FDA approval without reported NAION. In addition, the risk factors for NAION closely mimic risk factors for ED, including > 50 years of age, hypertension, hypercholesterolemia, diabetes mellitus, smoking, and heart disease. NAION is the most common acute optic nerve disease in people over the age of 50 years. Despite unclear evidence of direct association, the FDA is mandating new warning labels for PDE-5 inhibitors that include acute blindness as a potential adverse effect.

Vardenafil

Vardenafil (Levitra, Bayer Corp., West Haven, Connecticut) is a newer PDE-5 inhibitor that was FDA approved in 2003 for the treatment of ED. Like sildenafil, vardenafil is a selective PDE-5 inhibitor. It is > 1000-fold more selective for PDE-5 than PDE-3, the isoenzyme involved in regulation of cardiac contractility [23]. PDE-5 activity has also been established in the genitourinary tract, gastrointestinal tract, vascular, cerebral, and pulmonary tissues, and there is potential for vardenafil effects on these systems. By inhibiting PDE-5, vardenafil potentates the relaxant effects necessary for erection initiated by nitric oxide release from the NANC autonomic nerves of the parasympathetic system and the vascular endothelium during sexual stimulation. Specifically, vardenafil inhibits PDE-5, the enzyme responsible for degradation of cGMP thereby potentiating relaxantion of the corporeal arterial and sinusoidal smooth muscle.

Pharmacokinetics and pharmacodynamics

The absolute bioavailability of vardenafil is 15%, with a maximum plasma concentration achieved at 30 to 120 minutes in a fasting individual. Consumption of a high-fat meal before ingesting vardenafil decreases the maximum plasma concentration by 18% to 50%. Therefore, it is recommended that sildenafil be ingested 1 hour before sexual activity and not in association with heavy meals or the depressant effects of alcohol consumption. The terminal half life for vardenafil is 4.5 hours.

As with sildenafil, vardenafil is degraded in the liver by cytochrome P-450 3A4 and 2C9 [24]. Therefore, patients with hepatic dysfunction, >65 years of age, or taking cytochrome P-450 3A4 or 2C9 inhibitors have increased plasma levels of vardenafil. Potent cytochrome P-450 3A4 or 2C9 inhibitors include grapefruit, cimetidine, ketoconazole, and erythromycin. Patients taking ritonavir or indinavir, protease inhibitors with two metabolic pathways shared with vardenafil, should not be prescribed vardenafil doses >5 mg every 48 hours. Severe renal insufficiency is also associated with elevated serum levels of vardenafil [24]. Patients with the above conditions should be prescribed a starting dose of 5 mg and should not exceed a 10 mg dose secondary to their decreased metabolism of vardenafil [24].

Efficacy

Vardenafil was initially evaluated in four major double-blind, randomized, placebo-controlled fixed-dose, multicenter trials involving 2431 men with a mean age of 57 years (range 20–83 years). Efficacy was determined using the IIEF, global assessement question (GAQ), and Sexual Encounter Profile (SEP) for vaginal penetration and ability to engage in intercourse. In the North American study, 65%, 75%, and 80% of men receiving vardenafil at 5, 10, and 20 mg, respectively, were able to attain penetration as opposed to 52% of men receiving placebo. This improvement was maintained for >6 months. These results are supported by the improvement in men able to engage in intercourse: 51%, 64%, and 65% of men receiving placebo successfully engaged in intercourse opposed to 32% of men receiving placebo [25]. In response to the GAQ ("has the treatment improved your erections?"), 65%, 73%, and 81% of patients receiving 5, 10, and 20 mg of vardenafil responded affirmatively [26]. All dosages of vardenafil were superior to placebo across all primary efficacy variables in a broad range of patients with ED, regardless of etiology or severity of ED. Postmarketing safety and efficacy of vardenafil was evaluated in 29,358 men with ED as a multinational surveillance study. Patients were interviewed regarding both overall treatment success, and individual sexual attempts in a questionnaire; 73.6% of and 88.5% of patients experienced improved erections after the first and second tablet, respectively. Vardenafil dosages of 10 mg and 20 mg were evaluated with similar improvement rates for both dosages. Sexual attempts were successful with respect to partner penetration in 94.9% of patients and with respect to maintenance of erection during intercourse in 87.7% of patients [27]. Therefore, vardenafil has a similar onset of duration, administration, and efficacy as sildenafil.

Safety, contraindications, and precautions

The primary adverse effects of vardenafil in clinical trials include headache 8% to 18%, flushing 6% to 13%, rhinitis 1% to 8%, and dyspepsia 2% to 6% [28]. Altered vision can also occur infrequently with vardenafil. The fixed-dose, randomized, placebo-controlled trial determined that these adverse effects are dose related, and can therefore be minimized by using the lowest effective dose [27]. Additionally, vardenafil has been suggested in association with nonarteritic anterior ischemia optic neuropathy in four cases, but needs further evaluation to determine causality. Despite unclear evidence of direct association the FDA is mandating new warning labels for PDE-5 inhibitors that include acute blindness as a potential adverse effect.

The contraindications for vardenafil reflect those of sildenafil, and result from the vasodilatory action of PDE-5 inhibitors. This class of drug potentates the hypotensive effects of nitrates, and is therefore contraindicated in patients using organic nitrates or other nitric oxide donors including recreational nitric oxide use. Additionally, vardenafil should be taken with caution for patients with coronary ischemia, congestive heart failure, borderline low blood pressure, low cardiac output states, or an intensive multidrug regimen for systemic hypertension. Examination of cardiovascular effects of vardenafil during exercise in men with known coronary artery disease revealed that men with stable coronary artery disease had no adverse effects from vardenafil. There was no effect on symptoms, exercise duration, or exercise-induced ischemia as determined by exercise stress echocardiography [24].

Tadalafil

Tadalafil (Cialis, Lilly ICOS, Indianapolis, Indiana) is a PDE-5 inhibitor that was FDA approved in 2003 for the treatment of ED. Like sildenafil and vardenafil, tadalafil is a selective PDE-5 inhibitor. It is > 10,000-fold more selective for PDE-5 than PDE-3, the isoenzyme involved in regulation of cardiac contractility [29]. Therefore, tadalafil has less risk of cardiac side effects. Additionally, tadalafil is > 700-fold more selective for PDE-5 than PDE-6, the isoenzyme involved in phototransduction in the retina. PDE-5 activity has also been established in the genitourinary tract, gastrointestinal tract, vascular, cerebral, and pulmonary tissues, and there is potential for tadalafil effects on these systems. By inhibiting PDE-5, tadalafil potentates the relaxant effects necessary for erection initiated by nitric oxide release from the NANC autonomic nerves of the parasympathetic system and the vascular endothelium during sexual stimulation. Specifically, tadalafil inhibits PDE-5, the enzyme responsible for degradation of cGMP, thereby potentiating relaxantion of the corporeal arterial and sinusoidal smooth muscle.

Pharmacokinetics and pharmacodynamics

The absolute bioavailability of tadalafil has not yet been determined. Tadalafil reached maximum concentration at a median of 120 minutes (range 30 minutes to 6 hours). Tadalafil has a half-life of 17.5 hours [9]. Therefore, the length of effect is significantly longer for tadalafil than either vardenafil or sildenafil. The duration of tatadalfil clinical efficacy has been reported up to 36 hours after dosing. Additionally, the plasma concentration of tadalafil is unaffected by food or alcohol consumption, in contrast to vardenafil and sildenafil, which require fasting for maximum effect. Therefore, tadalafil can be administered without regard to dietary intake [9].

As with the other PDE-5 inhibitors, tadalafil is degraded in the liver by cytochrome P-450 3A4 and 2C9 [29]. Therefore, patients with hepatic dysfunction, > 65 years of age, or taking cytochrome P-450 3A4 or 2C9 inhibitors, have increased plasma levels of tadalafil. Potent cytochrome P-450 3A4 or 2C9 inhibitors include grapefruit, cimetidine, ketoconazole, ritonavir, and erythromycin. Patients taking

a cytochrome P450 3A4 inhibitor should not be prescribed tadalafil doses > 5 mg daily. Severe renal insufficiency is also associated with elevated serum levels of tadalafil. Patients with the above conditions should be prescribed a starting dose of 5 mg, and should not exceed a 10-mg dose every 48 hours secondary to their decreased metabolism of tadalafil [29].

Efficacy

The initial evaluation of tadalafil included 22 clinical trials involving 4000 patients. Seven randomized, multicenter, double-blinded, placebo-controlled, parallel-arm trials involving the general population were used to establish safety and efficacy. The primary outcomes used in evaluation of tadalafil included IIEF and SEP focusing on achieving both penetration and successful intercourse. One study involving 348 men taking 20 mg of tadalafil demonstrated sustained efficacy of at least 36 hours, representing a significantly longer duration of action that the other PDE-5 inhibitors [30]. At 24 and 36 hours postingestion, respectively, 57.3% and 60.4% of patients receiving tadalafil had successful intercourse in contrast to 31.3% and 29.9% of patients receiving placebo. In comparison to placebo tadalafil significantly increased all outcomes measures in comparison to placebo including IIEF, SEP, and GAQ [31].

Tadalafil is approved for treatment of ED in over 80 countries including the United States. Tadalafil was found to be safe and effective in integrated analyses of studies involving broad ED patient populations. In these studies, the incidence of severe baseline ED (IIEF EF domain score ≤ 10) was 36% and underlying preexisting hypertension and diabetes mellitus were 30% and 21%, respectively. In this largely primary-care population the severity of baseline ED and the incidence of comorbid ED-associated medical conditions were comparable to the demographic characteristics in the Massachusetts Male Aging Study and in other epidemiologic reviews of ED.

Safety, contraindications, and precautions

The trials evaluating Tadalafil revealed a favorable adverse effect profile, with headaches, flushing, dyspepsia, and back pain being the primary adverse effects [31]. Transient altered vision can also occur with tadalafil, although to a lesser extent than the other PDE-5 inhibitors, secondary to the highly selective nature of tadalafil. The fixed-dose, randomized, placebo-controlled trial determined that these adverse effects are dose related, and can therefore be minimized by using the lowest effective dose [32]. Despite the minimal activity of tadalafil for PDE-6 found in the retina, tadalafil has been suggested in association with nonarteritic anterior ischemia optic neuropathy in one case. Despite minimal evidence of direct association the FDA is mandating new warning labels for PDE-5 inhibitors that include acute blindness as a potential adverse effect.

The contraindications for tadalafil reflect those of the PDE-5 inhibitor class of drug, and result from the vasodilatory action of PDE-5 inhibitors. This class of drug potentates the hypotensive effects of nitrates, and is therefore contraindicated in patients using organic nitrates or other nitric oxide donors [33]. Additionally, tadalafil should be taken with caution for patients with coronary ischemia, congestive heart failure, borderline low blood pressure, low cardiac output states, or an intensive multidrug regimen for systemic hypertension. Examination of cardiovascular effects of tadalafil during exercise in men with known coronary artery disease revealed that men with stable coronary artery disease had no adverse effects from tadalafil. There was no effect on symptoms, exercise duration, or exercise-induced ischemia as determined by exercise stress echocardiography [29].

Special populations

Patients with diabetes mellitus

ED is common in men with diabetes mellitus, with diabetic men being three times as likely to have ED than their nondiabetic counterparts. In the Massachusetts Male Aging Study, a large population-based random sample cohort, diabetic men had a 28% age-adjusted prevalence of complete ED compared with the general population of men (10%) [34]. Additionally, the incidence of ED increased with increasing age, duration of diabetes, and deteriorating metabolic control, and was higher in individuals with type 2 diabetes than those with type 1. Many times, ED may even be the first manifestation of diabetes; in a study conducted by Solomon et al in the UK, they found that out of 174 men presenting to a urologist, 56 men (36%) were found to be diabetic, with six of these men being previously undiagnosed with diabetes [35]. The increased prevalence of diabetes and ED may be secondary to diabetic associations such as neuropathy, hyperlipidemia, and microvascular complications that may further influence endothelial dysfunction. Because of the unique pathophysiology of the diabetic patient, clinical recommendations for treatment of ED merit special consideration.

The PDE5 inhibitors sildenafil, tadalafil, and vardenafil have all been evaluated in diabetic men. However, there have been no comparative trials evaluating these medications, and therefore, efficacy comparisons cannot be ascertained.

An initial pilot study of 21 diabetic patients (types 1 and 2), with a mean age of 50 years and a 3-year median duration of ED, examined the efficacy of sildenafil in doses up to 50 mg [36]. ED improvement (measured by diary, questionnaire, and RigiScan) was noted in 48% and 52% of the men receiving 25 mg and 50 mg of sildenafil, respectively. More recently, a large study of 268 diabetic men (mean age of 57 years, mean diabetes duration of 12 years, 21% with type I and 79% with type 2) with a 12-year mean duration of ED was randomized for 12 weeks of treatment in a double-blind, placebo-controlled, flexible dose-escalation study [37]. The flexible dose study started at 50 mg sildenafil with dose adjustments (up and down) based on efficacy and adverse events. At the end of the 12-week study, improved erections were noted in 56% of sildenafil patients compared with 22% receiving placebo ($P < 0.001$). Likewise, sexual intercourse rates were 48% versus 12%.

Recently, a randomized, double-blind, placebo-controlled, fixed-dose study of 282 men with ED and diabetes transpired (mean age of 46.4, mean diabetes duration of 11 years), where patients were assigned to either 100 mg of sildenafil or placebo [38]. At the end of the 12-week study, positive clinical results were obtained in 51% of the patients in the sildenafil group compared with 11% of the patients in the placebo group. At least one successful attempt of sexual intercourse was noted in 59% of patients taking sildenafil compared with 21% of patients receiving placebo ($P < 0.002$). These three studies suggest that oral sildenafil may be a moderately effective treatment for men with diabetes.

The majority of these studies are conducted on the total diabetic population and mostly involve men with type 2 diabetes. There are few studies discussing treatment options on men with type 1 diabetes, and studies that do exist have small sample sets and tend to be inconclusive [39]. Despite the younger age of men with type 1 diabetes, the incidence of ED is substantial. A study conducted on diabetic men in Italy found that the age-adjusted prevalence of ED was indeed higher in men with type 1 diabetes (51%) compared with their type 2 counterparts (37%). Additionally, men with an elevated BMI and type 1 diabetes were found to have a significantly higher risk of ED compared with men with an elevated BMI and type 2 diabetes [40]. With 5% to 10% of diabetic men having type 1 diabetes, there is a need to focus on PDE-5 inhibition therapies in this special population.

Stuckey et al [41] performed a double-blind placebo-controlled flexible dose study on a total of 188 patients, type 1 patients were randomized to sildenafil (25–100 mg) or placebo for 12 weeks. Improvements in ED using IIEF question 3 (achieving an erection) and IIEF 4 question 4 (maintaining an erection) were found to be statistically significant in patients receiving sildenafil, and these improvements were irrespective of the degree of ED severity. Adjuvant therapy with oral propionyl-L-carnitine (PLC) and sildenafil was explored in a randomized, double-blind, fixed-dose study in 40 patients with diabetes and ED unresponsive to sildenafil monotherapy [42]. Efficacy was measured using the IIEF subscores for question 3 (Q3; achieving an erection) and question 4 (Q4; maintaining an erection). This study found a statistically significant difference in these scores in the patient group receiving sildenafil and PLC compared with the group receiving sildenafil alone. Although larger scale clinical trials are necessary before this regimen is deemed an acceptable option, salvage therapy with PLC plus sildenafil may be a worthwhile consideration for ED in diabetic patients refractory to sildenafil monotherapy.

Both tadalafil and vardenafil have been studied as therapies for diabetic men with ED; however, the results are promising for both alternative PDE5 inhibitors. Tadalafil was evaluated in a multicenter, randomized, double-blind, placebo-controlled trial involving 216 diabetic men (mean age 55.7) with a minimum 3-month history of ED [43]. Patients were randomized to placebo, tadalafil 10 mg, or tadalafil 20 mg for 12 weeks. Therapy with tadalafil (10 mg and 20 mg) significantly enhanced erectile function across IIEF erectile function domain, erection vaginal penetration rates, and successful intercourse rates. Nearly two-thirds (64%) of patients in the tadalafil 20-mg group and more than half (56%) in the tadalafil 10-mg group reported improved erections. Further, a retrospective analysis of pooled data from 12 placebo-controlled trials evaluating tadalafil for ED in diabetic men compared with that in men without diabetes included 637 men with diabetes (mean age 57 years) and 1681 men without diabetes (mean age 56 years) [44]. Compared with the placebo, both tadalafil 10 mg and 20 mg dosages improved all primary efficacy outcomes in both patient groups. Additionally, diabetic men receiving tadalafil 20 mg experienced a mean improvement of 7.4 in their IIEF erectile function domain score against baseline versus 0.9 for placebo. This group also reported on average that 53% of their attempts at intercourse were successful, compared with 22% for placebo.

Similar results have been identified with vardenafil. Goldstein et al [45] and the Vardenafil Diabetes Study Group conducted a multicenter, double-blind, placebo-controlled, fixed-dose study with 452 diabetic men (mean age 57) with a minimum 6-month history of ED. Patients were randomized to placebo, vardenafil 10 mg, or vardenafil 20 mg as needed for 12 weeks. This study reported a dose-dependent improvement in erections using a GAQ study tool of 57 and 72% for men taking 10 and 20 mg doses of vardenafil, respectively, compared with 13% for men taking placebo. Similar results were observed using the IIEF domain, with final scores for the 10 and 20 mg doses being 17.1 and 19.0, respectively, compared with 12.6 for the placebo group. Overall, vardenafil treatment was found to increase intercourse success rates at all levels of baseline ED severity, at each level of plasma HbA1c, and for type 1 and 2 diabetes.

Patients with spinal cord injury

Spinal cord injury (SCI), whether it be traumatic or medical, affects a considerable number of men who are otherwise young, active, and healthy. SCI results in many consequential comorbidities, including ED, impaired ejaculation, and changes in genital orgasmic perception. Men with SCI usually require treatment for ED, with first-line treatments being phosphodiesterase-5 inhibitors.

Sildenafil has been shown to be highly effective and well tolerated in men with ED and SCI [46]. The efficacy of sildenafil in the population of SCI individuals has been examined in several studies, including a single-dose, double-blinded, placebo-controlled study in 27 patients [47]. In that study, 75% of sildenafil patients compared with 7% of placebo patients reported that treatment had improved their erections. A significant improvement in satisfaction with their sex life was reported by patients taking sildenafil. No patients discontinued treatment due to adverse events. A larger randomized, double-blinded, placebo-controlled, crossover, flexible-dose study of 178 patients with ED and SCI employed the IIEF and partner questionnaires to assess efficacy of sildenafil [48]. In this study, 15% (27 of 178) of these patients had no pre-study erectile function. Erectile function improved in 83% of patients taking sildenafil versus 12% of those taking placebo. The sexual intercourse success rate was > 70% on sildenafil, and 0% for those taking placebo (n = 45).

A randomized, blinded, crossover clinical trial was conducted in Italy investigating sildenafil versus tadalafil for ED in men with SCI [49]. In this study of 28 patients, tadalafil allowed a majority of men to achieve a longer duration of satisfied sexual functioning of up to 24 hours postdosing compared with sildenafil. Additionally, patients on tadalafil reported improved overall sex life satisfaction as well as sexual relations with their partner compared with their experience on the sildenafil arm. Although further comparison trials are necessary in this special population of patients, this data suggests that tadalafil may have the potential to become an important treatment option for ED in SCI patients.

Patients with multiple sclerosis

Sexual problems in the multiple sclerosis (MS) patient include ED, ejaculatory disorders, and difficulty reaching orgasm. ED is the most common complaint, with the prevalence of ED in MS being approximately 70% [50,51]. First-line treatment includes the phosphodiesterase-5 inhibitors. A double-blind, placebo-controlled, flexible-dose study of sildenafil in men with ED and MS demonstrated improved erections in 90% of patients in the sildenafil group compared with 24% of patients in the placebo group [52]. Sildenafil was also found to be well tolerated in patients with MS doses of 25, 50, and 100 mg. The same group also demonstrated an improvement in quality of life with sildenafil for patients with ED and MS [53]. There have been no clinical trials to date administering tadalafil or vardenafil in this patient population.

Patients after radical prostatectomy

Unlike the traditional radical prostatectomy, the nerve-sparing approach has significantly improved postoperative erectile function.

Nonetheless, when objectively evaluated, up to 80% of men sustain some degree of ED following nerve-sparing surgery. There has been a substantial amount of research performed with this patient population and the safety and efficacy of phosphodiesterase-5 inhibitors, with the majority of clinical trials involving the use of sildenafil. In a subgroup analysis of men in American trials having had prostatectomies (n = 42), 42.5% of those receiving sildenafil demonstrated improved erections compared with 14.6% of patients receiving placebo [6,54]. The resulting intercourse success rate was nearly 30%, compared with 5% taking placebo. Because this study grouped all prostatectomy patients together (both nerve-sparing and nonnerve-sparing), a more accurate response rate can be provided based on a patient's specific operative outcome. Thus, Zippe et al [55] have demonstrated an improvement of erections in 71.7% (38 of 50), 50% (6 of 12), and 15.4% (4 of 26) of men following a bilateral nerve-sparing, unilateral nerve-sparing, and nonnerve-sparing procedure, respectively. A larger retrospective study out of the Cleveland Clinic reported similar results; out of 470 patients who underwent radical prostatectomy, 227 (48%) sought treatment for ED, and 174 (37%) were prescribed sildenafil citrate [56]. The starting dose was 50 mg, which was increased to 100 mg if the patient did not have a positive response. Stratifying the patient population by modality of treatment, after 1 year of treatment with sildenafil, 100 (57%) of 174 patients responded to the drug: 79 (76%) of 104 in the bilateral nerve-sparing group, 15 (53.5%) of 28 in the unilateral nerve-sparing group, and 6 (14.2%) of 42 in the nonnerve-sparing group. Using the Sexual Health Inventory for Men (SHIM) tool to analyze the data, this study reported that the magnitude of the improvement was greater in the bilateral nerve-sparing group (19.97 $\pm$ 1.12) than in the unilateral nerve-sparing (15.89 $\pm$ 3.38) or nonnerve-sparing (10.06 $\pm$ 2.0) groups. Factors that were statistically significant with a successful outcome included the presence of at least one neurovascular bundle, a preoperative SHIM score of 15 or greater, age 65 years old or younger, and interval from RP to drug use of more than 6 months.

In an attempt to preserve healthy corporal tissue, more recent studies have suggested expanding the use of PDE5i to include the immediate postoperative period. Recognizing that PDE5i acts to promulgate the effects of nitric oxide, then conceptually, it should work best when cavernous nerves are intact, to allow for its release and subsequent tumescence. In contrast, if neither cavernous nerve could be spared during a prostatectomy, sildenafil would have no effect on the severed nerve bundles. In this case, injectable vasoactive agents might work best. Reducing cavernosal fibrosis has been attempted with both sildenafil and prostaglandin injections. A study looked at corpora cavernosal biopsies during and 6 months following a bilateral nerve-sparing radical prostatectomy in 40 potent patients [57]. Every other night, patients took sildenafil (50 or 100 mg) every other night for 6 months beginning the day of catheter removal. This early sildenafil treatment resulted in preservation of corporal smooth muscle while preventing the development of corporal fibrosis. In fact, patients on the 100-mg sildenafil dose seemed to develop much less fibrosis and there was even a statistically significant increase in mean corporal smooth muscle content 6 months after prostatectomy.

Likewise, long-term follow up studies with sildenafil show equally promising data. Raina et al [58] reported 3-year follow-up data for 48 patients receiving sildenafil after radical prostatectomy. Sildenafil was prescribed at a dose of 50 mg and increased to 100 mg if needed. Based on self-administered questionnaire using the SHIM and the ED Inventory of Treatment Satisfaction tools, 71% of patients reported a positive response to sildenafil. No differences were found in the 1-year and 3-year SHIM and ED Inventory of Treatment Satisfaction scores between patients undergoing nerve-sparing surgery. The most common side effects at 3 years were headache (12%), flushing (10%), and blue or blurred vision (2%). No patient discontinued the drug at 3 years because of side effects. Therefore, this study shows that the majority of patients with ED following radical prostatectomy who initially respond to sildenafil will continue to do so at 3 years with minimal comorbidities.

Tadalafil has also demonstrated promising results when administered to patients who underwent radical prostatectomy. A randomized, double-blind, placebo-controlled, multicenter study from Italy administered tadalafil 20 mg or placebo, on demand, to 303 men with ED following bilateral nerve-sparing radical retropubic prostatectomy 12 to 48 months before the study [59]. Patients receiving tadalafil reported greater improvement based on their IIEF score compared with placebo. For those receiving tadalafil, the mean percentage of successful penetration attempts was 54% and the mean percentage of successful intercourse attempts was 41%. For the subgroup with evidence of postoperative tumescence these values were 69% and 52%, respectively. Patients receiving tadalafil reported greater treatment satisfaction on the ED Inventory of Treatment Satisfaction than those receiving placebo. The most common adverse effects were headache (21%), dyspepsia (13%), and myalgia (7%). As this was the only clinical trial to date in the stated literature investigating tadalafil to patients with ED following bilateral nerve-sparing radical retropubic prostatectomy, we conclude that Tadalafil 20 mg, taken on demand, was effective as well as well tolerated for this patient population.

Studies administering vardenafil to men with ED following radical prostatectomy have demonstrated similar results. A double-blind study from 58 centers out of the United States and Canada randomized 440 patients with ED after nerve-sparing radical prostatectomy to vardenafil 10 or 20 mg or placebo [60]. Assessing response after 12 weeks using the erectile function domain of the IIEF, diary questions measuring vaginal penetration and intercourse success rates, and a GAQ on erection, the study found that both vardenafil doses were significantly superior to placebo for all efficacy variables. Improved erections (based on GAQ) were reported by 65.2% and 59.4% of patients on 20 and 10 mg vardenafil, respectively, and by only 12.5% of patients on placebo. Among men with bilateral neurovascular bundle sparing, positive GAQ responses were reported by 71.1% and 59.7% of patients on 20 and 10 mg vardenafil, respectively, versus 11.5% of those on placebo. The average intercourse success rate per patient receiving 20 mg vardenafil was 74% in men with mild to moderate ED and 28% in men with severe ED, compared with 49% and 4% for placebo, respectively. Adverse events were few and variable, including incidents of mild to moderate headache, flushing, and rhinitis. For men with ED after nerve-sparing radical retropubic prostatectomy, this study showed that vardenafil significantly improved erectile function.

For patients who have suboptimal responses to PDE-5 inhibitors for ED following radical prostatectomy, future directions suggest combined regimens with various treatment modalities. One study by Mydlo et al [61] reported promising results for combined therapy using intracorporal injection (ICI) of alprostadil and oral PDE-5 inhibitors for 34 men achieving suboptimal responses to sildenafil and vardenafil. Assessing erectile function with the SHIM tool, 68% of patients had an improved in erectile function after ICI therapy. On follow-up, 36% of these patients used ICI therapy only intermittently. This study suggests that ICI therapy as an adjunct or maintenance therapy to their PDE-5 inhibitor may be another alternative in patients refractory to standard PDE-5 inhibitor treatment.

Patients after radiation therapy for prostate cancer

In contrast to the sudden onset of ED in men following radical prostatectomy, the development of ED in those receiving radiation therapy for prostate cancer is more insidious, with degrees of ED following radiation therapy to range from 34% to 62% [62–66]. Patient age, pretreatment erectile function, mode and dose of radiation delivery, neoadjuvant androgen deprivation, and the time point following radiation at which the patient is evaluated have all been identified as predictors of ED following pelvic radiation therapy [67].

PDE-5 inhibitors have been evaluated as a treatment option for men with ED and a history of pelvic radiation therapy. In one study out of Memorial Sloan Kettering, 50 patients with ED after three-dimensional conformal external beam radiotherapy with a median dose of 75.6 Gy were treated with 50 mg of sildenafil and instructed to use the medication for at least three occasions [68]. Significant improvement in the firmness and durability of erection after sildenafil was reported in 74% and 66% of study participants, respectively. Moreover, 90% of patients with erections classified as "partial" after radiotherapy had a significant response to sildenafil compared with only 52% with erections classified as "flaccid." Another study out of Switzerland looked at the response to sildenafil over time in 35 patients with ED following external-beam radiotherapy. Study participants received sildenafil 100 mg orally once a week for 6 consecutive weeks, and were assessed weekly using the International Index of Sexual Function, with response defined as a score of 18 or more. The time course of response was gradual with 40% of patients responding in the first week, while 77% responded in 6 weeks. This data suggests that not only can sildenafil reverse ED after radiotherapy in a substantial proportion of prostate cancer patients but also that it should not be discontinued prematurely for this group of individuals because of presumed ineffectiveness. Furthermore, similar results were ascertained for patients with ED after prostate brachytherapy. In a study by Merrick et al [69], 62 patients with ED and who underwent brachytherapy were treated with sildenafil in an open-label, nonrandomized study. A favorable response to sildenafil was observed in 80.6% of these patients, with only a history of diabetes being predictive of treatment failure with borderline statistical validity. This suggests that brachytherapy-induced ED can be treated with sildenafil with promising results.

Long-term follow-up using sildenafil shows equally efficacious results. A study out of Cornell provided treatment with sildenafil in 100 patients presenting with ED secondary to either three-dimensional conformal external beam irradiation or brachytherapy for prostate cancer and assessed the impact of the interval after radiation on success of this treatment [70]. Patients undergoing who achieved normalization of the IIEF erectile function domain at less than 12, 13, to 24 and 25 to 36 months for the brachytherapy/conformal external beam irradiation groups were 60%/50%, 48%/42%, and 26%/19%, respectively. Thus, although sildenafil improves erectile function in men with ED following radiation therapy for prostate cancer, there is a clear time dependence for the response with a serial stepwise decrease over a 3-year period.

Patients with depression

Beyond direct effects on sexual function, ED also leads to depressive symptoms, low self-esteem, and other signs of psychologic distress [71–74]. Several studies have assessed the effect of PDE-5 inhibitors on men with ED and depression. In one landmark study, a randomized, double-blind, placebo-controlled trial was conducted to evaluate the effects of sildenafil treatment in men with ED and mild-to-moderate comorbid depressive illness [75]. Out of the patients receiving sildenafil, 73% were considered responders, in contrast to 14% of patients receiving placebo. The study showed that regardless of the treatment received (placebo or sildenafil), patients who reported a positive treatment also a significant improvement in depression parameters! In those patients, it was suggested that depression was most likely a secondary factor to ED; regardless, the study demonstrated that sildenafil treatment resulted in improvements in both sexual and nonsexual aspects of quality of life.

Patients with increased age

ED represents an important quality of life concern for many aging men. Studies seem to conflict regarding the efficacy of PDE-5 inhibitors in this population of men. For instance, with respect to sildenafil, a study in 1998 compared IIEF responses in men younger to those older than 65 years of age; no difference in erectile function between the two age groups was demonstrated [76]. In contrast, a more recent study out of Japan found a statistically significant different between patients under and over 65 years of age (89.1% versus 65.8% efficacy, respectively) [77]. It is noteworthy, however, that this second study used a modified IIEF questionnaire (the IIEF-5, which asked only five questions), and used only 25 and 50 mg doses of sildenafil. The fact that the 100-mg dose of silde-nafil was not used may be significant in light of evidence that as men age, the resting tone of caver-nosal smooth muscle is reset to a higher level. This higher level of smooth muscle tone may require a greater degree of relaxation to permit tumescence [78]. Although the older patients in the Japan study showed a higher prevalence of diabetes mellitus, hypertension, and benign prostatic hyperplasic, only the diagnosis of diabetes appeared to decrease the efficacy of sildenafil. Another study out of Ja-pan evaluated the efficacy of sildenafil in elderly men over the age of 60 [79]. The study compared re-sponse using the IIEF-5 domain to men younger than 70 years to men 70 years and older. Although the study found that younger men had a higher rate of improvement compared with their older coun-terparts, the study still found promising a near nor-malization of erectile function and also excellent tolerability in the older group. The most commonly experienced adverse events were flushing and dyspepsia, which occurred in 6.8% and 2.3%, res-pectively. No patients discontinued sildenafil treat-ment due to adverse events. Thus, this study suggests that sildenafil is efficacious and well toler-ated by elderly men with ED, even among those older than 70 years. Potential predictors of a poor response to sildenafil treatment of ED in elderly pa-tients were investigated by a study in Korea involv-ing 162 patients aged 60 or older [80]. Efficacy was assessed using the self-administered IIEF, with the overall efficacy to sildenafil being 47% in this study population. On univariate analysis, uncontrolled di-abetes, current smoking, hypogonadism (<3 μg/L testosterone) and low pretreatment EF domain score (<17) were selected as predictors of a poor re-sponse. On multivariate logistic regression, a low pretreatment EF domain score was the strongest in-dependent prognostic factor for a poor response (odds ratio 2.25, 95% confidence interval, 1.45–7.33), and this was followed by hypogonadism (1.89, 1.12–3.16) and current smoking (1.34, 1.04–3.52). Althought the results of this study on elderly men is not nearly as promising as that for a younger population of men, these results suggest that mod-ifying reversible risk factors, may be beneficial in augmenting the efficacy of sildenafil in elderly men. Further studies with tadalafil and vardenafil also need to elderly men so that more data on this special population can be ascertained.

Alpha-blockers

PDE-5 interaction with alpha-blockers has been recognized as a possible source of hypoten-sion. Alpha-blockers are used widely in the treatment of symptomatic benign prostatic hyper-trophy, and may be used in treating hypertension. The FDA has recently approved changes in the labeling of PDE-5 inhibitors to address these interactions. The new labels suggest that the concomitant use of alpha blockers and PDE-5 inhibitors is no longer considered a contraindica-tion. Details of precautions are the concomitant use of alpha-blockers with PDE-5 inhibitors'are available in the individual package inserts of the three currently available drugs.

Management of phosphodiesterase-5 inhibitor initial failure

The introduction of PDE-5 inhibitors has revolutionized the treatment of ED, reducing the reliance on more invasive therapeutic options. PDE-5 inhibitors have been demonstrated to be effective and well tolerated in men with a broad range of severity and etiology of ED. However 30% to 35% of men will fail to respond to an adequate trial of a PDE-5 inhibitor, and many may be lost to further treatment despite the availability of other therapeutic options. There are several options available for the treatment of oral therapy failure. The options discussed in-clude: (1) patient education; (2) dose optimiza-tion; (3) switching to another oral agent; (4) improvement of comorbid conditions; (5) combi-nation with testosterone in patients with hypogo-nadism; (6) sex therapy and marital counselling; (7) combination with a vacuum device, other oral medications, intraurethral, or intracavernosal therapy; (8) switching to intracavernosal injection therapy or penile prosthesis.

Summary

PDE-5 inhibitors are a well-established, first-line therapy for ED. Extensive clinical trials and clinical experience established the highly significant efficacy and the safety of this class of drugs in the treatment of ED. Furthermore, the efficacy of PDE-5 inhibitors has been established in men with ED with broad range of etiologies and comorbidities. The future of PDE-5 inhibitors includes the expansion of indications such as the treatment of pulmonary hypertension and the potential of treatment of symptomatic BPH.

References

[1] Jardin A, Wagner G, Khoury S, et al. Erectile dysfunction—the First International Consultation. Plymouth (United Kingdom): Health Publication Ltd.; 2000.

[2] Broderick G. Oral pharmacotherapy for male sexual dysfunction. Totowa (NJ): Humana Press Inc.; 2005.

[3] Matsumot T, Kobayashi T, Kamata K. Phosphodiesterase in the vascular system. J Smooth Muscle Res 2003;39:67–86.

[4] Corbin JD, Francis SH. Molecular biology and pharmacology of PDE-5-inhibitor therapy of erectile dysfunction. J Androl 2003;24(6 suppl):S38–41.

[5] Viagra labeling information, NDA submission. New York: Pfizer; 1997.

[6] Boolell M, Allen MJ, Ballard SA, et al. Sildenafil: an orally active type 5 cyclic GMP-specific phosphodiesterase inhibitor for the treatment of penile erectile dysfunction. Int J Impot Res 1996;8:47–52.

[7] Kloner RA, Zusman RM. Cardiovascular effects of sildenafil citrate and recommendations for its use. Am J Cardiol 1999;84:11n–7n.

[8] Kloner RA. Erectile dysfunction and cardiovascular risk factors. Hosp Pract 2001;36:41–51.

[9] Porst H. IC351 (tadalafil, Cialis): update on clinical experience. Int J Impot Res 2002;14(1 suppl):57–64.

[10] Goldstein I, Lue T, Padma-Nathan H, et al. Oral sildenafil in the treatment of erectile dysfunction. N Engl J Med 1998;338:1397–404.

[11] Shabsigh R, Anastasiadis AG. Erectile dysfunction. Annu Rev Med 2003;54:153–68.

[12] Rosen RC, Riley A, Wagner G, et al. The international index of erectile dysfunction (IIEF): a multidimensional scale for assessment of erectile dysfunction. Urology 1997;49:822–30.

[13] Padma-Nathan H, Steere WD, et al. Efficacy and safety of oral sildenafil in the treatment of erectile dysfunction: A double blind, placebo-controlled study of 329 patients. Int J Clin Pract 1998;52:1–4.

[14] Steers W, Guay AT, Leriche A, et al. Assessment of the efficacy and safety of Viagra (sildenafil citrate) in men with erectile dysfunction during long-term treatment. Int J Impot Res 2001;13:261–7.

[15] Sklar GN, Szostak MJ. Urology salvage of sildenafil failures from primary care physicians [abstract 712]. J Urol 2002;28:177.

[16] Morales A, Gingell C, Collins M, et al. Clinical safety of oral sildenafil citrate (VIAGRA) in the treatment of erectile dysfunction. Int J Impot Res 2002; 10:69–73.

[17] Padma-Nathan H. The Sildenafil Study Group. A 24-week, fixed-dose study to assess the effeicacy and safety of sildenafil (Viagra) in men with erectile dysfunction. J Urol 1998;159(suppl):238A.

[18] Morales A, Gingell C, Collins M, et al. Clinical safety of sildenafil citrate (Viagra) in the treatment of erectile dysfunction. Urol Clin North Am 2001;28: 321–34.

[19] NIH Consensus Development Panel on Impotence. Impotence. JAMA 1993;270:83–90.

[20] Padma-Nathan F, Guiliano F. Oral drug therapy for erectile dysfunction. Urol Clin N Am 2001;28: 321–34.

[21] Wespes E, Amar E, Hatzichristou D, et al. Guidelines on erectile dysfunction. Eur Urol 2002;41:1–5.

[22] Arruda-Olson AM, Mahoney DW, Nehra A, et al. Cardiovascular effects of sildenafil during exercise in men with known or probable coronary artery disease: a randomized crossover trial. JAMA 2002;287: 719–25.

[23] Federal Drug Administration Vardenafil information.

[24] Levitra labeling information, NDA submission. West Haven (CT): Bayer; 2003.

[25] Hellstrom WJ, Gittelman M, Padma-Nathan H, et al. Sustained efficacy and tolerability of vardenafil, a highly potent selective PDE-5 inhibitor, in men with erectile dysfunction: results of a randomized, double-blind 26 week placebo-controlled pivotal trial. Urology 2003;62(1 suppl):8–14.

[26] Hellstrom WJ, Gittelman M, Padma-Nathan H, et al. Vardenafil for treatment of men with erectile dysfunction: efficacy and safety in a randomized, double-blind, placebo-controlled trial. J Androl 2002;23:763–71.

[27] Van Ahlen H, Zumbe J, Stauch K, et al. The real-life safety and efficacy of vardenafil: an international post-marketing surveillance study—results from 29 358 German patients. J Int Med Res 2005;33:337–48.

[28] Donatucci C, Eardley I, McVary KT, et al. Vardenafil improves erectile function regardless of etiology or baseline severity in men with erectile dysfunction [abstract 715]. J Urol 2002;167(1 suppl):178.

[29] Cialis labeling information, NDA submission. Indianapolis (IN): Lilly ICOS; 2003.

[30] Porst H, Padma-Nathan H, Guiliano F, et al. Efficacy of tadalafil for the treatment of erectile dysfunction at 24 and 36 hours after dosing: a randomized controlled trial. Urology 2003;62:121–5.

[31] Brock GB, McMahon CG, Chen KK, et al. Efficacy and safety of tadalafil for the treatment of erectile dysfunction: results of integrated analyses. J Urol 2002;168:1332–6.

[32] Brock GB, McMahon CG, Chen KK, et al. Efficacy and safety of tadalafil for the treatment of erectile dysfunction: results of integrated analyses [abstract 708]. J Urol 2002;167(1 suppl):176.

[33] Kloner RA, Hutter AM, Emmick JT, et al. Time course of the interaction between tadalafil and nitrates. J Am Coll Cardiol 2003;42:1855–60.

[34] Feldman HA, Goldstein I, Hatzichristou DG, et al. Impotence and its medical and psychosocial correlates: results of the Massachusetts Male Aging Study. J Urol 1994;151:54–61.

[35] Solomon H, Man J, Wierzbicki AS, et al. Erectile dysfunction: cardiovascular risk and the role of the cardiologist. Int J Clin Pract 2003;57:96–9.

[36] Price DE, Gingell JC, Gepi-Attee S, et al. Sildenafil: study of a novel oral treatment for erectile dysfunction in diabetic men. Diabet Med 1998;15:821–5.

[37] Rendell MS, Rajfer J, Wicker PA, et al. Sildenafil for treatment of erectile dysfunction in men with diabetes: a randomized controlled trial. Sildenafil Diabetes Study Group. JAMA 1999;281:421–6.

[38] Safarinejad MR. Oral sildenafil in the treatment of erectile dysfunction in diabetic men: a randomized double-blind and placebo-controlled study. J Diabetes Complications 2004;18:205–10.

[39] Klein R, Klein BE, Lee KE, et al. Prevalence of self-reported erectile dysfunction in people with long-term IDDM. Diabetes Care 1999;19:135–41.

[40] Fedele D, Coscelli C, Cucinotta D, et al. Incidence of erectile dysfunction in Italian men with diabetes. J Urol 2001;166:1368–71.

[41] Stuckey BG, Jadzinsky MN, Murphy LJ, et al. Sildenafil citrate for treatment of erectile dysfunction in men with type 1 diabetes: results of a randomized controlled trial. Diabetes Care 2003;26:279–84.

[42] Gentile V, Vicini P, Prigiotti G, et al. Preliminary observations on the use of propionyl-L-carnitine in combination with sildenafil in patients with erectile dysfunction and diabetes. Curr Med Res Opin 2004;20:1377–84.

[43] Saenz de Tejada I, Anglin G, Knight JR, et al. Effects of tadalafil on erectile dysfunction in men with diabetes. Diabetes Care 2002;25:2159–64.

[44] Fonseca V, Seftel A, Denne J, et al. Impact of diabetes mellitus on the severity of erectile dysfunction and response to treatment: analysis of data from tadalafil clinical trials. Diabetologia 2004;47:1914–23.

[45] Goldstein I, Young JM, Fischer J, et al. Vardenafil, a new phosphodiesterase type 5 inhibitor, in the treatment of erectile dysfunction in men with diabetes: a multicenter double-blind placebo-controlled fixed-dose study. Diabetes Care 2003;26:777–83.

[46] Derry F, Hultling C, Seftel AD, et al. Efficacy and safety of sildenafil citrate (Viagra) in men with erectile dysfunction and spinal cord injury: a review. Urology 2002;60(2 suppl):49–57.

[47] Derry FA, Dinsmore WW, Fraser M, et al. Efficacy and safety of oral sildenafil (Viagra) in men with erectile dysfunction caused by spinal cord injury. Neurology 1998;51:1629–33.

[48] Giuliano F, Hultling C, El Masry WS, et al. Randomized trial of sildenafil for the treatment of erectile dysfunction in spinal cord injury. Sildenafil Study Group. Ann Neurol 1999;46:15–21.

[49] Del Popolo G, Li Marzi V, Mondaini N, et al. Time/duration effectiveness of sildenafil versus tadalafil in the treatment of erectile dysfunction in male spinal cord-injured patients. Spinal Cord 2004;42:643–8.

[50] Betts C, D'Mellow M, Fowler C, et al. Erectile dysfunction in multiple sclerosis: associated neurological and neurophysiological deficits, and treatment of the condition. Brain 1994;117:1303–10.

[51] Zorzon M, Zivadinov R, Bosco A, et al. Sexual dysfunction in multiple sclerosis: a case–control study. I. Frequency and comparison of groups. Mult Scler 1999;5:418–27.

[52] Fowler C, Miller J, Sharief M. Viagra (sildenafil citrate) for the treatment of erectile dysfunction in men with multiple sclerosis. Ann Neurol 1999;46:497.

[53] Miller J, Fowler C, Sharief M. Effect of sildenafil citrate (Viagra) on quality of life in men with erectile dysfunction and multiple sclerosis. Ann Neurol 1999;46:496–7.

[54] Padma-Nathan H. and the Sildenafil Study Group. Efficacy of Viagra (sildenafil citrate) in the treatment of erectile dysfunction (ED) in men with transurethral or radical prostatectomy. J Urol annual meeting; 1999.

[55] Zippe CD, Jhaveri FM, Klein EA, et al. Role of Viagra after radical prostatectomy. Urology 2000;55:241–5.

[56] Raina R, Lakin MM, Agarwal A, et al. Efficacy and factors associated with successful outcome of sildenafil citrate use for erectile dysfunction after radical prostatectomy. Urology 2004;65:960–6.

[57] Schwartz EJ, Wong P, Graydon RJ. Sildenafil preserves intracorporeal smooth muscle after radical retropubic prostatectomy. J Urol 2004;171(2 Pt 1):771–4.

[58] Raina R, Lakin MM, Agarwal A, et al. Long-term effect of sildenafil citrate on erectile dysfunction after radical prostatectomy: 3-year follow-up. Urology 2003;62:110–5.

[59] Montorsi F, Nathan HP, McCullough A, et al. Tadalafil in the treatment of erectile dysfunction following bilateral nerve sparing radical retropubic prostatectomy: a randomized, double-blind, placebo controlled trial. J Urol 2004;172:1036–41.

[60] Brock G, Nehra A, Lipshultz LI, et al. Safety and efficacy of vardenafil for the treatment of men with erectile dysfunction after radical retropubic prostatectomy. J Urol 2003;170(4 Pt 1):1278–83.

[61] Mydlo JH, Viterbo R, Crispen P. Use of combined intracorporal injection and a phosphodiesterase-5 inhibitor therapy for men with a suboptimal response to sildenafil and/or vardenafil monotherapy after radical retropubic prostatectomy. BJU Int 2005;95:843–6.

[62] Mulhall JP, Yonover P, Sethi A, et al. Radiation exposure to the corporeal bodies during 3-dimensional conformal radiation therapy for prostate cancer. J Urol 2002;167:539–43.

[63] Beard CJ, Propert KJ, Reiker PP, et al. Complications after treatment with external-beam irradiation in early-stage prostate cancer patients: a prospective multiinstitutional outcomes study. J Clin Oncol 1997;15:223–9.

[64] Crook J, Esche B, Futter N. Effect of pelvic radiotherapy for prostate cancer on bowel, bladder, and sexual function: the patient's perspective. Urology 1996;47:387–94.

[65] Beard CJ, Lamb C, Buswell L, et al. Radiation-associated morbidity in patients undergoing small-field external beam irradiation for prostate cancer. Int J Radiat Oncol Biol Phys 1998;41:257–62.

[66] Mantz CA, Song P, Farhangi E, et al. Potency probability following conformal megavoltage radiotherapy using conventional doses for localized prostate cancer. Int J Radiat Oncol Biol Phys 1997;37:551–7.

[67] Turner SL, Adams K, Bull CA, et al. Sexual dysfunction after radical radiation therapy for prostate cancer: a prospective evaluation. Urology 1999;54: 124–9.

[68] Zelefsky MJ, McKee AB, Lee H, et al. Efficacy of oral sildenafil in patients with erectile dysfunction after radiotherapy for carcinoma of the prostate. Urology 1999;53:775–8.

[69] Merrick GS, Butler WM, Lief JH, et al. Efficacy of sildenafil citrate in prostate brachytherapy patients with erectile dysfunction. Urology 1999;53:1112–6.

[70] Ohebshalom M, Parker M, Guhring P, et al. The efficacy of sildenafil citrate following radiation therapy for prostate cancer: temporal considerations. J Urol 2005;174:258–62.

[71] Althof SE, Turner LA, Levine SB, et al. Intracavernosal injection in the treatment of impotence: a prospective study of sexual, psychological, and marital functioning. J Sex Marital Ther 1987;13:155–67.

[72] Derogatis LR, Meyer JK. A psychological profile of the sexual dysfunctions. Arch Sex Behav 1979;8: 201–23.

[73] Jonler M, Moon T, Brannan W, et al. The effect of age, ethnicity and geographical location on impotence and quality of life. Br J Urol 1995;75:651–5.

[74] Krane RJ, Goldstein I. Saenz de Tejada I. Impotence. N Engl J Med 1989;321:1648–59.

[75] Seidman SN, Roose SP, Menza MA, et al. Treatment of erectile dysfunction in men with depressive symptoms: results of a placebo-controlled trial with sildenafil citrate. Am J Psychiatry 2001;158: 1623–30.

[76] Wagner G, Maytom M, Smith M, et al. Analysis of the efficacy of sildenafil (Viagra) in the treatment of male erectile dysfunction in elderly patients. J Urol 1998;159(suppl):238A.

[77] Tsujimura A, Yamanaka M, Takahashi T, et al. The clinical studies of sildenafil for the ageing male. Int J Androl 2002;25:28–33.

[78] Melman A, Gingell JC. The epidemiology and pathophysiology of erectile dysfunction. J Urol 1999;161: 5–11.

[79] Fujisawa M, Sawada K. Clinical efficacy and safety of sildenafil in elderly patients with erectile dysfunction. Arch Androl 2004;50:255–60.

[80] Park K, Ku JH, Kim SW, et al. Risk factors in predicting a poor response to sildenafil citrate in elderly men with erectile dysfunction. Br J Urol Int 2005;95: 366–70.

ELSEVIER
SAUNDERS

Urol Clin N Am 32 (2005) 527–545

UROLOGIC
CLINICS
of North America

Cumulative Index 2005

Note: Page numbers of article titles are in **boldface** type.

A

Ablation, tissue, office-based procedures for, in benign prostatic hyperplasia, **327–335**

Accountants, role of in urologic practice, **263–269**
    capital improvements, 265
    choice of business entity, 263–264
        C corporation, 263
        limited liability company or partnership, 263
        partnership, 263
        S corporation, 264
        sole proprietor, 263
    depreciation methods, 265–266
    other tax considerations, 268–269
        alternative minimum tax planning, 269
        in divorce, 268–269
    practice compensation models, 264–265
        base salary plus incentive, 264–265
        compensation divided equally, 264
        part equal, part productivity, 264
        productivity, 264
    tax laws and tax strategies, 266–268
        capital gains rates, 267
        charitable deductions of vehicles, 266–267
        health savings accounts, 267–268
        marriage relief penalty, 267

Accrual basis accounting, 296

Acupuncture, neuromodulation with, in pediatric patients, 103–104

Acute scrotum, office-based ultrasound of, 348

Adjuvant chemotherapy, systemic, after cystectomy for bladder cancer, **217–229**
    approaches to, 219–221
    historical review of, 218–219
    in patients with high risk of relapse and death, 221–222
    in patients with premorbid conditions and toxicities, 222–223
    molecular markers of outcome, 224–225

    new cisplatin-based combinations for, 223
    with radiation therapy, 223–224

Afferent nerves, of the bladder, neuroanatomy and neurophysiology, 12–13

Age Discrimination in Employment Act, 258

Aging, use of PDE-5 inhibitors in men with increased age, 522

Alcohol consumption, role of lifestyle factors in erectile dysfunction, 412–416

Algorithm concept, in targeted therapy for bladder cancer, 243

Alpha-blockers, use of PDE-5 inhibitors in men taking, 522

Alternative minimum tax planning, 269

American Academy of Professional Coders, 289

American Health Information Management System, 289

American Urological Association, services for coding and reimbursement, 287–288

Americans with Disabilities Act, 256–257

Amino acids, in treatment of erectile dysfunction, 491

Aminolevulinic acid, 5-, with phototherapy for high-risk patients with superficial bladder cancer, 127

Androgen deficiency, in etiology and treatment of erectile dysfunction, **457–468**
    alternative androgen supplements, 462–463
    evaluation of, 459–460
    in the aging male, 458–459
    testosterone replacement therapy, forms of, 460–462
        monitoring patients on, 464
        risks and benefits of, 463–464
        testosterone and erectile function, 457–458

Androgen supplements, alternative, 462–463

Angina pectoris, expanding indications for neuromodulation in, 62

Apomorphine, in treatment of erectile dysfunction, 488–490

Arteriogenic causes, of erectile dysfunction, 389–390

Autonomic nervous system, innervation of pelvic organs, 165–166

Autonomic pathways, neuroanatomy of penile erection, 380–381

B

Bacillus Calmette-Guérin (BCG), intravesical immunotherapy with, in high-risk patients with superficial bladder cancer, 123–127
  in T1G3 bladder cancer, 135–138
    options after failure of, 136–138

Balloon-based thermotherapy, urethral fluid, for benign prostatic hyperplasia, 331–332

Benefits, retirement plans, for physicians and employees, 269, **309–317**

Benign prostatic hyperplasia, office-based procedures for, **327–335**
  interstitial laser coagulation, 331
  intraprostatic injection for, 330–331
  transrectal ultrasound (TRUS), 332–333
  transurethral microwave thermotherapy (TUMT), 327–328
  transurethral needle ablation (TUNA), 328–330
  urethral fluid balloon-based thermotherapy, 331–332

Bilateral sacral neuromodulation, European experience with, **51–57**
  clinical application of, 52–55
  scientific basis of, 51–52

Bion-r device, pudendal nerve neuromodulation using, **111–114**

Bladder, lymphatic drainage of, 188–189
  neuroanatomy and neurophysiology, 11–15
    afferent and efferent pathways, 12–13
    guarding reflexes, 13–14
    micturition reflexes, 11–12
    reflexes that promote micturition, 14
  neurogenic due to spinal cord injury, sacral neuromodulation for, 20–21, 60–61
  office-based ultrasound of, 342–344
    masses, 343–344

residual urine, 344
urodynamics, 344
office-based urodynamic studies of, **353–370**
overactive, detrusor overactivity incontinence, pudendal nerve neuromodulation for, **111–114**
  injectable botulinum toxin therapy for neurogenic and nonneurogenic, 92–93
  percutaneous neuromodulation for, in pediatric patients, 76
  sacral nerve stimulation indicated for, 20

Bladder cancer, 121–246
  cystectomy for, adjuvant systemic chemotherapy after, **217–229**
    approaches to, 219–221
    historical review of, 218–219
    in patients with high risk of relapse and death, 221–222
    in patients with premorbid conditions and toxicities, 222–223
    molecular markers of outcome, 224–225
    new cisplatin-based combinations for, 223
    with radiation therapy, 223–224
  neobladder with prostatic capsule and seminal-sparing, **177–185**
    arguments against, 183
    functional outcomes, 181–183
    oncologic factors, 179
    patient selection for, 177–179
    prostate cancer and, 179–181
  nerve-sparing, **165–175**
    anatomic and physiologic considerations, 165–168
    outcomes after, 169–174
    patient selection for, 168
    tips to minimize nerve damage during, 168–169
  quality of life after urinary diversion and, **207–216**
    challenges in, 209–210
    studies on, 210–215
    tools for measurement of, 208–209
  radical, early intervention with, **147–155**
    in invasive disease, 152–153
    in noninvasive disease, 147–152
  urethral transitional cell carcinoma occurring after radical, **199–206**
    monitoring for, 201–202
    orthotopic diversion and risk for, 201
    rate in men, 199–200
    risk factors in men, 200
    risk factors in women, 200–201

survival after, 202–204
treatment of, 202
intravesical chemotherapy and
immunotherapy in superficial, **121–131**
chemotherapy, 121–123
emerging technologies, 126–127
immunotherapy, 123–125
salvage programs, 125–126
invasive, neoadjuvant chemotherapy for,
231–237
surgical factors in, **157–164**
lymphadenectomy, role in high-grade invasive,
187–197
anatomy of lymphatic drainage, 188–189
historical perspective, 187–188
incidence of lymph node metastasis at
autopsy, 189–190
incidence of metastasis following radical
cystectomy, 190
morbidity and mortality of, 192–193
number of lymph nodes assessed, 191
number of lymph nodes removed, 191–192
prognostic factors, 193–195
surgical boundaries of, 190–191
neoadjuvant chemotherapy for invasive,
231–237
downstaging with, 233
impact on survival, 233–234
importance of surgical factors in evaluating
results of, 235
in perspective, 235–236
lessons from INT-0080 trial, 234–235
versus adjuvant chemotherapy, 232–233
superficial, indicators of high risk, 147–148
carcinoma in situ, 148
cell cycle regulators, 148
chromosomal alterations, 148
high-grade disease, 148
tumor stage, 148
surgical factors in, **157–164**
surgical factors in superficial and invasive,
157–164
T1G3, optimal management of, **133–145**
cystectomy in, early *versus* deferred,
138–139
diagnosis and initial management, 133–134
intravesical therapy, 135–136
prognostic factors, 134–135
recent advances, 139–140
newer intravesical agents, 139
sequential intravesical therapy, 139
treatment options after BCG failure,
136–138

targeted therapy, clinical applications in,
239–246
Bladder stimulation, historical overview of,
direct detrusor, 2–3
transurethral, 2
Bladder substitution, orthotopic, nerve-sparing
cystectomy and, 168–173
Botulinum toxin, urologic neuromodulation
with injectable, **91–101**
adverse events and contraindications, 98–99
commercially available toxins, 92
for detrusor sphincter dyssynergia and
urinary retention, 94–96
for neurogenic and nonneurogenic
overactive bladder, 92–93
in prostate, 94–96
injection techniques, 97–98
mechanism of action, 91–92
Bowel function, preservation of, with nerve-
sparing cystectomy for bladder cancer,
167–168
Budgeting, for urologic practices, **294–297**
budget components, 295–296
capital, 296
expense, 295
operating, 295–296
revenue, 295
cash *versus* accrual basis accounting, 296
reasons for, 294–295
using the budget and financial statements,
296–297
Budgets, components of, 295–296
capital, 296
expense, 295
operating, 295–296
revenue, 295
Business entity, choice of, for urologic practice,
263–264
C corporation, 263
limited liability company or partnership,
263
partnership, 263
S corporation, 264
sole proprietor, 263

C

C corporation, basic elements of, 263
Canada, sacral neuromodulation in, **41–49**

Cancer, role of comorbidities in erectile dysfunction, 409–412

Capital budget, 296

Capital gains tax rates, 267

Capital improvements, in urologic practice, 265

Carcinoma in situ, indicating high-risk superficial bladder cancer, 148

Cardiovascular risk factors, erectile dysfunction and, **397–402**
    as an early marker of vascular disease, 398–399
    can PDE-5 inhibitors improve vascular function, 400–401
    endothelial dysfunction and, 397–398
    in patients with known coronary artery disease, 400
    initial workup for patient with ED related to, 399–400
    role in epidemiology of, 409–412

Carnitine, oral, for therapy of Peyronie's disease, 473

Cash basis accounting, 296

Cavernosal (venogenic) causes, of erectile dysfunction, 390–391

Cell cycle regulators, indicating high-risk superficial bladder cancer, 148

Centers for Medicare and Medicaid Services, coding information from, 289

Central nervous system agents, in treatment of erectile dysfunction, **487–501**
    amino acids, 491
    apomorphine, 488–490
    dopamine, 487–488
    growth hormone-releasing peptide, 491
    melanocortin receptors, 492–496
    nitric oxide, 492
    noradrenaline, 490–491
    opioid peptides, 492
    oxytocin, 491–492
    serotonin, 490

Certification Commission for Health Information Technology, 281

Charitable deductions, of vehicles, 266–267

Chemotherapy, adjuvant, after cystectomy for bladder cancer, **217–229**
    approaches to, 219–221
    historical review of, 218–219
    in patients with high risk of relapse and death, 221–222
    in patients with premorbid conditions and toxicities, 222–223
    molecular markers of outcome, 224–225
    new cisplatin-based combinations for, 223
    with radiation therapy, 223–224
  intravesical, in high-risk patients with superficial bladder cancer, **121–131**
    adequate resection prior to, 121–122
    emerging technologies with, 126–127
    maintenance, 123
    newer agents for, 126
    postsurgical, in previously untreated patients, 122–123
  intravesical, in T1G3 bladder cancer, 136, 137, 139–140
  neoadjuvant, for invasive bladder cancer, **231–237**
    downstaging with, 233
    impact on survival, 233–234
    importance of surgical factors in evaluating results of, 235
    in perspective, 235–236
    lessons from INT-0080 trial, 234–235
    versus adjuvant chemotherapy, 232–233

Chemothermotherapy, in therapy of high-risk patients with superficial bladder cancer, 127

Children. *See* Pediatrics.

Chromosomal alterations, indicating high-risk superficial bladder cancer, 148

Chronic illness, role in erectile dysfunction, 409–412

Chronic pain, genitourinary. *See* Pain, chronic.

Chronic voiding dysfunction. *See* Voiding dysfunction.

Cialis. *See* Tadalafil.

Cisplatin, systemic adjuvant chemotherapy with combinations based on, after cystectomy for bladder cancer, 223

Civil Rights Act of 1964, 258

Classification, pathophysiology of erectile dysfunction, 385–392
    arteriogenic, 389–390
    cavernosal (venogenic), 390–391
    endocrinologic, 387–389
    endothelium, 391–392
    fibroelastic component, 391
    gap junction, 391

impaired endothelium-dependent
vasodilatation, 390
neurogenic, 386–387
psychogenic, 385–386
smooth muscle, 391
structural changes, 390
vasogenic, 390

Cleveland Clinic Foundation, complications of
sacral neuromodulation in patients at, 66–68

Coders, certifications for, *286–287*

Coding, for urodynamic studies, 365–368
reimbursement and, **285–290**
basics resources for urology practices,
287–288
books, newsletters and software for,
288–289
certifications for coders, 286–287
grace period eliminated, 286
hiring essential staff, 286
history of *Current Procedural Technology*
(CPT) coding, 286
internal audit process, 287
Medicare resources on, 289
National Correct Coding Initiative coding
edits, 288
resources for, 286

Colchicine, oral, for therapy of Peyronie's
disease, 472

Collagenase, intralesional therapy for Peyronie's
disease, 474

Comorbidities, role in erectile dysfunction,
409–412

Compensation models, for urologic practice,
264–265
base salary plus incentive, 264–265
compensation divided equally, 264
part equal, part productivity, 264
productivity, 264

Compliance, office-based urodynamic study of,
360–361

Complications, of sacral neuromodulation
therapy, troubleshooting for, **65–69**

Computerized records. *See* Electronic health
records.

Condyloma, genital, office-based treatment for,
325–326

Constipation, sacral neuromodulation for, 61,
81–89

Contracts, insurance, how to negotiate, **271–273**

Coronary artery disease, erectile dysfunction in
patients with known, 400

Corpora cavernosa, in hemodynamics of penile
erection and detumescence, 379–380

Corpus spongiosum, in hemodynamics of penile
erection and detumescence, 380

Council on the Application of Health
Information Technology, 282

Current Procedural Terminology (CPT), for
coding, history of, 286

Cyclic GMP, cellular, impact of regulation of
PDE-5 on signaling and inhibitor potency,
425
modulation of, in penile erectile function and
dysfunction, 422–423

Cystectomy, for bladder cancer, adjuvant
systemic chemotherapy after, **217–229**
early *versus* deferred in T1G3 tumors,
138–139
neobladder with prostatic capsule and
seminal-sparing, **177–185**
arguments against, 183
functional outcomes, 181–183
oncologic factors, 179
patient selection for, 177–179
prostate cancer and, 179–181
nerve-sparing, **165–175**
anatomic and physiologic
considerations, 165–168
outcomes after, 169–174
patient selection for, 168
tips to minimize nerve damage during,
168–169
quality of life after urinary diversion and,
207–216
challenges in, 209–210
studies on, 210–215
tools for measurement of, 208–209
radical, early intervention with,
147–155
in invasive disease, 152–153
in noninvasive disease, 147–152
radical, with pelvic lymph node dissection,
for locally advanced, 159–163
urethral management after radical, **199–206**
monitoring urethra after, 201–202
orthotopic diversion and risk for
urethral transitional cell carcinoma,
201

Cystectomy (*continued*)
    rate of urethral transitional cell
      carcinoma in men, 199–200
    risk factors in men, 200
    risk factors in women, 200–201
    survival after urethral transitional
      cell carcinoma following,
      202–204
    treatment of urethral transitional cell
      carcinoma after, 202

Cystitis, interstitial, sacral nerve stimulation for,
  20–21, 59–60

Cystometry, filling, office-based urodynamic
  study of, 358–360

Cystoscopes, flexible, office-based procedures
  with, 320–325
    characteristics of, 320–321
    diagnostic and therapeutic procedures with,
      322–325
    techniques with, 321–322

Cystoscopic procedures, office-based, **319–326**
  flexible cystoscopes, 320–325
    characteristics of, 320–321
    diagnostic and therapeutic procedures
      with, 322–325
    techniques with, 321–322
  history, 319–320

Cytopenias, systemic adjuvant chemotherapy
  after cystectomy for bladder cancer in
  patients with, 222–223

D

Deductions, charitable, of vehicles, 266–267

Defined contribution plans, for physicians and
  employees, 310–313
    401(k) plans, 311–312
    age-weighted profit-sharing plans, 311
    money purchase pension plans, 310
    new comparability plans, 311
    profit-sharing plans, 310
    savings incentive match plans for employees
      (SIMPLE), 312–313

Depreciation methods, in urologic practice,
  265–266

Depression, role of comorbidities in erectile
  dysfunction, 409–412
  use of PDE-5 inhibitors in men with, 521

Detrusor overactivity, office-based urodynamic
  study of, 360

Detrusor overactivity incontinence, pudendal
  nerve neuromodulation using the *bion*-r
  device for, **111–114**

Detrusor sphincter dyssynergia, injectable
  botulinum toxin therapy for, 94–96

Diabetes mellitus, use of PDE-5 inhibitors in
  men with, 517–518

Disabilities, Americans with Disabilities Act,
  256–257

Discrimination, against employees, Age
  Discrimination in Employment Act, 258
  Americans with Disabilities Act, 256–257
  Civil Rights Act of 1964, 258

Diversion. *See* Urinary diversion.

Divorce, tax planning for, 268–269

Doctors' Office Quality-Information Technology
  project, 281

Dopamine, in treatment of erectile dysfunction,
  487–488

Dysfunctional elimination syndrome, in
  pediatric patients, neuromodulation
  techniques for, **103–109**
  See also Voiding dysfunction.

E

E-Health Initiative, 281

Early intervention, radical cystectomy for
  bladder cancer, **147–155**

Efferent nerves, of the bladder, neuroanatomy
  and neurophysiology, 12–13

Electromotive intravesical therapy, with
  mitomycin C, in high-risk patients with
  superficial bladder cancer, 126

Electromyography, in clinical evaluation of
  voiding dysfunction, 24
  in office-based urodynamic studies, 363–364

Electronic health records, 276–283
  applications options for, 277–278
  barriers to adoption of, 278–279
  compliance issues associated with, 280–281
  potential improvements due to, 278
  potential return on investment in, 277
  product selection process, 279–280
  professional and government efforts to foster
    adoption of, 281–282
  progress toward, 276–277
  vision of, in urologic practice, 282–283

Employees, personnel issues, **253–262**
  Age Discrimination in Employment Act,
    258
  Americans with Disabilities Act, 256–257
  Civil Rights Act of 1964, 258
  Family and Medical Leave Act, 253–256
  how to handle, 258–261
    employee handbooks, 258–259
    employee terminations, 260–261
    investigations, 259–260

Endocrinologic causes, of erectile dysfunction,
  387–389

Endothelium, in pathophysiology of erectile
  dysfunction, 391–392, 397–398

Epidemiology, of erectile dysfunction, **403–417**
  prevalence and incidence, 404–409
  role of comorbidities and chronic illness,
    409–412
  role of lifestyle factors, 412–416
  of Peyronie's disease, 470–471

Epidermal growth factor receptor, in targeted
  therapy for bladder cancer, **239–246**

erbB family, in targeted therapy for bladder
  cancer, **239–246**

Erectile dysfunction, 379–525
  androgen deficiency in etiology and treatment
    of, **457–468**
    alternative androgen supplements, 462–462
    evaluation of, 459–460
    in the aging male, 458–459
    testosterone replacement therapy, forms of,
      460–462
      monitoring patients on, 464
      risks and benefits of, 463–464
    testosterone and erectile function, 457–458
  cardiovascular risk factors and, as an early
    marker of vascular disease, 398–399
  can PDE-5 inhibitors improve vascular
    function, 400–401
  endothelial dysfunction and, 397–398
  in patients with known coronary artery
    disease, 400
  initial workup for patient with, 399–400
  clinical evaluation of, **447–455**
    clinical assessment, 450–451
      basic laboratory testing, 451
      medical and sexual history, 450–451
      physical examination, 451
      symptom scales, 450
    identification of risk factors, 447–450
    specialized, 451–453

    neurologic, 453
    psychologic, 453
    vascular, 452–453
  epidemiology of, **403–417**
    prevalence and incidence, 404–409
    role of comorbidities and chronic illness,
      409–412
    role of lifestyle factors, 412–416
  molecular biology of, **419–429**
  pathophysiology of, **379–395**
    classification, 385–392
      arteriogenic, 389–390
      cavernosal (venogenic), 390–391
      endocrinologic, 387–389
      endothelium, 391–392
      fibroelastic component, 391
      gap junction, 391
      impaired endothelium-dependent
        vasodilatation, 390
      neurogenic, 386–387
      psychogenic, 385–386
      smooth muscle, 391
      structural changes, 390
      vasogenic, 390
  Peyronie's disease, etiology, epidemiology, and
    medical treatment, **469–478**
    surgical treatment, **479–485**
  psychosocial evaluation and treatment of,
    431–445
    etiology, 433–434
    evaluation and diagnosis, 434–439
    nosology and definition, 433
    referral, 442–443
    Sexual Tipping Point and combination
      treatment, 432–433
    treatment, 439–442
  treatment of, central nervous system agents,
    487–501
    phosphodiesterase-5 (PDE-5) inhibitors
      current status and future trends,
        511–525
      molecular biology of, **419–429**
    surgical implants, **503–509**

Erection, penile, molecular biology of, **419–429**
  pathophysiology of. *See* Erectile dysfunction.
  physiology of, **379–395**
    hemodynamics and mechanism of,
      379–380
    molecular mechanism of smooth muscle
      contraction and relaxation, 384–385
    neuroanatomy and neurophysiology of,
      380–384

Expense budget, 295

External energy therapy, for Peyronie's disease,
    475–476
        iontophoresis, 475–476
        shock wave therapy, 475

F

Family and Medical Leave Act, 253–256

Family history, in psychosocial evaluation of
    erectile dysfunction, 439

Fecal incontinence, sacral neuromodulation for,
    61, **81–89**

Fibroelastic componenet, erectile dysfunction
    due to, 391

Filling cystometry, office-based urodynamic
    study of, 358–360

Financial statements, how to use budgets and,
    296–297

Flexible cystoscopes, office-based procedures
    with, 320–325
        characteristics of, 320–321
        diagnostic and therapeutic procedures with,
            322–325
        techniques with, 321–322

G

Gap junction, in pathophysiology of erectile
    dysfunction, 391

Gemcitabine, in intravesical chemotherapy in
    high-risk patients with superficial bladder
    cancer, 126

Genital condyloma, office-based treatment for,
    325–326

Genitourinary pain, chronic, sacral
    neuromodulation for, 60

Glans penis, in hemodynamics of penile erection
    and detumescence, 380

Grade, tumor, indicating high-risk superficial
    bladder cancer, 148

Growth hormone-releasing peptide, in treatment
    of erectile dysfunction, 491

H

Handbooks, employee, 258–259

Health Insurance Portability and Accountability
    Act of 1996, compliance issues with, using
    electronic health records, 280–281

Health Level Seven Functional Standard (HL7),
    282

Health records. *See* Electronic health records
    and Medical records.

Health savings accounts, 267–268

Health-related quality of life. *See* Quality of life.

Heart failure, systemic adjuvant chemotherapy
    after cystectomy for bladder cancer in
    patients with, 222

Hemodynamics, of penile erection and
    detumescence, 379–380

History taking, in psychosocial evaluation of
    erectile dysfunction, 434–436

Human epidermal growth factor receptors, in
    targeted therapy for bladder cancer, **239–246**

Human papillomavirus, office-based treatment
    for genital warts, 325–326

Hydroceles, office-based ultrasound of scrotum,
    347–348

Hydronephrosis, office-based ultrasound of
    kidney, 340–341

Hypercholesterolemia, role of comorbidities in
    erectile dysfunction, 409–412

Hypertension, role in erectile dysfunction,
    409–412

Hyperthermia, localized, chemothermotherapy
    for high-risk patients with superficial bladder
    cancer, 127

I

Illness, chronic, role in erectile dysfunction,
    409–412

Imiquimod 5% cream, office-based treatment for
    genital warts, 325–326

Immunotherapy, intravesical, for T1G3 bladder
    cancer, 135–136
        options after BCG failure, 136–138
            interferon therapy, 137
            radiation and photodynamic therapy,
                137–138
            repeat BCG treatment, 137
        recent advances in, 139–140
            newer agents, 139–140
            sequential therapy, 139
        intravesical, in high-risk patients with
            superficial bladder cancer, **121–131**

emerging technologies, 126–127
optimized administration of bacillus
    Calmette-Guérin, 124–125
salvage program, 125–126
when treatment fails, 125

Implantable pulse generator, surgical technique
    for implantation of, **27–35**

Implants. *See* Penile prosthesis implantation.

Incontinence, fecal, sacral neuromodulation for,
    61, **81–89**

Incontinence, urinary, due to detrusor
    overactivity, pudendal nerve
    neuromodulation for, **111–114**

Information technology, electronic health
    records, 276–283

Injection, intraprostatic, office-based, for benign
    prostatic hyperplasia, 330–331

Insurance companies, negotiating
    reimbursement contracts with, **271–273**

Interferon, salvage therapy with, after
    intravesical immunotherapy, in high-risk
    patients with superficial bladder cancer,
    125–126
        in T1G3 bladder cancer, 137

Interferons, intralesional therapy for Peyronie's
    disease, 474–475

Internet marketing, 302–303

Interstim. *See* Implantable pulse generator.

Interstitial cystitis, sacral nerve stimulation for,
    20–21, 59–60

Interstitial laser coagulation, office-based, for
    benign prostatic hyperplasia, 331

Intralesional therapy, for Peyronie's disease,
    473–475
        collagenase, 474
        interferons, 474–475
        steroids, 473–474
        verapamil, 474

Intraprostatic injection, office-based, for benign
    prostatic hyperplasia, 330–331

Intravesical therapy, for T1G3 bladder cancer,
    135–140
        chemotherapy, 136
        immunotherapy, 135–136
        options after BCG failure, 136–138
            interferon therapy, 137

radiation and photodynamic therapy,
    137–138
repeat BCG treatment, 137
recent advances in, 139–140
    newer agents, 139–140
    sequential therapy, 139
in high-risk patients with superficial bladder
    cancer, **121–131**
    chemotherapy, 121–123, 126–127
        adequate resection prior to, 121–122
        emerging technologies with, 126–127
        maintenance, 123
        newer agents for, 126
        postsurgical, in previously untreated
            patients, 122–123
    immunotherapy, 123–127
        emerging technologies, 126–127
        optimized administration of bacillus
            Calmette-Guérin, 124–125
        salvage program, 125–126
        when treatment fails, 125

Invasive bladder cancer. *See* Bladder cancer,
    invasive.

Investigations, of personnel issues, 259

Iontophoresis, for Peyronie's disease, 475–476

K
Kidneys, office-based ultrasound of, 340–342
    hydronephrosis, 340–341
    masses, 341–342
    perirenal and renal pelvis processes, 342

L
Laser coagulation, interstitial, office-based, for
    benign prostatic hyperplasia, 331

Leak-point pressures, office-based urodynamic
    study of, 361–362

Leave of absence, for employees, Family and
    Medical Leave Act, 253–256

Left ventricular impairment, systemic adjuvant
    chemotherapy after cystectomy for bladder
    cancer in patients with, 222

Levitra. *See* Vardenafil.

Lifestyle factors, role in epidemiology of in
    erectile dysfunction, 412–416

Limited liability company, basic elements of, 263

Limited liability partnership, basic elements of,
    263

Locally advanced bladder cancer. *See* Bladder cancer, invasive.

Lower urinary tract disease, role in erectile dysfunction, 409–412

Lymphadenectomy, extended, potential impact on nerve-sparing in cystectomy for bladder cancer, 168
  role in high-grade invasive bladder cancer, **187–197**
    anatomy of lymphatic drainage, 188–189
    historical perspective, 187–188
    incidence of lymph node metastasis at autopsy, 189–190
    incidence of metastasis following radical cystectomy, 190
    morbidity and mortality of, 192–193
    number of lymph nodes assessed, 191
    number of lymph nodes removed, 191–192
    prognostic factors, 193–195
    surgical boundaries of, 190–191

M

Maintenance chemotherapy, intravesical, in high-risk patients with superficial bladder cancer, 123

Management, of urologic practice, 253–317
  accountants, role of, **263–269**
    capital improvements, 265
    choice of business entity, 263–264
      C corporation, 263
      limited liability company or partnership, 263
      partnership, 263
      S corporation, 264
      sole proprietor, 263
    depreciation methods, 265–266
    other tax considerations, 268–269
      alternative minimum tax planning, 269
      in divorce, 268–269
    practice compensation models, 264–265
      base salary plus incentive, 264–265
      compensation divided equally, 264
      part equal, part productivity, 264
      productivity, 264
    tax laws and tax strategies, 266–268
      capital gains rates, 267
      charitable deductions of vehicles, 266–267
      health savings accounts, 267–268
      marriage relief penalty, 267
  budgeting, **294–297**
    budget components, 295–296
      capital, 296
      expense, 295
      operating, 295–296
      revenue, 295
    cash *versus* accrual basis accounting, 296
    reasons for, 294–295
    using the budget and financial statements, 296–297
  coding and reimbursement, **285–290**
    basics resources for urology practices, 287–288
    books, newsletters and software for, 288–289
    certifications for coders, 286–287
    grace period eliminated, 286
    hiring essential staff, 286
    history of *Current Procedural Technology* (CPT) coding, 286
    internal audit process, 287
    Medicare resources on, 289
    National Correct Coding Initiative coding edits, 288
    resources for, 286
  marketing, **299–308**
    attracting new patients, 302–303
    four pillars of success, 299
    improving communication with referral sources, 306–308
      intraspecialty referrals, 307–308
      nontraditional referrals, 308
    motivating staff for, 303–306
    to patients already in the practice, 299–302
  medical records, **275–284**
    electronic health records, 276–283
      applications options for, 277–278
      barriers to adoption of, 278–279
      compliance issues associated with, 280–281
      potential improvements due to, 278
      potential return on investment in, 277
      product selection process, 279–280
      professional and government efforts to foster adoption of, 281–282
      progress toward, 276–277
      vision of, 282–283
    historical perspective, 275
    typical model for, 275–276
  negotiating insurance contracts, **271–273**
  personnel issues, **253–262**
    Age Discrimination in Employment Act, 258
    Americans with Disabilities Act, 256–257
    Civil Rights Act of 1964, 258

Family and Medical Leave Act, 253–256
  how to handle, 258–261
    employee handbooks, 258–259
    employee terminations, 260–261
    investigations, 259–260
  retirement plans for physicians and employees,
    269, **309–317**
    avoiding early retirement penalty, 317
    choosing a plan, 313–316
    defined benefit plans, 309–310
    defined contribution plans, 310–313
      401(k) plans, 311–312
      age-weighted profit-sharing plans, 311
      money purchase pension plans, 310
      new comparability plans, 311
      profit-sharing plans, 310
      savings incentive match plans for
        employees (SIMPLE), 312–313
    four steps for qualified plan distributions,
      316–317
    implementing a plan, 313, 316
  strategic planning, **291–294**
    assessment of strengths, weaknesses,
      opportunities, and threats, 293
    determining group's readiness for, 292
    example of, 293–294
    having the right people present for,
      292–293
    identifying major issues threatening the
      group, 292
    importance of, 291–292

Marketing, for urologic practices, **299–308**
  attracting new patients, 302–303
  four pillars of success, 299
  improving communication with referral
    sources, 306–308
    intraspecialty referrals, 307–308
    nontraditional referrals, 308
  motivating staff for, 303–306
  to patients already in the practice, 299–302

Marriage relief penalty, 267

Masses, urologic, office-based ultrasound of, in
  bladder, 343–344
  in kidney, 341–342
  in scrotum, 348

Maternity leave, for employees, Family and
  Medical Leave Act, 253–256

Medical leave, for employees, Family and
  Medical Leave Act, 253–256

Medical records, management of, in urologic
  practice, **275–284**

electronic health records, 276–283
  applications options for, 277–278
  barriers to adoption of, 278–279
  compliance issues associated with,
    280–281
  potential improvements due to, 278
  potential return on investment in, 277
  product selection process, 279–280
  professional and government efforts to
    foster adoption of, 281–282
  progress toward, 276–277
  vision of, 282–283
  historical perspective, 275
  typical model for, 275–276

Medicare, coding for, informational resources,
  289

Melanocortin system, in treatment of erectile
  dysfunction, 492–496
  mechanisms of action, 495
  preclinical studies, 495–496
  receptor subtypes, 493–494
  sites of action, 494–495

Metastasis, of bladder cancer to lymph nodes,
  incidence of, at autopsy, 189–190
  incidence of, following radical cystectomy,
    190

Microwave thermotherapy, transurethral, for
  benign prostatic hyperplasia, 327–328

Micturition reflexes, neuroanatomy and
  neurophysiology of, 11–12

Migraine, chronic, expanding indications for
  neuromodulation in, 62

Mitomycin C, intravesical chemotherapy with,
  in high-risk patients with superficial bladder
  cancer, 122–123
  electromotive, 127

Molecular biology, of erectile function and
  dysfunction and phosphodiesterase
  inhibition, **419–429**

Molecular markers, of outcome of systemic
  adjuvant chemotherapy after cystectomy for
  bladder cancer, 224–225

Molecular mechanisms, of penile erection,
  384–385

Multiple sclerosis, use of PDE-5 inhibitors in
  men with, 519

Muscle dysfunction, pelvic floor, sacral nerve
  stimulation indicated for, 21

N

National Correct Coding Initiative, coding edits from, 288

Needle ablation, transurethral, office-based, for benign prostatic hyperplasia, 328–330

Negotiations, for insurance contracts, **271–273**

Neoadjuvant chemotherapy, for invasive bladder cancer, **231–237**
   downstaging with, 233
   impact on survival, 233–234
   importance of surgical factors in evaluating results of, 235
   in perspective, 235–236
   lessons from INT-0080 trial, 234–235
   versus adjuvant chemotherapy, 232–233

Neobladder, with prostatic capsule and seminal-sparing cystectomy for bladder cancer, **177–185**
   arguments against, 183
   functional outcomes, 181–183
   oncologic factors, 179
   patient selection for, 177–179
   prostate cancer and, 179–181

Nerve-sparing cystectomy, for bladder cancer, **165–175**
   anatomic and physiologic considerations, 165–168
   outcomes after, 169–174
   patient selection for, 168
   tips to minimize nerve damage during, 168–169

Nerves, pelvic, afferent and efferent, of the bladder, neuroanatomy and neurophysiology, 12–13
   stimulation of, historical overview of, 3–4

Neuroanatomy, of penile erection, 380–384

Neurogenic bladder, injectable botulinum toxin therapy for, 92–93
   sacral nerve stimulation for, 20–21, 60–61

Neurogenic causes, of erectile dysfunction, 386–387

Neuromodulation, pelvic, 1–117
   bilateral, European experience with, **51–57**
      clinical application of, 52–55
      scientific basis of, 51–52
   Canadian experience with, **41–49**
   complications and troubleshooting, **65–69**
   current indications for, **37–40**
      urge incontinence, 38–39

      urgency frequency, 38–39
      urinary retention, 39
   expanding indications for, **59–63**
      chronic genitourinary pain, 60
      fecal incontinence and constipation, 61
      in children, 61–62
      interstitial cystitis, 59–60
      neurogenic bladder due to spinal cord injury, 60–61
      nonurologic uses, 62
         angina pectoris, 62
         chronic migraine, 62
   for constipation and fecal incontinence, 61, **81–89**
      evolution of technique, 82–83
      patient selection for, 82
   future directions in, **115–117**
   historical overview, **1–10**
      direct detrusor stimulation, 2–3
      pelvic floor stimulation, 4
      pelvic nerve stimulation, 3–4
      sacral root stimulation, 5–8
      spinal cord stimulation, 4–5
      transurethral bladder stimulation, 2
   how it works, **11–18**
      afferent and efferent pathways, 12–13
      effect of sacral afferent input, 14–15
      guarding reflexes, 13–14
      micturition reflexes, 11–12
      reflexes promoting micturition, 14
   in pediatric patients, **103–109**
      acupuncture, 103–104
      expanding indications for, 61–62
      percutaneous, for overactive bladder, 76
      posterior tibial nerve stimulation, 105
      sacral nerve root stimulation, 106–108
      transurethral electric bladder stimulation, 105–106
   percutaneous, **71–79**
      early experiences with, 72–73
      in pediatrics, 76
      other indications, 76–77
      rationale for, 71–72
      recent evidence, 73–76
   selecting patients for, **19–26**
   surgical techniques for sacral implantation, **27–35**
   with injectable botulinum toxin, **91–101**
   with the *bion*-r device, **111–114**

Neurophysiology, of penile erection, 380–384
   related to sacral nerve stimulation, **11–18**
      afferent and efferent pathways, 12–13
      effect of sacral afferent input, 14–15

guarding reflexes, 13–14
how it SNS works, 15–17
micturition reflexes, 11–12
reflexes promoting micturition, 14

Neurostimulation. *See* Neuromodulation.

Nitric oxide, in treatment of erectile dysfunction, 492

Noradrenaline, in treatment of erectile dysfunction, 490–491

O

Obesity, role of lifestyle factors in erectile dysfunction, 412–416

Office-based procedures, for genital condyloma, 325–326
general and cystoscopic procedures, **319–326**
prostate procedures, **327–335**
urodynamics, **353–370**
urologic ultrasound, **337–352**

Operating budget, 295–296

Opioid peptides, in treatment of erectile dysfunction, 492

Orthotopic bladder substitution, nerve-sparing cystectomy and, 168–173

Overactive bladder, detrusor overactivity incontinence, pudendal nerve neuromodulation for, **111–114**
in pediatric patients, percutaneous neuromodulation for, 76
injectable botulinum toxin therapy for neurogenic and nonneurogenic, 92–93
office-based urodynamic study of, 360
peripheral nerve stimulation for refractory, 39–40
sacral nerve stimulation indicated for, 20

Oxytocin, in treatment of erectile dysfunction, 491–492

P

Pain, chronic genitourinary, sacral neuromodulation for, 60

Pain, pelvic, sacral nerve stimulation indicated for, 20–21

Paperless office. *See* Electronic health records.

Partner issues, in psychosocial evaluation of erectile dysfunction, 439

Partnerships, basic elements of, 263

Pathophysiology, of erectile dysfunction, 379–525

Patient selection, for sacral nerve stimulation, **19–26**

Pediatrics, neuromodulation in, **103–109**
acupuncture, 103–104
expanding indications for, 61–62
percutaneous, for overactive bladder, 76
posterior tibial nerve stimulation, 105
sacral nerve root stimulation, 106–108
transurethral electric bladder stimulation, 105–106

Pelvic floor, stimulation of, historical overview of, 4

Pelvic floor muscle dysfunction, sacral nerve stimulation indicated for, 21

Pelvic lymph node dissection, with radical cystectomy, for locally advanced bladder cancer, 159–163

Pelvic nerves, stimulation of, historical overview of, 3–4

Pelvic neuromodulation. *See* Neuromodulation, pelvic.

Pelvic organs, autonomic innervation of, 165–167

Pelvic pain, sacral nerve stimulation indicated for, 20–21

Penile prosthesis implantation, for erectile dysfunction, **503–509**
complications following, 507
design of, 504–505
patient selection, 503–504
surgical technique, 505–506
for Peyronie's disease, 483–484

Penis, office-based ultrasound of, 349–350

Pensions. *See* Retirement plans.

Percutaneous nerve evaluation, and sacral neuromodulation, Canadian experience with, **41–49**

Percutaneous neuromodulation, **71–79**
early experiences with, 72–73
in pediatrics, 76
other indications, 76–77
rationale for, 71–72
recent evidence, 73–76

Peripheral nerve stimulation, for refractory overactive bladder, 39–40

Peripheral pathways, neuroanatomy of penile erection, 380

Perirenal processes, office-based ultrasound of kidney, 340–341

Personnel issues, **253–262**
  Age Discrimination in Employment Act, 258
  Americans with Disabilities Act, 256–257
  Civil Rights Act of 1964, 258
  Family and Medical Leave Act, 253–256
  how to handle, 258–261
    employee handbooks, 258–259
    employee terminations, 260–261
    investigations, 259–260

Peyronie's disease, **469–478, 479–485**
  epidemiology, 470–471
  etiology, 469–470
  medical therapy, 471–476
    combination therapies, 476
    external energy therapy, 475–476
    intralesional, 473–475
    oral, 472–473
    topical, 473
  office-based ultrasound of, 349–350
  surgical therapy of, **479–485**
    penile prosthetic implantation, 483–484
    plication, 481–482
    tunica lengthening procedures, 482–483
    tunica shortening, 481

Phosphodiesterase-5 (PDE-5) inhibitors, clinical evaluation of erectile dysfunction in the era of, **447–455**
  current status and future trends, **511–525**
    management of initial PDE-5 failure, 522–523
    selectivity of, 512
    sildenafil, 512–514
    tadalafil, 516–517
    use in special populations, 517–523
      after radiation therapy for prostate cancer, 521
      after radical prostatectomy, 519–521
      depression, 521
      diabetes mellitus, 517–518
      increased age, 522
      multiple sclerosis, 519
      patients taking alpha-blockers, 522
      spinal cord injury, 518–519
    vardenafil, 514–516
  improvement of vascular function due to, 400–401
  molecular biology of erectile function and dysfunction, **419–429**

cessation of inhibitor effects, 425–426
impact of regulation of PDE-5 on cyclic GMP signaling and inhibitor potency, 425
mechanism of action, 423–425
modulation of cellular cyclic GMP level, 422–423
signaling pathways in penile erection, 419–422
tissues affected by action of, 426

Photodynamic therapy, for high-risk patients with superficial bladder cancer, 127
  salvage therapy with, after BCG failure in T1G3 bladder cancer, 137–138

Physicians' Electronic Health Record Coalition, 281

Planning. See Strategic planning.

Plication, for Peyronie's disease, 481–482

Posterior tibial nerve stimulation, in pediatric patients, 105

Postvoid residual volume, office-based urodynamic study of, 357–358

Potassium aminobenzoate, oral, for therapy of Peyronie's disease, 472

Practice management. See Practice.

Pressure-flow analysis, office-based urodynamic study of, 362–363

Productivity, in practice compensation models, 264

Profit-sharing plans, 310–311

Prognostic factors, in bladder cancer patients, with lymph node metastases after radical cystectomy, 193–195
  with T1G3 tumors, 134–135

Prostate, office-based procedures for benign prostatic hyperplasia, **327–335**
  interstitial laser coagulation, 331
  intraprostatic injection for, 330–331
  transrectal ultrasound (TRUS), 332–333
  transurethral microwave thermotherapy (TUMT), 327–328
  transurethral needle ablation (TUNA), 328–330
  urethral fluid balloon-based thermotherapy, 331–332
  office-based ultrasound of, **344–347**
    cancer, 346–347
    future of, 347
    prostate volume, 345–346

Prostate cancer, in cystoprostatectomy specimens performed for bladder cancer, 179–181
use of PDE-5 inhibitors after radiation therapy for, 521

Prostate conditions, injectable botulinum toxin therapy for, 96–97

Prostate-sparing cystectomy, for bladder cancer, **177–185**
arguments against, 183
functional outcomes, 181–183
oncologic factors, 179
patient selection for, 177–179
prostate cancer and, 179–181

Prostatectomy, radical, use of PDE-5 inhibitors in men after, 519–521

Prosthesis, penile. *See* Penile prosthesis implantation.

Psychiatric considerations, in psychosocial evaluation of erectile dysfunction, 438

Psychogenic causes, of erectile dysfunction, 385–386

Psychosocial evaluation, of erectile dysfunction, **431–445**
etiology, 433–434
evaluation and diagnosis, 434–439
exploring other psychosocial issues, 437–438
family and early psychosexual history, 439
history taking, 434–436
partner/relationship issues, 439
previous treatment approaches, 438
psychiatric considerations, 438
questionnaires, 439
sex status examination, 436–437
the single patient, 439
nosology and definition, 433
referral, 442–443
Sexual Tipping Point and combination treatment, 432–433
treatment, 439–442
combination therapy, 442
follow-up and therapeutic probe, 440–441
weaning and relapse prevention, 441–442

Pudendal nerve neuromodulation, using the *bion*-r device, **111–114**

Q

Quality of life, in bladder cancer patients after cystectomy and urinary diversion, **207–216**
challenges in, 209–210
studies on, 210–215
tools for measurement of, 208–209

R

Radiation therapy, for prostate cancer, use of PDE-5 inhibitors in men after, 519–521
salvage therapy with, after BCG failure in T1G3 bladder cancer, 137–138
with systemic adjuvant chemotherapy after cystectomy for bladder cancer, 223

Radical cystectomy, for bladder cancer, early intervention with, **147–155**
in invasive disease, 152–153
in noninvasive disease, 147–152
neobladder with prostatic capsule and seminal-sparing, **177–185**
arguments against, 183
functional outcomes, 181–183
oncologic factors, 179
patient selection for, 177–179
prostate cancer and, 179–181
nerve-sparing, with orthotopic bladder substitution, **165–175**
urethral transitional cell carcinoma occurring after, **199–206**
monitoring for, 201–202
orthotopic diversion and risk for, 201
rate in men, 199–200
risk factors in men, 200
risk factors in women, 200–201
survival after, 202–204
treatment of, 202
with pelvic lymph node dissection, for locally advanced, 159–163

Radical prostatectomy, use of PDE-5 inhibitors in men after, 519–521

Records. *See* Electronic health records and Medical records.

Referral sources, marketing urologic practice to, 306–308
intraspecialty referrals, 307–308
nontraditional referrals, 308

Referrals, to a sex therapist, for patients with erectile dysfunction, 442–443

Reimbursement, for services, coding and, **285–290**
negotiating insurance contracts, **271–273**

Relationship issues, in psychosocial evaluation of erectile dysfunction, 439

Renal impairment, systemic adjuvant chemotherapy after cystectomy for bladder cancer in patients with, 222

Renal pelvis processes, office-based ultrasound of kidney, 340–341

Residual urine, office-based ultrasound of bladder, 344
    postvoid, office-based urodynamic study of, 357–358

Retention. *See* Urinary retention.

Retirement plans, for physicians and employees, 269, **309–317**
    avoiding early retirement penalty, 317
    choosing a plan, 313–316
    defined benefit plans, 309–310
    defined contribution plans, 310–313
        401(k) plans, 311–312
        age-weighted profit-sharing plans, 311
        money purchase pension plans, 310
        new comparability plans, 311
        profit-sharing plans, 310
        savings incentive match plans for employees (SIMPLE), 312–313
    four steps for qualified plan distributions, 316–317
    implementing a plan, 313, 316

Revenue budget, 295

RF-*bion* device, 113

Risk factors, for erectile dysfunction, 447–450
    cardiovascular, **397–402**
    medical comorbidities and chronic illness, **403–417**

S

S corporation, basic elements of, 264

Sacral nerve root stimulation, in pediatric patients, 106–108

Sacral nerve stimulation, pelvic neuromodulation with, 1–117
    Canadian experience with, **41–49**
    complications and troubleshooting, **65–69**
    current indications for, 20–21, **37–40**
    European experience with, **51–57**
    expanding indications for, **59–63**
    for constipation and fecal incontinence, **81–89**

historical overview, **1–10**
how it works, **11–18**
in pediatrics, **103–109**
neurophysiology related to, **11–18**
    afferent and efferent pathways, 12–13
    effect of sacral afferent input, 14–15
    guarding reflexes, 13–14
    how it SNS works, 15–17
    micturition reflexes, 11–12
    reflexes promoting micturition, 14
percutaneous, **71–79**
selecting patients for, **19–26**
surgical techniques for sacral implantation, **27–35**
using injectable botulinum toxin, **91–101**

Sacral root, stimulation of, historical overview of, 5–8

Salvage therapy, after failure of intravesical therapy in bladder cancer, in T1G3 tumors, 136–138
    with interferon in high-risk patients with superficial bladder cancer, 125–126

Scrotum, office-based ultrasound of, 347–349
    acute, 348
    hydroceles, 347–348
    masses, 348
    trauma, 348–349

Sedentary lifestyle, role of lifestyle factors in erectile dysfunction, 412–416

Seminal-sparing cystectomy. *See* Prostate-sparing cystectomy.

Sequential intravesical therapy, for T1G3 bladder tumors, 139

Serotonin, in treatment of erectile dysfunction, 490

Sex status examination, in psychosocial evaluation of erectile dysfunction, 436–437

Sex therapists, referrals to, for patients with erectile dysfunction, 442–443

Sexual arousal, central neural activation during, 382–384

Sexual function, preservation of, with nerve-sparing cystectomy for bladder cancer, 167
    outcome of, 172–174
    with prostatic capsule and seminal-sparing cystectomy for bladder cancer, **177–185**
    arguments against, 183
    outcome of, 181–183

Sexual history, in psychosocial evaluation of erectile dysfunction, 434–436

Sexual Tipping Point, and combination treatment for erectile dysfunction, 432–433

Shock wave therapy, for Peyronie's disease, 475

Signaling pathways, providing for penile erection, 419–422

Sildenafil (Viagra), 512–514
pharmacokinetics and pharmacodynamics, 513–514
safety, contraindications, and precautions, 514

Single patients, with erectile dysfunction, psychosocial evaluation of, 439

Smoking, role of lifestyle factors in erectile dysfunction, 412–416

Smooth muscle, in pathophysiology of erectile dysfunction, 391

molecular mechanisms of contraction and relaxation during penile erection, 384–385

Sole proprietors, 263

Somatic pathways, neuroanatomy of penile erection, 381

Spinal cord, stimulation of, historical overview of, 4–5

Spinal cord injury, neurogenic bladder due to, sacral neuromodulation for, 20–21, 60–61
use of PDE-5 inhibitors in men with, 518–519

Staff, motivation of, to market and promote practice, 303–304

Stage, tumor, indicating high-risk superficial bladder cancer, 148

Steroids, intralesional therapy for Peyronie's disease, 473–474

Stoller afferent nerve stimulator, for refractory overactive bladder, 39–40

Strategic planning, for urologic practices, **291–294**
assessment of strengths, weaknesses, opportunities, and threats, 293
determining group's readiness for, 292
example of, 293–294
having the right people present for, 292–293
identifying major issues threatening the group, 292
importance of, 291–292

Stroke, role of comorbidities in erectile dysfunction, 409–412

Structural changes, erectile dysfunction due to, 390

Superficial bladder cancer. *See* Bladder cancer, superficial.

Supraspinal pathways, neuroanatomy of penile erection, 381–382

Surgery, techniques for sacral implantation for neuromodulation, **27–35**

Surgical factors. *See also* Cystectomy.
in invasive bladder cancer, **159–164**
in superficial bladder cancer, **157–159**

Surgical therapy, of Peyronie's disease, **479–485**
penile prosthetic implantation, 483–484
plication, 481–482
tunica lengthening procedures, 482–483
tunica shortening, 481

Systemic therapy. *See* Chemotherapy.

T

T1G3 bladder cancer. *See* Bladder cancer.

Tadalafil (Cialis), 516–517

Tamoxifen citrate, oral, for therapy of Peyronie's disease, 472–473

Targeted therapy, in bladder cancer, clinical applications of, **239–246**
potential of, using systemic adjuvant chemotherapy after cystectomy, 224–225

Tax laws, and tax strategies for urologic practice, 266–268
alternative minimum tax planning, 269
capital gains rates, 267
charitable deductions of vehicles, 266–267
health savings accounts, 267–268
marriage relief penalty, 267
planning for divorce, 268–269

Termination, of employment, 260–261

Testosterone, erectile function and, 457–458

Testosterone replacement therapy, for erectile dysfunction, forms of, 460–462
monitoring patients on, 464
risks and benefits of, 463–464

Thermotherapy, for benign prostatic hyperplasia, transurethral microwave, 327–328
urethral fluid balloon-based, 331–332

Tissue ablation, office-based procedures for, in benign prostatic hyperplasia, **327–335**

Topical therapy, for Peyronie's disease, 473

Transitional cell carcinoma, of prostate, in cystoprostatectomy specimens performed for bladder cancer, 179–181
   urethral, occurring after radical cystectomy for bladder cancer, 201–204
      monitoring for, 201–202
      orthotopic diversion and risk for, 201
      rate of in men, 199–200
      risk factors in men, 200
      risk factors in women, 200–201
      survival after, 202–204
      treatment of, 202

Transitional cell carcinoma. *See* Bladder cancer.

Transrectal ultrasound, of the prostate, 332–333

Transurethral bladder stimulation, historical overview of, 2

Transurethral electric bladder stimulation, in pediatric patients, 105–106

Transurethral microwave thermotherapy, for benign prostatic hyperplasia, 327–328

Transurethral needle ablation, office-based, for benign prostatic hyperplasia, 328–330

Transurethral resection, of bladder tumors, in optimal management of T1G3 tumors, 133–134
   intravesical chemotherapy and immunotherapy after, **121–131**
   surgical factors, **157–164**
      second or restaging, 158–159

Trauma, scrotal, office-based ultrasound of, 348–349

Tunica lenthening procedures, for Peyronie's disease, 482–483

Tunica shortening procedures, for Peyronie's disease, 481

U

Ultrasound, urologic, office-based, **337–352**
   bladder, 342–344
      masses, 343–344
      residual urine, 344
      urodynamics, 344
   instrumentation, 338–339
   kidneys, 340–342
      hydronephrosis, 340–341
      masses, 341–342
      perirenal and renal pelvis processes, 342
   penis and urethra, 349–350
      Peyronie's disease, 349–350
   physics of, 337–338
   prostate, transrectal, 332–333, 344–347
      cancer, 346–347
      future of, 347
      in benign prostatic hyperplasia, 332–333
      volume, 345
   scrotum, 347–349
      acute, 348
      hydroceles, 347–348
      masses, 348
      trauma, 348–349
   training, 339–340

Urethra, management of, after radical cystectomy for bladder cancer, **199–206**
      urethral transitional cell carcinoma occurring after, 201–204
      monitoring for, 201–202
      orthotopic diversion and risk for, 201
      rate of in men, 199–200
      risk factors in men, 200
      risk factors in women, 200–201
      survival after, 202–204
      treatment of, 202
   office-based ultrasound of, 349–350

Urge incontinence, peripheral nerve evaluation in patients with, **41–49**
   sacral nerve stimulation for, 38–39

Urgency frequency, peripheral nerve evaluation in patients with, **41–49**
   sacral nerve stimulation for, 38–39

Urinary diversion, quality of life in bladder cancer patients after cystectomy and, **207–216**
      challenges in, 209–210
      studies on, 210–215
      tools for measurement of, 208–209

Urinary retention, nonobstructive, peripheral nerve evaluation in patients with, **41–49**
   sacral nerve stimulation indicated for, 21
   results of clinical trials, 38–39

Urinary tract disease, lower, role in erectile dysfunction, 409–412

Urine, residual, office-based ultrasound of bladder, 344

postvoid, office-based urodynamic study of, 357–358

Urodynamic assessment, in clinical evaluation of voiding dysfunction, 24–25

Urodynamics, office-based, 344, **353–370**
    coding for, 365–368
    compliance, 360–361
    detrusor overactivity, 360
    electromyography, 363–364
    equipment, 355
    filling cystometry, 358–360
    indications, 354
    initial approaches, 354–355
    leak-point pressures, 361–362
    postvoid residual volume, 357–358
    pressure-flow analysis, 362–363
    uroflowmetry, 355–357
    videourodynamics, 364–365

Uroflowmetry, office-based, 355–357

Urothelial cancer. *See* Bladder cancer, Prostate cancer, and Urethra.

V

Valrubicin, in intravesical chemotherapy in high-risk patients with superficial bladder cancer, 126

Vardenafil (Levitra), efficacy, 515
    pharmacokinetics and pharmacodynamics, 515
    safety, contraindications, and precautions, 515–516

Vascular disease, erectile dysfunction as an early marker of, 398–399
    improvements in function due to PDE-5 inhibitors, 400–401

Vasoconstriction, erectile dysfunction due to, 390

Vasodilatation, impaired endothelium-dependent, erectile dysfunction due to, 390

Ventricular impairment, left, systemic adjuvant chemotherapy after cystectomy for bladder cancer in patients with, 222

Verapamil, intralesional therapy for Peyronie's disease, 474

Viagra. *See* Sildenafil.

Videourodynamics, in office-based urodynamic studies, 364–365

Vitamin E, oral, for therapy of Peyronie's disease, 472

Voiding dysfunction, clinical evaluation of, 21–25
    history, 22
    pelvic floor muscle electromyogram, 24
    physical examination, 22–24
    urodynamic assessment, 24–25
    pelvic neuromodulation for, 1–117
        Canadian experience with, **41–49**
        complications and troubleshooting, **65–69**
        current indications for, **37–40**
        European experience with, **51–57**
        expanding indications for, **59–63**
        historical overview, **1–10**
            direct detrusor stimulation, 2–3
            pelvic floor stimulation, 4
            pelvic nerve stimulation, 3–4
            sacral root stimulation, 5–8
            spinal cord stimulation, 4–5
            transurethral bladder stimulation, 2
        how it works, **11–18**
        in pediatric patients, **103–109**
        percutaneous, **71–79**
        selecting patients for, **19–26**
        surgical techniques for sacral implantation, **27–35**

Volume, of urine, postvoid residual, office-based urodynamic study of, 357–358

W

Warts, genital, office-based treatment for, 325–326

Workgroup for Electronic Data Interchange, 282

United States Postal Service
Statement of Ownership, Management, and Circulation

1. Publication Title	2. Publication Number	3. Filing Date
Urologic Clinics of North America	0 0 9 4 - 0 1 4 3	9/15/05

4. Issue Frequency	5. Number of Issues Published Annually	6. Annual Subscription Price
Feb, May, Aug, Nov	4	$195.00

7. Complete Mailing Address of Known Office of Publication (Not printer) (Street, city, county, state, and ZIP+4)

Elsevier Inc.
6277 Sea Harbor Drive
Orlando, FL 32887-4800

Contact Person
Gwen C. Campbell

Telephone
215-239-3685

8. Complete Mailing Address of Headquarters or General Business Office of Publisher (Not printer)

Elsevier Inc., 360 Park Avenue South, New York, NY 10010-1710

9. Full Names and Complete Mailing Addresses of Publisher, Editor, and Managing Editor (Do not leave blank)

Publisher (Name and complete mailing address)

Tim Griswold, Elsevier Inc., 1600 John F. Kennedy Blvd., Suite 1800, Philadelphia, PA 19103-2899

Editor (Name and complete mailing address)

Catherine Bewick, Elsevier Inc., 1600 John F. Kennedy Blvd., Suite 1800, Philadelphia, PA 19103-2899

Managing Editor (Name and complete mailing address)

Heather Cullen, Elsevier Inc., 1600 John F. Kennedy Blvd., Suite 1800, Philadelphia, PA 19103-2899

10. Owner (Do not leave blank. If the publication is owned by a corporation, give the name and address of the corporation immediately followed by the names and addresses of all stockholders owning or holding 1 percent or more of the total amount of stock. If not owned by a corporation, give the names and addresses of the individual owners. If owned by a partnership or other unincorporated firm, give its name and address as well as those of each individual owner. If the publication is published by a nonprofit organization, give its name and address.)

Full Name	Complete Mailing Address
Wholly owned subsidiary of	4520 East-West Highway
Reed/Elsevier Inc., US holdings	Bethesda, MD 20814

11. Known Bondholders, Mortgages, and Other Security Holders Owning or Holding 1 Percent or More of Total Amount of Bonds, Mortgages, or Other Securities. If none, check box ☐ None

Full Name	Complete Mailing Address
N/A	

12. Tax Status (For completion by nonprofit organizations authorized to mail at nonprofit rates) (Check one)
The purpose, function, and nonprofit status of this organization and the exempt status for federal income tax purposes:
☐ Has Not Changed During Preceding 12 Months
☐ Has Changed During Preceding 12 Months (Publisher must submit explanation of change with this statement)

(See Instructions on Reverse)

PS Form 3526, October 1999

13. Publication Title	14. Issue Date for Circulation Data Below
Urologic Clinics of North America	August 2005

15.	Extent and Nature of Circulation	Average No. Copies Each Issue During Preceding 12 Months	No. Copies of Single Issue Published Nearest to Filing Date
a.	Total Number of Copies (Net press run)	5475	5100
b. Paid and/or Requested Circulation	(1) Paid/Requested Outside-County Mail Subscriptions Stated on Form 3541. (Include advertiser's proof and exchange copies)	2655	2622
	(2) Paid In-County Subscriptions Stated on Form 3541 (Include advertiser's proof and exchange copies)		
	(3) Sales Through Dealers and Carriers, Street Vendors, Counter Sales, and Other Non-USPS Paid Distribution	1539	1595
	(4) Other Classes Mailed Through the USPS		
c.	Total Paid and/or Requested Circulation [Sum of 15b. (1), (2), (3), and (4)]	4194	4217
d. Free Distribution by Mail (Samples, complimentary, and other free)	(1) Outside-County as Stated on Form 3541	101	132
	(2) In-County as Stated on Form 3541		
	(3) Other Classes Mailed Through the USPS		
e.	Free Distribution Outside the Mail (Carriers or other means)		
f.	Total Free Distribution (Sum of 15d. and 15e.)	101	432
g.	Total Distribution (Sum of 15c. and 15f.)	4295	4349
h.	Copies not Distributed	1180	751
i.	Total (Sum of 15g. and h.)	5475	5100
j.	Percent Paid and/or Requested Circulation (15c. divided by 15g. times 100)	98%	97%

16. Publication of Statement of Ownership
☐ Publication required. Will be printed in the November 2005 issue of this publication. ☐ Publication not required

17. Signature and Title of Editor, Publisher, Business Manager, or Owner

[signature]
Elsevier Executive Director of Subscription Services

Date
9/15/05

I certify that all information furnished on this form is true and complete. I understand that anyone who furnishes false or misleading information on this form or who omits material or information requested on the form may be subject to criminal sanctions (including fines and imprisonment) and/or civil sanctions (including civil penalties).

Instructions to Publishers

1. Complete and file one copy of this form with your postmaster annually on or before October 1. Keep a copy of the completed form for your records.

2. In cases where the stockholder or security holder is a trustee, include in items 10 and 11 the name of the person or corporation for whom the trustee is acting. Also include the names and addresses of individuals who are stockholders who own or hold 1 percent or more of the total amount of bonds, mortgages, or other securities of the publishing corporation. In item 11, if none, check the box. Use blank sheets if more space is required.

3. Be sure to furnish all circulation information called for in item 15. Free circulation must be shown in items 15d, e, and f.

4. Item 15h., Copies not Distributed, must include (1) newsstand copies originally stated on Form 3541, and returned to the publisher, (2) estimated returns from news agents, and (3), copies for office use, leftovers, spoiled, and all other copies not distributed.

5. If the publication had Periodicals authorization as a general or requester publication, this Statement of Ownership, Management, and Circulation must be published; it must be printed in any issue in October or, if the publication is not published during October, the first issue printed after October.

6. In item 16, indicate the date of the issue in which this Statement of Ownership will be published.

7. Item 17 must be signed.

Failure to file or publish a statement of ownership may lead to suspension of Periodicals authorization.

PS Form 3526, October 1999 (Reverse)

Changing Your Address?

Make sure your subscription changes too! When you notify us of your new address, you can help make our job easier by including an exact copy of your Clinics label number with your old address (see illustration below.) This number identifies you to our computer system and will speed the processing of your address change. Please be sure this label number accompanies your old address and your corrected address—you can send an old Clinics label with your number on it or just copy it exactly and send it to the address listed below.

We appreciate your help in our attempt to give you continuous coverage. Thank you.

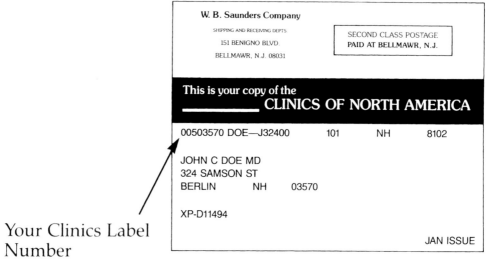

Your Clinics Label Number
Copy it exactly or send your label
along with your address to:
W.B. Saunders Company, Customer Service
Orlando, FL 32887-4800
Call Toll Free 1-800-654-2452

Please allow four to six weeks for delivery of new subscriptions and for processing address changes.